DIABETES MELLITUS AND HUMAN HEALTH CARE

A Holistic Approach to Diagnosis and Treatment

DIABETES MELLITUS AND HUMAN HEALTH CARE

A Holistic Approach to Diagnosis and Treatment

Edited by

Anne George, Robin Augustine, and Mathew Sebastian

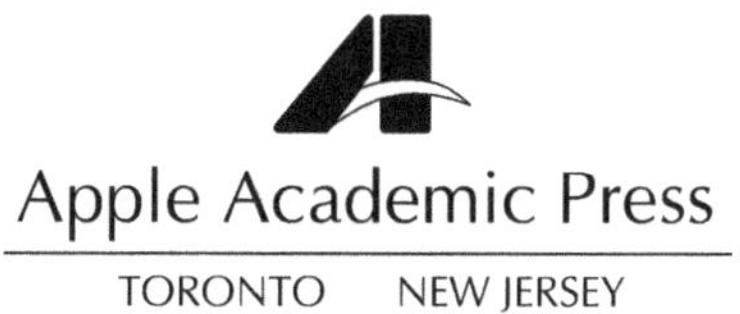

Apple Academic Press Inc.
3333 Mistwell Crescent
Oakville, ON L6L 0A2
Canada

Apple Academic Press Inc.
9 Spinnaker Way
Waretown, NJ 08758
USA

First issued in paperback 2021

Exclusive worldwide distribution by CRC Press, a member of Taylor & Francis Group

ISBN 13: 978-1-77463-303-8 (pbk)
ISBN 13: 978-1-926895-76-5 (hbk)

Library of Congress Control Number: 2013952512

Library and Archives Canada Cataloguing in Publication

Diabetes mellitus and human health care: a holistic approach to diagnosis and treatment/ edited by Anne George, Robin Augustine, and Mathew Sebastian.

Includes bibliographical references and index.
ISBN 978-1-926895-76-5
1. Diabetes--Diagnosis. 2. Diabetes--Treatment. 3. Diabetes--Alternative treatment.
I. George, Anne, 1961-, editor of compilation II. Augustine, Robin, editor of compilation
III. Sebastian, Mathew, editor of compilation

RC660.D553 2013 616.4'62 C2013-907308-6

Apple Academic Press also publishes its books in a variety of electronic formats. Some content that appears in print may not be available in electronic format. For information about Apple Academic Press products, visit our website at **www.appleacademicpress.com** and the CRC Press website at **www.crcpress.com**

ABOUT THE EDITORS

Anne George

Anne George, MD, is an Associate Professor at Government Medical College, Kottayam, Kerala, India. She did her MBBS (Bachelor of Medicine, Bachelor of Surgery) at Trivandrum Medical College, University of Kerala, India. She acquired a DGO (Diploma in Obstetrics and Gynaecology) from the University of Vienna, Austria; Diploma Acupuncture from the University of Vienna; and an MD from Kottayam Medical College, Mahatma Gandhi University, Kerala, India. She has organized several international conferences, is a fellow of the American Medical Society, and is a member of many international organizations. She has five publications to her name and has presented 25 papers.

Robin Augustine

Mr. Robin Augustine is a research fellow working at International and Interuniversity Centre for Nanoscience and Nanotechnology, Mahatma Gandhi University, Kottayam, Kerala, India. He received a bachelor's degree in botany from the University of Calicut, Kerala, India, and a master's degree in bioengineering from Madurai Kamaraj University, Tamil Nadu, India. He is experienced in developing smart biomaterials such as wound dressings, tissue engineering scaffolds, and suture matrials. Presently he is engaged in the design and development of nanotechnology-based smart wound dressing materials for chronic diabetic wounds. He has publications in international journals and conference proceedings in his credit.

Mathew Sebastian

Mathew Sebastian, MD, has a degree in surgery (1976) with specialization in Ayurveda. He holds several diplomas in acupuncture, neural therapy (pain therapy), manual therapy, and vascular diseases. He was a missionary doctor in Mugana Hospital, Bukoba in Tansania, Africa (1976–1978), and underwent surgical training in different hospitals in Austria, Germany, and India for more than

10 years. Since 2000 he is the doctor in charge of the Ayurveda and Vein Clinic in Klagenfurt, Austria. At present he is a Consultant Surgeon at Privatclinic Maria Hilf, Klagenfurt. He is a member of the scientific advisory committee of the European Academy for Ayurveda, Birstein, Germany, and the TAM advisory committee (Traditional Asian Medicine, Sector Ayurveda) of the Austrian Ministry for Health, Vienna. He conducted an International Ayurveda Congress in Klagenfurt, Austria, in 2010. He has several publications to his name.

CONTENTS

LIST OF CONTRIBUTORS

M. Abhilash
School of Biosciences, Mahatma Gandhi University, Priyadarshini Hills, Kottayam–686560, Kerala, India.

Shamima Akter
Health and Disease Research Center for Rural Peoples (HDRCRP), Dhaka–1207, Bangladesh.

Gangadhara Angajala
Chemistry Research Laboratory, School of Advanced Sciences, VIT University, Vellore–632014, Tamil Nadu, India.

Robin Augustine
International and Interuniversity Centre for Nanoscience and Nanotechnology, Mahatma Gandhi University, Priyadarshini Hills, Kottayam–686560, Kerala, India.

P. V. Bharatam
Department of Medicinal Chemistry, National Institute of Pharmaceutical Education and Research (NIPER), Sector-67, S. A. S. Nagar, Mohali–160062, Punjab, India.

Harshal Bhitkar
Department of Medicine, Dr. S. C. Government Medical College, Nanded–431601, Maharashtra, India.

Rahul Chandran
Bioprospecting Laboratory, Department of Botany, Bharathiar University, Coimbatore–641046, Tamil Nadu, India.

B. N. Das
Shoe Design and Development Centre, Council of Scientific and Industrial Research–Central Leather Research Institute, Adyar, Chennai–600020, Tamil Nadu, India.

S. D. Dubey
Department of Dravaguna, Institute of Medical Sciences, Banaras Hindu University, Varanasi–221005, India.

Satyanarayan Durgam
Department of Medicine, Dr. S. C. Government Medical College, Nanded–431601, Maharashtra, India.

Debapriya Garabadu
Neurotherapeutics Lab, Department of Pharmaceutics, Indian Institute of Technology, Banaras Hindu University, Varanasi–221005, India.

Gautham Gopalakrishna
Shoe Design and Development Centre, Council of Scientific and Industrial Research–Central Leather Research Institute, Adyar, Chennai–600020, Tamil Nadu, India.

S. Hemalatha
Department of Pharmaceutics, Institute of Technology, Banaras Hindu University, Varanasi–221005, India.

Michiaki Hiroe
National Center for Global Health and Medicine (NCGM), Tokyo, Japan.

Yoshio Iwashima
Graduate School of Medicine, Faculty of Medicine, University of Tsukuba, Tsukuba, Ibaraki–305 8575, Japan.

Prasant Kumar Jena
Institute of Science, Nirma University, S. G. Highway, Chharodi, Ahmedabad–382481, Gujarat, India.

Subrina Jesmin
Health and Disease Research Center for Rural Peoples (HDRCRP), Dhaka–1207, Bangladesh.

Nandakumar Kalarikkal
International and Interuniversity Centre for Nanoscience and Nanotechnology, Mahatma Gandhi University, Priyadarshini Hills, Kottayam–686560, Kerala, India.

Sairam Krishnamurthy
Neurotherapeutics Lab, Department of Pharmaceutics, Indian Institute of Technology, Banaras Hindu University, Varanasi–221005, India.

Manish Kumar
Department of Pharmaceutics, Institute of Technology, Banaras Hindu University, Varanasi–221005, India.

Abdullah Al Mamun
Health and Disease Research Center for Rural Peoples (HDRCRP), Dhaka–1207, Bangladesh.

Thamilvaani Manaharan
School of Medicine and Health Sciences, Monash University, Sunway Campus, 46150, Bandar Sunway, Malaysia.

Dilip Mhaisekar
Department of Pulmonary Medicine, TB and Chest, Dr. S. C. Government Medical College, Vazirabad, Nanded–431601, Maharashtra, India.

Taro Mizutani
Graduate School of Medicine, Faculty of Medicine, University of Tsukuba, Tsukuba, Ibaraki–305 8575, Japan.

Masao Moroi
National Center for Global Health and Medicine (NCGM), Tokyo, Japan.

Meenakshi Narkhede
48, Dashmeshnagar, Kushalnagar, Osmanpura, Aurangabad–431005, Maharashtra, India.

Uma D. Palanisamy
School of Medicine and Health Sciences, Monash University, Sunway Campus, 46150 Bandar Sunway, Malaysia.

Thangaraj Parimelazhagan
Bioprospecting Laboratory, Department of Botany, Bharathiar University, Coimbatore–641046, Tamil Nadu, India.

Satyendra K. Prasad
Department of Pharmaceutics, Institute of Technology, Banaras Hindu University, Varanasi–221005, India.

Arifur Rahman
Health and Disease Research Center for Rural Peoples (HDRCRP), Dhaka–1207, Bangladesh.

G. Saraswathy
Shoe Design and Development Centre, Council of Scientific and Industrial Research–Central Leather Research Institute, Adyar, Chennai–600020, Tamilnadu, India.

Sriram Seshadri
Institute of Science, Nirma University, S. G. Highway, Chharodi, Ahmedabad–382481, Gujarat, India.

Nobutake Shimojo
Graduate School of Medicine, Faculty of Medicine, University of Tsukuba, Tsukuba, Ibaraki, 305 8575, Japan.

Shilpa Singh
Institute of Science, Nirma University, S. G. Highway, Chharodi, Ahmedabad–382481, Gujarat, India.

Farzana Sohael
Health and Disease Research Center for Rural Peoples (HDRCRP), Dhaka–1207, Bangladesh.

Radhakrishnan Subashini
Chemistry Research Laboratory, School of Advanced Sciences, VIT University, Vellore–632 014, Tamil Nadu, India.

Nikhil Taxak
Department of Medicinal Chemistry, National Institute of Pharmaceutical Education and Research (NIPER), Sector-67, S. A. S. Nagar, Mohali–160062, Punjab, India.

Sabu Thomas
International and Interuniversity Centre for Nanoscience and Nanotechnology, Mahatma Gandhi University, Priyadarshini Hills, Kottayam–686560, Kerala, India.

Vijay Viswanathan
MV Hospital for Diabetes, Diabetes Research Centre, Royapuram, Chennai–600013, Tamilnadu, India.

Swapnil Yadav
Department of Medicine, Dr. S. C. Government Medical College, Nanded–431601, Maharashtra, India.

Naoto Yamaguchi
Graduate School of Medicine, Faculty of Medicine, University of Tsukuba, Tsukuba, Ibaraki–305 8575, Japan.

LIST OF ABBREVIATIONS

AAS	Atomic absorption spectroscopy
ABTS	2,2′-Azino-bis(3-ethylbenzthiazoline-6-sulphonic acid)
ACC	Acetyl-CoA carboxylase
ACD	Acid citrate dextrose
ACE	Angiotensin converting enzyme
ADA	American Diabetes Association
ADI	Acceptable daily intake
AEAC	Ascorbic acid equivalent antioxidant capacity
AFO	Ankle-foot orthosis
AGEs	Advanced-glycation end-products
AL	Alginate
ALP	Alkaline phosphate
ALT	Alanine aminotransferase
AMI	Acute myocardial infarction
AMPK	5' Adenosine monophosphate-activated protein kinase
AMY	Amygdala
Ang-1	Angiopoietin-1
ANOVA	Analysis of variance
ANS	Autonomic nervous system
APC	Antigen presenting cells
AR	Activities of recombinant
AR	Aldose reductase
ARBs	Angiotensin receptor blockers
AST	Aspartate transaminase
ATP	Adenosine triphosphate
AVF	Adjustable velcro fasteners
AWD	Active wound dressing

BB	Biobreeding
BHA	Butylated hydroxyl anisole
BHT	Butylated hydroxyl toluene
BMI	Body mass index
BS	Broad spectrum
BSA	Bovine serum albumin
cAMP/PKA	Cyclic adenosine monophosphate/protein kinase A
CARDS	Collaborative atorvastatin diabetes study
CAT	Catalase
CDK5	Cyclin-dependent kinase 5
CdTe	Cadmium telluride
CGM	Continuous glucose monitoring
CGRP	Calcitonin-gene-related peptide
CHD	Coronary heart disease
CLI	Critical limb ischemia
CMC	Carboxymethylcellulose
CNS	Central nervous system
CNT	Carbon nanotube
CO	Cardiac output
CORT	Corticosterone
CPCSEA	Committee for the Purpose of Control and Supervision of Experiments on Animals
CPY	Cytochromes P450
CREB	Calcium responsive element binding
CRP	C-Reactive protein
CRS	Cold restraint stress
CS	Chitosan
CSIR	Central Leather Research Institute
CTLA-4	Cytotoxic T-lymphocyte-associated antigen 4
CVD	Cardiovascular disease
D_2O	Deuterium oxide
DA	Dopamine
DAN	Diabetic autonomic neuropathy
DEX	Dexamethasone
DFT	Density functional theory

DFU	Diabetic foot ulcers
DFZ	Diformazan
DIAMOND	Diabetes mondiale
DIM	Differentiation initiation medium
DM	Diabetes mellitus
DMEM	Dulbecco's modified Eagle's medium
DMF	Dimethylformamide
DMSO	Dimethyl sulfoxide
DNA	Deoxyribonucleic acid
DNS	Dextrose and sodium chloride
DOPAC	3,4-Dihydroxyphenylacetic acid
DPIs	Dry-powder inhalers
DPM	Differentiation progression medium
DPP	Diabetes Prevention Program
DPP-4	Dipeptidyl peptidase-4
DPPH	2,2-Diphenyl-1-picrylhydrazyl
DTT	Dithiothreitol
EAC	Erythrocyte-antibody-complement
ECD	Electrochemical detection
ECG	Electrocardiography
ECM	Extracellular matrix
EDTA	Ethylenediamine tetracetic acid
EGF	Epidermal growth factor
ELISA	Enzyme-linked immunosorbent assay
eNOS	Endothelial nitric oxide synthase
EPC	Endothelial progenitor cell
ESBL	Extended-spectrum beta-lactamases
ET	Endothelin
ETC	Electron transport chain
EVA	Ethylene vinyl acetate
FBS	Fetal calf serum
FDA	Food and drug administration
FDPS	Finnish diabetes prevention study
$FeCl_3$	Ferric chloride
FFA	Free fatty acids

FGF	Fibroblast growth factor
FLI	Foam layer
FLK-1	Fetal liver kinase 1
FLT-1	Fms-like tyrosine kinase 1
FMOs	Flavoprotein monooxygenases
FPG	Fasting plasma glucose
FRAP	Ferric reducing ability of plasma
FRIM	Forest Research Institute of Malaysia
FRS	Free radical scavenging
GAD	Glutamic acid decarboxylase
GD	Gestational diabetes
GDH	Glucose dehydrogenase
GDM	Gestational diabetes mellitus
GIP	Glucose-dependent insulinotropic peptide
GL	Glycemic load
Glide	Grid-based ligand docking with energetics
GLP-1	Glucagon-like peptide-1
GLUT4	Glucose transporter type 4
GM-CSF	Granulocyte-macrophage colony-stimulating factor
GN	Gram negative
GOLD	Genetic optimization for ligand docking
GOx	Glucose oxidase
GP	Gram positive
GSH	Glutathione
GSK-3	Glycogen-synthase kinase-3
GUV	Giant unilamellar vesicle
GWA	Genome wide association
H_2O_2	Hydrogen peroxide
HAV	Hallux abducto valgus
HbA1c	Hemoglobin A1c
HDL	High density lipoprotein
HDL-C	High-density lipoprotein cholesterol
HFD	High fat diet
HGM	Home glucose monitoring
HGP	Hepatic glucose production

5-HIAA	5-Hydroxyindoleacetic acid
HIP	Hippocampus
HLA	Human leukocyte antigen
HNF4A	Hepatocyte nuclear factor-4 alpha
HPA	Hypothalamic pituitary adrena
HPLC	High performance liquid chromatography
HPTLC	High performance thin layer chromatography
5-HT	5-Hydroxytryptamine
HTN	Hypertension
HUVEC	Human umbilical vein endothelial cell
HVA	Homovanillic acid
HYP	Hypothalamus
IA-2	Insulinoma-associated antigen-2
IAA	Insulin autoantibody
IAEC	Institutional Animal Ethics Committee
IAPP	Islet-amyloid polypeptide
IBD	Inflammatory bowel disease
IBMX	3-Isobutyl-1-methylxanthine
ICCU	Intensive cardiac care unit
ICP-OES	Inductively coupled plasma-optical emission spectrometry
IDDM	Insulin-dependent diabetes mellitus
IFG	Impaired fasting glucose
IGF	Insulin-like growth factor
IGT	Impaired glucose tolerance
IL-1β	Interleukin-1β
IL2RA	Interleukin-2 receptor alpha
IL-6	Interleukin 6
ILs	Interleukins
INS	Insulin gene
INS-VNTR	Insulin gene variable number tandem repeat
IPF-1	Insulin promoter factor-1
IRS	Insulin-receptor substrates
ISC	Isocyanate
ISF	Interstitial fluid

$K_3Fe\ (CN_6)$	Potassium ferricyanate
LD	Linkage disequilibrium
LDH	Lactate dehydrogenase
LDL	Low density lipoprotein
LEA	Lower extremity amputation
LI	Large intestine
LJM	Limited joint mobility
LPO	Lipid peroxidation
LV	Left ventricular
LVFS	Left ventricular fractional shortening
MACCE	Major adverse cardiac and cerebrovascular event
MCP	Monocyte chemoattractant protein
MCR	Micro cellular rubber
MDA	Mitochondrial malondialdehyde
MDIs	Metered dose inhalers
MFB	Myofibroblasts
MHC	Major histocompatibility complex
MI	Myocardial infarction
MMP	Mitochondrial membrane potential
MMPs	Matrix metalloproteases
MO	Molecular orbital
mRNAs	Messenger ribonucleic acid
MRSA	Methicillin-resistant *Staphylococcus aureus*
MTT	5-Diphenyltetrazolium
MVTR	Moisture vapor transmission rate
NAC	Nucleus accumbens
NAD^+	Nicotinamide adenine dinucleotide
NADH	Nicotinamide adeninine dinucleotide
NADPH	Nicotinamide adenine dinucleotide phosphate
2-NBDG	Fluorescent deoxyglucose analog
NBT	Nitro blue tetrazolium
NE	Norepinephrine
NEFA	Nonesterified fatty acid
NGM	Noninvasive glucose monitor

NHS	Nurse's Health Study
NIDDM	Non-insulin dependent diabetes mellitus
NIR	Near-infrared radiation
NMDA	N-methyl-D aspartate
NMR	Nuclear magnetic resonance
NO	Nitric oxide
NOD	Nonobese diabetic
NPH	Neutral protamine hagedorn
NPWT	Negative pressure wound therapy
NSTEMI	Non-ST elevated myocardial infarction
OBD	On-board diagnostics
OECD	Organization of Economic Co-operation and Development
OGTT	Oral glucose tolerance test
OHAs	Orally administered antihyperglycemic agents
OLETF	Otsuka Long Evans Tokushima fatty
OPLS	Optimized potential for liquid simulations
P12A	Pro12-to-Ala
PAD	Peripheral arterial disease
PAI	Plasminogen activator inhibitor
PBS	Phosphate buffered saline
PCR	Polymerase chain reaction
PDGF	Platelet-derived growth factor
PEC	Personal ear clip
PFC	Pre-frontal cortex
PG	Propylene glycol
PGA	Poly(γ-glutamic acid)
PGZ	Pioglitazone
PH	Pleckstrin homology
PHMB	Polyhexamethylene biguanide
PI3-K	Phosphatidylinositol 3-kinase
PKA	Protein kinase A
PKB	Protein kinase B
PKC	Protein kinase C

pMDIs	Pressurized metered-dose inhalers
PNPG	4-Nitrophenyl-β-D-glucopyranoside
PPARγ	Peroxisome proliferator-activated receptor gamma
PPP	Peak plantar pressure
PPRE	Peroxisome proliferator response element
PQQ	Pyrroloquinoline quinine
PTPN22	Protein tyrosine phosphatase nonreceptor 22
PU	Polyurethane
PVPP	Polyvinyl polypyrrolidine
QDs	Quantum dots
QFD	Quality function deployment
RCS	Rigid counter stiffener
RGZ	Rosiglitazone
RNA	Ribonucleic acid
ROS	Reactive oxygen species
RPG	Random plasma glucose
RS	Runescape
SCFA	Short-chain fatty acids
SD	Statistical difference
SDH	Succinate dehydrogenase
SDS	Sodium dodecyl sulfate
SDT	Spontaneously diabetic Torii
SEM	Scanning electron microscopy
SEM	Standard error of the mean
SGOT	Serum glutamic oxaloacetic transaminase
SGPT	Serum glutamic-pyruvic transaminase
SI	Small intestine
SIRIM	Standards and Industrial Research Institute of Malaysia
SK	Streptokinase
SMRT	Skin moisture rebalancing technology
SNPs	Single nucleotide polymorphisms
SOD	Superoxide dismutase

SOM	Site of metabolism
SPSS	Statistical package for social sciences
STEMI	ST-elevated myocardial infarction
STR	Striatum
STZ	Streptozotocin
SUR1	Sulfonylurea receptor 1
TAG	Triacylglycerol
T1DM	Type 1 diabetes mellitus
T2DM	Type 2 diabetes mellitus
TBA	Thiobarbituric acid
TC	Total cholesterol
TCA	Trichloroacetic acid
TCCs	Total contact casts
TCR	T cell receptor
TFW	Therapeutic footwear
TG	Triglycerides
TGF-β1	Transforming growth factor
Tie-2	Tyrosine kinase 2
TMRM	Tetra methyl rhodamine methylester
TNFα	Tumor necrosis factor alpha
TPC	Total phenolic content
TPTZ	2,4,6-Tripyridyl-s-triazine
TRIZ	Teoriya Resheniya Izobretatelskikh Zadatch
Trolox	6-Hydroxy-2,5,7,8-tetramethylchroman-2-carboxylic acid
Trx1	Thioredoxin-1
TZD	Thiazolidinedione
TZDSO	Thiazolidinedione ring sulfoxide
USDA	U.S. Department of Agriculture
UV	Ultraviolet
VEGF	Vascular endothelial growth factor

VEGFR-2	Vascular endothelial growth factor receptor 2
VLDL	Very low density lipoprotein
WHO	World Health Organization
ZDF	Zucker diabetic fatty

PREFACE

This book, *Diabetes Mellitus and Human Health Care,* contains cutting-edge chapters by leading researchers and practitioners who deal with critical issues concerning diagnosis, treatment, and management of diabetes. This book also enlightens on some of the recent progress in diabetic care and therapy. The topics range from on recent trends in traditional medicine used to control diabetes to advanced biosensor technology to detect this devastating disease. Each chapter follows a holistic approach that integrates the science behind the diabetes, engineering approaches to detect and treat it, and the medical practices to be adopted to eradicate it. This book offers a wealth of valuable data and discussions that will be of use to researchers as well as practicing physicians concerned with the diagnosis, treatment, and management of diabetes and other ailments related to diabetes.

Recent attention has been focused on plant extracts and plant-derived compounds to treat type 2 diabetes. The book also focuses on the phytomedicines used for the treatment of diabetes such as *Withania coagulans* with up-to-date information on the various investigations conducted confirming the antidiabetic potential of this plant. Another medicinal plant *Glycosmis pentaphylla* which is used in traditional medicine for a long time for cough, rheumatism, an anemia, jaundice, and other ailments, is evaluated for its free radical quenching activity. Plants that serve both as antioxidant scavengers as well as antidiabetic agents would be ideal to treat diabetic and its complications. In this light antioxidant, antidiabetic, and chemical composition of the plant *Syzygium aqueum* leaf extracts are also included as a separate chapter.

The chapters, some of which include basic studies in the molecular mechanism of diabetes, provide rich insights into our experiences today with a broad range of modern approaches toward diabetes care. Understanding of genetics of any disease can provide a better choice of the treatment and easy management of them from the root cause. Pathway analysis of the type 2 diabetes highlights the mechanism of the causality of diabetes and different genes and processes involved in it. Controlling the pathways at the important junctures can regulate the diabetes either by enhancing insulin production or increasing its efficiency. In one chapter, the microcirculatory disturbances in diabetic heart and the therapeutic strategies to restore them are discussed in detail. Although, growth factor or cell-based angiogenic therapies are an attractive therapeutic option for diabetic patients, a better understanding of pro- and antiangiogenic influences in diabetic patients is crucial to maximize the outcome of such therapies.

There are many classes of drugs used to treat type-2 diabetes. Thiazolidinediones are an important class among them. In one chapter novel 2, 4-thiazolidinedione derivatives containing aryl sulphonyl urea moieties have been successfully evaluated for the antihyperglycemic activity. Molecular mechanism of S-oxidation of anti-diabetic thiazolidinedione class of drugs is evaluated by computational approaches in another chapter. The process of S-oxidation of thiazolidinedione ring was studied using different oxidants like H_2O_2, HOONO, and C_4a-hydroperoxyflavin using density functional theory. Thus, the chapter describes the molecular mechanism of S-oxidation which paves the pathway for further improvements and efficiency in drug discovery.

People with diabetes are at increased risk for complications of wound healing for several reasons. A greater understanding of the molecular mechanism of diabetes and advances in biomaterial research has led to significant advancements in the management of diabetic wounds. One chapter outlines how current advances in molecular biology, polymer technology, and biomaterials can be incorporated into a multidisciplinary translational research approach for formulating novel smart wound dressings for diabetic wound treatment. Diabetic foot ulcers are the major cause of hospitalization of patients with diabetes. Foot ulcers and their subsequent complications are an important cause of morbidity and mortality in patients with diabetes. This provides an insight to the importance of diabetic foot care, especially the role of footwear and orthosis in the management of chronic diabetic wounds. A chapter is devoted to the research to be carried out to improve the design and need of customized therapeutic footwear for patients with diabetes.

Type-2 diabetes mellitus patients are susceptible to stresses. The study in the book evaluates the temporal effect of repeated stress in the pathophysiology of T2DM. The aggravation of diabetes-induced metabolic parameters by repeated stress was more pronounced after diabetes induction compared to before diabetes induction. Thus, different treatment paradigms may have to be developed other than conventional therapies to treat these conditions.

In another chapter the role of sugar–rich diet in the insulin resistance and alteration in gut microflora is extensively discussed. The correlation between diabetes mellitus and acute myocardial infarction is also a matter of discussion in this book. The prevention of cardiac complication in diabetes patients is a great challenge. Development of therapeutic strategy to restore coronary microcirculation and VEGF signaling cascade in diabetes is a novel approach to prevent cardiac complication in diabetes at the molecular level. One of the chapters discusses the above aspects in detail.

In this book, topics on the molecular mechanism, diagnosis, prevention, and treatment options of diabetes are discussed in a lucid manner and in a readily accessible form. As a result, each chapter provides an in-depth array of knowledge satisfying to professional colleagues interested in diabetes care. Further this book focuses on the recent advances in the management of diabetes, by focusing on a holistic approach. We have given great attention on global trends in diabetes, epidemiology of diabetes, inhibitors in diabetes, and diabetes therapy in this book. The book will be extremely useful in the sense that it covers the recent trends in modern medicine (allopathy), Ayurveda and other traditional practices. The book emphasizes interdisciplinary research and holistic approach to the diagnosis and treatment of diabetes.

— Anne George, Robin Augustine, and Mathew Sebastian

CHAPTER 1

DIABETES AND HEALTH CARE: AN OVERVIEW

M. ABHILASH and ROBIN AUGUSTINE

CONTENTS

ABSTRACT

The diabetes has emerged as a major health problem worldwide, with serious health-related and socioeconomic impacts on individuals and populations. Diabetes is a complex disease linked with multiple factors and is associated with significant mortality and morbidity, leads to loss of quality of life. Apart from glucose dysregulation, both type 1 diabetes mellitus (T1DM) and type 2 diabetes mellitus (T2DM) are associated with damaging effects on tissues, with eventual progression to devastating complications. Diabetes increases the risk of macrovascular diseases (stroke and peripheral vascular disease), microvascular diseases (retinopathy and nephropathy), neuropathies, and the consequences that stem from these (congestive heart failure, diabetic foot). Individuals with the disease have to make major lifestyle changes and learn to live with timely monitoring of blood glucose, using multidrug treatment and insulin therapy, and proper dealing with complications of the disease. Several potentially modifiable risk factors are related to diabetes including obesity, physical inactivity, and dietary factors. Many of the factors associated with diabetes are modifiable, and research is currently focused on ways to prevent diabetes. Several efficacious and economically acceptable treatment strategies are currently available to reduce the burden of diabetes complications.

1.1 INTRODUCTION

The diabetes mellitus (DM) is a complex metabolic disorder resulting from either insulin insufficiency or insulin dysfunction. It is frequently associated with the development of micro and macro vascular diseases which include nephropathy, retinopathy, neuropathy, cerebrovascular, and cardiovascular diseases (CVD) (Kumar and Clark, 2005). Hypertension (HTN) and abnormal lipoprotein metabolism are often found in people with diabetes. The management of diabetes is a major health challenge, and its prevalence is increasing at an alarming rate worldwide. As per the statistics of International Diabetes Federation, diabetes currently affects more than 285 million people worldwide, a figure that is expected to rise to 435 million by 2030 (Shaw et al., 2010). Advances in clinical science during the second half of the 20th Century have led to improvements in understanding the aetiology and complications of diabetes, combined with the alleviation of suffering considerably. Several pathogenic processes are involved in the development of diabetes, ranging from the destruction of the β-cells of the pancreas with a subsequent insulin deficiency to abnormalities that result in insulin resistance. Alterations in fat, carbohydrate, and protein metabolism in diabetes are associated with insufficient action of insulin on target tissues. Impairment of insulin secretion and defects in insulin action frequently coexists, and it is often unclear which abnormality is the primary cause of the hyperglycemia. The management of diabetes is a major health challenge. Meanwhile, treatment options are expanding dramatically. The different classes of antidiabetic agents include biguanides, α-glucosidase inhibitors, sulphonylureas, rapid-acting insulin analogues, long-acting basal insulin analogues, incretin mimetics, and amylin mimetics. The use of insulin pumps has increased dramatically. The continuous glucose monitoring (CGM) has made glucose measurement easy. An attempt to develop an artificial pancreas is underway. The diabetes is a lifelong disease that seriously affects a person's well being. People with the disease have to make major lifestyle changes in addition to treatment strategies. This chapter describes an overview on diabetes; pathogenesis, risk factors, prevention, complications, management, and modern treatment strategies.

1.1.1 EPIDEMIOLOGY

The global prevalence of DM is rapidly increasing as a result of ageing, urbanization, and associated lifestyle modifications. The incidence of people with DM worldwide has doubled over the past three decades. This effect is most probably due to the pronounced changes in the human environment, and in human lifestyle and behavior that have related to globalization, leading into rapidly escalating rates of both obesity and diabetes (Zimmet et al., 2001). Globally, it was estimated that diabetes accounted for 12% of health expenditures in 2010, or at least $376 billion-a figure expected to hit $490 billion in 2030 (Zhang et al., 2010). The T1DM accounts for 5–10% of all cases of diabetes. The (T2DM) accounts for

90–95% of all diagnosed diabetes cases. This type of diabetes usually begins as insulin resistance (Thomson, 2007). Ethnic minority women, obese women, women with a risk of family history of diabetes, and women with gestational diabetes (GD) in a previous pregnancy are at higher risk than other women for developing GD (Deshpande et al., 2008). Women who have had GD have a 20–50% increased risk for developing T2DM later in life. Estimates of current and future diabetes suggest that globally, amidst 1995 and 2025, the adult population will increase by 64%, the incidence of diabetes in adults will increase by 35%, and the number of people with diabetes will rise up to 122% (King et al., 1998). In developed countries, there will be an 11% increase in the adult population, a 27% increase in the prevalence of adult diabetes, and a 42% increase in the number of people with diabetes. Regarding to developing countries, there will be an 82% increase in diabetes in the adult population and a 170% increase in the number of people with diabetes. The global prevalence of diabetes among adults (aged 20–79 years) will be 6.4%, affecting 285 million adults, in 2010, and will increase to 7.7%, and 439 million by 2030. There will be a 69% increase in numbers of adults with diabetes in developing countries and a 20% increase in developed countries between 2010 and 2030 (Shaw et al., 2010; Wild et al., 2004).

The diabetes mondiale (DIAMOND) project initiated by the World Health Organization (WHO) in 1990 addresses the public health implications of T1DM, especially the incidence of T1DM in children (Maahs et al., 2010). An initial report in 2000 described the incidence of T1DM in children ≤ 14 years of age in 50 countries worldwide from 1990–1994 (DIAMOND Project Group, 2006). A greater than 350-fold difference in the incidence of T1DM among the 100 populations worldwide was reported with age-adjusted incidences ranging from a lowest of 0.1/100,000 yearly in China and Venezuela to a highest of 36.5/100,000 in Finland and 36.8/100,000 in Sardinia. Populations in northern Africa had intermediate incidence rates of T1DM. Most of the Asian population showed very low incidences (Karvonen et al., 2000). Israel and Kuwait were exceptions with high and intermediate incidences respectively. Incidence rates were high in North America. In Canada, especially in Alberta and Prince Edward Island had very high incidence rates: 24 and 24.5/100,000 respectively. The US populations included in the DIAMOND study were drawn from the states of Illinois, Alabama and Pennsylvania reported incidences of 10–20/100,000 per year. Close to half of the European populations found to have an incidence between 5–10 in 100,000 per year with the remainder having higher rates (Maahs et al., 2010).

REGIONAL PREVALENCE

The diabetes and its complications are a major cause of morbidity and mortality in the United States and, like many of the countries experiencing such an increase in cases; it contributes substantially to health care costs (Zhang et al., 2010). The SEARCH for Diabetes in Youth study, in 2002–03, 1,905 youth with T1DM were diagnosed from a population of more than 10 million person-years under surveillance (Paris et al., 2009). Rates were highest in non-Hispanic white youth as compared to other races/ethnicities and were slightly higher in females as compared to males. It is expected that a continued rise will occur as the population continues to age and obesity increases.

The Asia-Pacific region contains some of the most populous countries in the world. Thus, the Asia-Pacific region is of prime importance to the epidemiology of diabetes. Predictions of WHO indicate that figure will rise to 300 million by the year 2025. The major burden of DM is now taking place in developing rather than in developed countries. Compared with developed countries, the proportion of young to middle-aged individuals with T2DM is higher in developing countries (Cockram, 2000). Furthermore, T2DM is not necessarily less prevalent in rural than in urban areas of developing countries, as is generally believed. The rural urban difference in prevalence is predicted to narrow owing to urbanization, rural to urban migration and its associated lifestyle changes. Asia has emerged as the 'diabetes epicenter' in the world, as a result of rapid economic development, urbanization, and the nutrition transition over a relatively short period of time (Gu et al., 2003). Among the 10 countries with the largest numbers of people predicted to have DM in 2030, five are in Asia (China, India, Pakistan, Indonesia, and Bangladesh) (Rahim et al., 2007; Sadikot et al., 2004). Of these, more than 150 million will be in Asia. For China, current estimates are 15 to 20 million, with an approximate rise to 50 million by 2025. Studies conducted in India in the last decade have highlighted that the prevalence of T2DM is increasing rapidly in the urban population (Mohan et al., 2007). The National Urban Diabetes Survey, carried out in six cities in 2001, found age - standardized prevalence rates of 12% for diabetes (with a slight male preponderance) and 14% for impaired glucose tolerance (IGT); subjects under 40 years of age had a prevalence of 5% (diabetes) and 13% (IGT) (Boddula et al., 2008). Thus, more than 30% of the global number of people with diabetes in 2025 will be in these two countries alone. In Japan prevalence rates approaching 10% for T2DM and more than 20% for IGT (Hidaka et al., 1996). Incidence rate estimates for T2DM range from 5 to 7 per 1000 person-years (Tajima, 1999).

Until about 40 years ago, diabetes was considered a rare disease in sub-Saharan Africa. The reported prevalence, in localised settings in a number of countries, including, Lesotho, Uganda, Ethiopia, Ghana, and Malawi, between 1960–1985 was around 1% (Sierra, 2009). There were two exceptions, Ivory Coast (5.7%) and South Africa (2.2–2.7%). In contrast, moderate prevalences were reported from South African studies undertaken in different cities and one peri-urban area (4–8%). These differences could be largely due to considerably higher rates of obesity in the South African population compared with other countries in the region (Levitt, 2008). In a recent systematic review of prevalence data from Ghanaians and Nigerians, diabetes was rare at 0.2% in urban Ghana in 1963 and 1.65% in urban Nigeria in 1985 (Amoah et al., 2002). The prevalence of diabetes had risen to 6.8% in Nigeria in 2000 (for adults aged ≥40 years) and 6.3% in Ghana in 1998 (for adults aged ≥ 25 years) (Motala, 2002). In Cameroon (West Africa), adults aged 24–74 years had an overall diabetes prevalence of 1.1%, with an IGT rate of 2.7%. Prevalence rates in the capital of Cameroon were 1.3% for diabetes and 1.8% for IGT, compared with rural prevalences of 0.8% for diabetes and 3.9% for IGT (Mbanya et al., 1997). Prevalence rates in North Africa especially in Sudan and Tunisia as well as Egypt are relatively high (4.2–9.3) (Shaw et al., 2010).

1.2 CLASSIFICATION OF DIABETES

The DM is a metabolic disorder characterized by hyperglycemia and insufficiency of secretion or action of endogenous insulin (Maritim et al.,

2003). Several pathogenic mechanisms are involved in the development of diabetes, range from lack of insulin secretion due to the destruction of the pancreatic β-cells with consequent insulin deficiency to abnormalities that result in resistance to insulin action (George and Alberti, 2010).The DM comprises a heterogeneous group of disorders characterized by high blood glucose levels. The disease can be divided into two major subclasses: insulin-dependent diabetes mellitus (IDDM) or T1DM, and non-insulin-dependent diabetes mellitus (NIDDM) or T2DM together with other less common types and GD (Aljasem et al., 2001).

1.2.1 TYPE 1 DIABETES

The T1DM results from insulin deficiency caused by cell-mediated autoimmune destruction of pancreatic β cells, and generally develop in the young (Bach et al., 1994). It accounts for approximately 10–15% of the diabetic population worldwide (American Diabetes Association (ADA), 2009). Markers of the immune destruction of the β-cell include autoantibodies to islet cell, insulin, glutamic acid decarboxylase (GAD) (GAD65), and autoantibodies to the tyrosine phosphatase, insulinoma-associated antigen 2 (IA-2) (Kuzuya and Matsuda, 1997). One and usually more of these autoantibodies are present in 85–90% of individuals when fasting hyperglycemia is initially detected. It shows strong association with specific alleles at the DQ- A and DQ - B loci of the human leukocyte antigen (HLA) complex, with linkage to the *DQA* and *DQB* genes, and it is influenced by the *DRB* genes (Pearson et al., 2003).

Some forms of T1DM observed in non-Europid populations, up to 80% may show no measurable autoantibodies; these are referred as idiopathic T1DM (McLarty et al., 1990). As with autoimmune diabetes, however, there is a clear loss of β-cell function as measured by low or absent C-peptide secretion. Some of these patients have permanent insulinopenia and are prone to ketoacidosis, but have no evidence of autoimmunity. Only a few patients with T1DM fall into this category, most of them belong to Asian or African ancestry (Patterson et al., 2009).

In addition to the typical young people with acute-onset T1DM, there is an older group with slower onset disease. They may present in middle age with apparent T2DM but have evidence of autoimmunity as assessed by GAD antibody measurements and ultimately become insulin-dependent. This is referred to as latent autoimmune diabetes of adults (Tuomi et al., 1993).

1.2.2 TYPE 2 DIABETES

The T2DM accounts for over 90% of the diabetic population globally (Gonzalez et al., 2009). In this type of diabetes, usually individuals do not need insulin treatment throughout their lifetime to survive. There are many different causes of this form of diabetes. Thus, insulin secretion is defective in these patients and insufficient to compensate for insulin resistance (Fowler, 2010; Grant et al., 2006). The risk of developing this form of diabetes increases with obesity, lack of physical activity and age. It occurs more common in women with prior GD and in people with HTN or dyslipidemia, and its incidence varies in different ethnic groups (George and Alberti, 2010).

1.2.3 GESTATIONAL DIABETES

The GD is defined as carbohydrate intolerance that begins or is first diagnosed during pregnancy (Metzger et al, 1998). The GD occurs in around 4–10% of pregnancies; however, its incidence varies as a function of nutritional habits and differences in genetic patterns between populations (Metzger et al., 2007). Besides, immediate pregnancy complications, women who have had GD also face increased risks of the development of T2DM in the years that follow their pregnancy.

1.3 PATHOPHYSIOLOGY

1.3.1 TYPE 1 DIABETES

The T1DM is a chronic inflammatory disease caused by a selective destruction of the insulin producing β-cells in the islets of Langerhans

(Atkinson and Eisenbarth, 2001).The incidence of T1DM has consistently increased globally during the last decades, particularly in children and developed countries (Gale, 2002). The T1DM is associated with the appearance of humoral and cellular islet autoimmunity, and a defective immunoregulation appears to be involved (Mathis and Benoist, 2004). The T1DM develops as a consequence of a combination of genetic susceptibility and environmental factors with limited knowledge and stochastic events. The studies in nonobese diabetic (NOD) mice have demonstrated that the disease occurs as a consequence of a breakdown in the regulation of the immune system, resulting in the expansion of autoreactive CD4 and CD8 T cells, B lymphocytes capable of autoantibody-production, and activation of the innate immune system that collaborate to destroy the insulin producing β-cells1 (Delli et al., 2010;. Roep, 1991; Wicker et al., 2005). These attributes of the disease are consistent with studies of human T1DM.

Genetic susceptibility is important in the development of T1DM. There has been much progress in the identification of genes and molecular pathways involved in the pathogenesis of T1DM. The genetic basis of T1DM is multifactorial (Maier and Wicker, 2005). Human histocompatibility (HLA) complex genes are the most powerful susceptibility determinants (Nerup et al., 1974). The HLA complex is the strongest susceptibility determinant and likely controls presentation of islet antigens to T cells. The stronger effect is from alleles coding for selected HLA class I and class II antigen-presenting molecules, which are restricting elements for autoreactive CD8 and CD4 T cells, respectively (Noble et al., 2002; Erlich et al., 2008). The HLA class II family molecules are expressed on the surface of antigen presenting cells (APC) such as dendritic cells and macrophages but also on activated B and T lymphocytes or even activated endothelial cells. High-risk HLA molecules on APC are likely to facilitate activation of $CD8^+$ T lymphocytes by $CD4^+$ T lymphocytes (Seyfert-Margolis et al., 2006; Pinkse et al., 2005). The HLA class II molecules on APC are responsible for antigen presentation to T-helper lymphocytes. The APC presenting β-cell autoantigens may thus be actively involved in the anti-self autoimmune response that may result from failure to sustain self-recognition or from promoting an anti-self response. Several of the genes linked to T1DM risk are not disease-specific but rather predispose to multiple diseases. Amongst these are protein tyrosine phosphatase nonreceptor 22

(PTPN22), cytotoxic T-lymphocyte-associated antigen 4 (CTLA-4), and interleukin-2 receptor alpha (IL2RA) (Bottini et al., 2006; Vella et al., 2005; Teft et al., 2006). In the last decade, genome wide studies have indicated that there are at least 15 other loci associated with T1DM.

Several silent immune events occur before the clinical symptoms of T1DM become apparent. Most importantly, autoantibodies are produced and self-reactive lymphocytes become activated and infiltrate the pancreas to destroy the insulin-producing beta-cells in the islets of Langerhans (Di Lorenzo et al., 2007). It was recognized that antibodies in sera from patients with T1DM could bind to sections of pancreatic islets. These antibodies were termed islet cell antibodies (Pinkse et al., 2005). The early presence of autoantibodies implicates a role for antibody-producing plasma B cells in the initial immunological events. Indeed, B cells clearly contribute to the pathogenesis of human T1DM (Pescovitz et al., 2009).

Both humoral and cellular autoimmune responses target multiple islet autoantigens, including (pro) insulin, GAD65, IA-2 and the cation efflux transporter zinc transporter 8 (ZnT8) (Bonifacio et al., 1995; Payton et al., 1995).The most highly specific autoantigens of β-cells are insulin and its precursor proinsulin because they are expressed only in β-cells. Insulin is a crucial autoantigen (insulin autoantibody (IAA)) in T1DM because it is the only β-cell-specific auto antigen in postnatal life. The IAAs are the first or among the first auto antibodies to appear when the disease process leading to T1DM is initiated in young children (Lu et al., 1996). The frequency of IAAs is also substantially higher among young children at the diagnosis of T1DM than among older children and adults (Willcox et al., 2009). The IAA, which are able to react with both insulin and proinsulin, tends to be the earliest marker of islet autoimmunity but their levels are often fluctuating and present in low titers (Castano et al., 1993). The zinc transporter (ZnT8 isoform-8 transporter) has recently been described as a second novel β-cell-specific auto antigen, in addition to insulin (Torn et al., 2008).

Considerable progress has been made in the understanding of T1DM pathogenesis as it relates to the appearance of islet autoimmunity prior to the clinical onset of the disease. The identification of exogenous factors triggering and driving β-cell destruction offers potential means for intervention aimed at the prevention of T1DM. So, it is necessary to pursue studies on the role of environmental factors in the pathogenesis of this disease.

1.3.2 TYPE 2 DIABETES

The NIDDM is a heterogeneous disorder characterized by abnormalities in insulin action and impaired insulin secretion. These abnormalities interact in a complex manner to lead to the development of hyperglycemia. The T2DM subjects manifest multiple disturbances in glucose homeostasis that include impaired insulin secretion, insulin resistance in liver, muscle, and adipocytes and abnormalities in splanchnic glucose uptake (Waldhausl et al., 1982; Staiger et al., 2009). Genetic factors are strongly involved in the development of NIDDM. Although, numerous candidate genes responsible for insulin resistance and insulin secretion have been studied, no specific gene(s) accounting for the majority of cases of the common type of T2DM has been identified (DeFronzo, 2010). Much evidence indicates that environmental factors play an important role in the development of NIDDM in genetically susceptible subjects. Obesity is a major factor which has been linked to NIDDM, and age, physical activity, and diet also contribute to the development of the disease. Impaired insulin secretion is found uniformly in T2DM patients in all ethnic populations (Spellman, 2010). This dynamic interaction between insulin secretion and insulin resistance has been well documented. The natural history of T2DM, starting with normal glucose tolerance, insulin resistance, and compensatory hyperinsulinemia, with progression to IGT and overt DM (Weyer et al., 1999).

1.3.3 β-CELL DYSFUNCTION

Beta-cell dysfunction plays an important role in the transition from normal glucose tolerance to hyperglycemia (Lebovitz, 1999; Gastaldelli, 2011). The T2DM develops when the beta-cell secretory capacity is not sufficient to overcome the insulin resistance of the tissues. In subjects with T2DM, several studies have reported decreased both beta-cell mass and insulin secretory granules (Butler et al., 2003). Although, little is known about the cause of the reduction in β cell mass, some changes in islet morphology, such as islet fibrosis and islet amyloid deposition, have been observed (Cooper et al., 1987). Islet amyloid consists of fibrils formed by islet-amyloid polypeptide (IAPP), which has homology with the calcitonin-gene-related peptide (CGRP) and is co-secreted with insulin (Kahn et al., 1990). Although, the role of IAPP in the pathogenesis of NIDDM is not clear, amyloid deposits have been suggested to have a toxic effect on β cells and/or to inhibit β cell function. In response to a change in glucose concentration (e.g. after meal ingestion), insulin is released in two phases. Insulin is secreted in pulses of rapid frequency in both humans and animals (Lang et al., 1979). In NIDDM patients, the regular, rapid oscillations are impaired and decreased amplitude and irregular cycles are observed. The defects in the oscillatory pattern of insulin secretion may be the earliest marker in the natural history of NIDDM (O'Rahilly et al., 1988; Clark, 1989).

The T2DM is a polygenic disorder, genes may affect β-cell apoptosis, regeneration, glucose sensing, glucose metabolism, ion channels, energy transduction, microtubules/microfilaments and other islet proteins necessary for the synthesis, packaging, movement, and release of secretory granules (Hales, 1994). To date, only a few polymorphisms have been identified as risk factors with confidence one involves an amino acid polymorphism (Pro12Ala) in the peroxisome proliferator-activated receptor-γ (PPAR-γ), which is expressed in insulin target tissues and β-cells (Stefan et al., 2001); this apparently conveys susceptibility to adverse effects of free fatty acid (FFA) on insulin release. More recently, variants of the transcription factor 7- like 2 gene (*TCF7L2)* were found to be associated with increased risk of T2DM (Grant et al., 2006). A list of candidate genes associated with T2DM is presented in Table.1.

TABLE 1 Candidate genes for predisposition to T2DM

Gene name	Probable effects
CDKAL1	Decreased glucose-stimulated insulin secretion
CDKN2A/B	Decreased glucose-stimulated insulin secretion
FTO	Increased overall fat mass

TABLE 1 *(Continued)*

HHEX	Decreased glucose-stimulated insulin secretion
KCNJ11	Decreased insulin secretion
KCNQ1	Decreased insulin and incretin secretion
PPAR-γ	Decreased whole-body insulin sensitivity
WFS1	Decreased incretin-stimulated insulin secretion
IGF2BP2	Decreased glucose-stimulated insulin secretion
ENPP1	Decreased whole-body insulin sensitivity
IRS-1	Insulin resistance
TNF-α	Insulin resistance
HNF4A	B-cell dysfunction
CAPN10	Glucose transport/insulin resistance.
IGF2BP2	mRNA processing in the β–cell.
S LC30A8	B- cell dysfunction/Zn transport.
JAZF1	B-cell dysfunction.
NOTCH2	Pancreatic development.

The several acquired and/or environmental factors have been identified that may increase the risk for developing T2DM by impairing β-cell function. Many studies have provided evidence that an acquired defect in insulin secretion is related to glucose toxicity. It was found that prolonged exposure of β cells to a high glucose level impairs insulin gene transcription, leading to decreased insulin secretion (Rossetti et al., 1990). Hyperglycemia may down-regulate the glucose transport system, leading to a reduction in insulin sensitivity (Robertson et al., 1994).

In addition to elevated levels of plasma glucose, individuals with T2DM have increased circulating levels of FFA as do people who are obese leading to a condition termed lipotoxicity (Schrauwen et al., 2004; Summers et al., 2006). Lipotoxicity describes the detrimental cellular effects of chronically elevated concentrations of fatty acids and excess lipid accumulation in tissues other than adipose tissue. The relation between lipotoxicity and hyperglycemia is shown in Figure 1. Excess adiposity is well known to promote the onset and severity of insulin resistance, contributing to the initiation and progression of IGT and T2DM. Evidence suggests that fatty acids inhibit glucose stimulated insulin secretion, impair insulin gene expression and, more importantly, promote β-cell apoptosis (Shimabukuro et al., 1998).

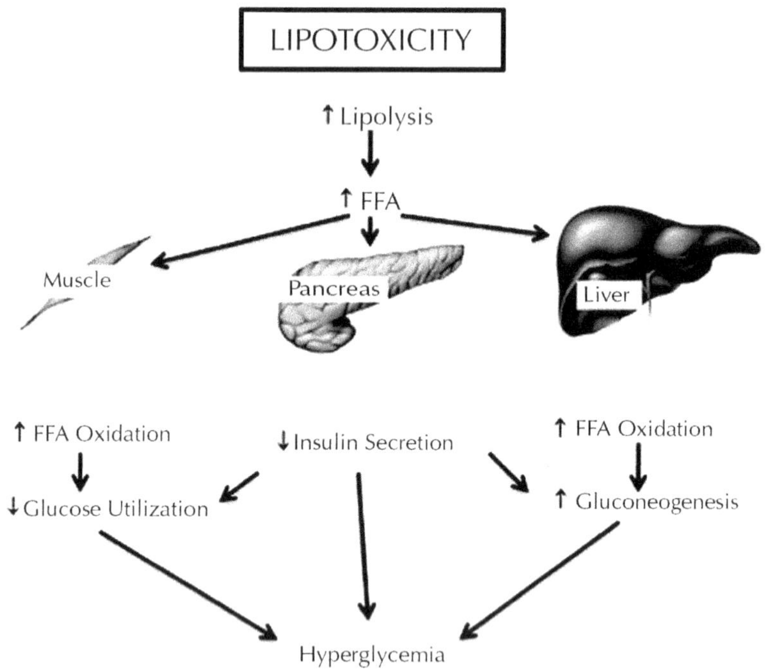

FIGURE 1 Relation between lipotoxicity and hyperglycemia.

The β-cell function and life cycle are known to be influenced by cytokines especially the proinflammatory cytokine interleukin-1β (IL-1β). Recently, it has received attention for its role in the pathogenesis of T2DM (Larsen et al., 2007). At low concentrations, IL-1β enhances human β-cell proliferation and decreases its apoptosis, whereas at higher concentration it impairs β-cell insulin release and increases its apoptosis (Maedler et al., 2002).

Recently, deficiency of or resistance to incretins (glucose-dependent insulinotropic peptide (GIP) and glucagon-like peptide-1 (GLP-1)) have been implicated in the pathogenesis of beta-cell dysfunction in T2DM patients (Vilsboll et al., 2001). Antibodies that neutralize GIP and GLP-1 impair glucose tolerance in a variety of animal species, including primates (Ahren et al., 1997).

Abnormalities in glucagon secretion have also been demonstrated in NIDDM. Plasma glucagon levels are elevated in NIDDM patients after glucose infusion as compared with normal subjects (Frank et al., 1998). In addition, the secretion of glucagon in response to hypoglycemia is abnormal in NIDDM patients (Shah et al., 2000). Therefore, alpha cell function may be abnormal in most NIDDM subjects.

1.3.4 INSULIN RESISTANCE

Insulin resistance appears to play a primary role in the development of NIDDM, and is the most important trait in the pathogenesis of NIDDM because it detects one to two decades prior to diagnosis of the disease. Insulin resistance may be best described as the loss of insulin regulation by the normal amount of insulin, which is a condition of reduced insulin sensitivity (Yki-Jarvinen, 1995). It has been reported that hyperinsulinemia precedes the development of NIDDM (Warram et al., 1990), and the progression from normal to IGT is associated with the development of severe insulin resistance (Unger and Grundy, 1985; Martin et al., 1992). Insulin resistance is a condition in which insulin in the body does not exert sufficient action proportional to its blood concentration. The impairment of insulin action in major target organs such as liver and muscles is a common pathophysiological feature of T2DM. Although, genetically influenced, insulin resistance is closely associated with obesity and ectopic fat accumulation, and may be mediated by increased FFAs (Gastaldelli et al., 2011).

The skeletal muscle is responsible for the major part (80%) of insulin-stimulated whole body glucose disposal, plays an important role in the development of insulin resistance (Pan et al., 1997). Insulin resistance in the muscle determines a reduced muscle uptake of glucose, mainly because of defects in intracellular insulin signaling. It has been observed that insulin resistance in skeletal muscle during FFA infusion rises when triglycerides start to accumulate inside muscle fibres in excess of their oxidation (Kelley et al., 1994).

Insulin resistance at the level of adipose tissue is also important. Besides promoting glucose uptake into adipocytes, insulin has two other important roles: promoting fatty acid re-esterification into triglyceride, and inhibiting triglyceride hydrolysis and release of FFA into the circulation (i.e. lipolysis) (Bergman et al., 1998). Triglyceride breakdown is increased and plasma nonesterified fatty acid (NEFA) concentrations are higher in patients with T2DM than in normal subjects studied at comparable insulin levels, suggesting that adipose tissue is also affected by insulin resistance (Roden et al., 1996).

Insulin acts at the level of the liver through a direct and/or indirect effect (i.e. on glucose transport and/or intracellular enzymes). The maintenance of normal glucose homeostasis is dependent upon three factors: hepatic glucose production (HGP), glucose uptake by muscle and adipocytes, and glucose-stimulated insulin secretion (Fery et al., 1994; Vaag et al., 1995). Insulin resistant subjects have increased fasting gluconeogenesis compared to their lean counterpart, despite normal endogenous glucose production (Meyer et al., 1998). This can be considered as an early manifestation of hepatic insulin resistance. It has been suggested that hepatic insulin resistance may be directly related to visceral adiposity, independent of total fat mass (Chen et al., 1995, Gastaldelli et al., 2007).

Insulin resistance clearly has a genetic component in NIDDM, as shown by the comparison of NIDDM subjects and non-diabetic subjects. The NIDDM is a complex disease that is currently thought to be influenced by more than a single gene or environmental factor (Busch and Hegele, 2001). Familial aggregation and the high concordance rate for the disease (60–100%) in identical twins suggest that genetic factors play an important role in the pathogenesis of NIDDM (Doria et al., 2008; Hanis et al., 1996). Such genes may affect β-cell apoptosis, regeneration, glucose sensing, glucose metabolism, ion channels, energy transduction, microtubules/microfilaments, and other islet proteins necessary for the synthesis, packaging, movement, and release of secretory granules (Bell et al., 2001). The advent of modern molecular biological techniques has been an invaluable resource for the genetic study of various diseases, including T2DM.

Inflammatory mediators are also important as the mechanisms of impaired insulin secretion and insulin signaling impairment. Recent attention has focused on the involvement of adipocyte-derived bioactive substances (adipokines) in insulin resistance (Donath et al., 2008). β-Cell function and life cycle are known to be influenced by cytokines especially the pro-inflammatory cytokine IL-1β (Larsen et al., 2007). The IL-1β is known for its cytokine-meditated β-cell destruction in T1DM but, more recently, it has received attention for its role in the pathogenesis of T2DM (Maedler et al., 2002).

The T2DM patients are under conditions of an increased oxidative stress and that the complications of DM are partially mediated by oxidative stress (Rains and Jain, 2011). Several mechanisms seem to be involved in the genesis of oxidative stress in diabetic patients (Ceriello, 2006). Among these, glucose autoxidation, non enzymatic protein glycation as well as the formation of advanced-glycation end products (AGEs) have been demonstrated in patients with diabetes and a direct relationship with the circulating blood glucose levels and glucose variability has been repeatedly demonstrated (Basta et al., 2004).The interplay between oxidative stress and AGEs is very complex.

Obesity has been shown to have a clear association with NIDDM (DeFronzo et al., 1997). An excess of the total amount of fat in the body and the distribution of body fat can each exert a negative effect on insulin sensitivity. This may be mediated by a variety of factors released from adipose tissue that can adversely affect β-cell function, including elevated levels of FFA, tumour necrosis factor alpha (TNF-α), resistin, leptin, and amylin as well as tissue accumulation of lipid (Carpentier et al., 2000; Hotamisligil and Spiegelman, 1994; Sanke et al., 1991). A central pattern of fat distribution (male-type obesity), manifested by an increase in waist/hip ratio, is particularly associated with insulin resistance. In contrast, the peripheral pattern of fat distribution (female-type obesity) has a relatively minor effect on insulin sensitivity (Kotronen et al., 2008). The reduced binding of insulin to target tissues in obesity is another possible mechanism for insulin resistance.

1.4 GENETICS AND MOLECULAR BASIS OF DIABETES

1.4.1 TYPE 1 DIABETES

The T1DM represents one of more than 80 diseases considered to have an autoimmune aetiology. The disease develops as a manifestation of the organ-specific immune destruction of the insulin-producing β-cells in the islets of Langerhans within the pancreas. There has been much progress in the identification of genes and molecular pathways involved in the pathogenesis of T1DM.

The human histocompatibility (HLA) complex contributes 40–50% of the overall susceptibility (Schranz, 1998). The strongest effect is from alleles coding for selected HLA class I and class II antigen-presenting molecules, which are restricting elements for autoreactive CD8 and CD4 T cells, respectively. The HLA complex is located on the short arm of chromosome 6 and is divided into three main regions: class I, class II and class III, harbouring genes involved in antigen presentation and the regulation of the immune response (Lie et al., 2005). Several class I alleles are independently associated with susceptibility, including HLA-A*0101, HLAA* 3002 and HLA-B39 (Noble et al., 2002; Valdes et al., 2005). The genotype that confers the highest risk of T1DM is the heterozygosity of the two high - risk HLA class II haplotypes: DR3 - DQ2 (DRB1 * *03 - DQA1 * 0501 - B1 * 0201)* and DR4 - DQ8 (*DRB1 * 04 - DQA1 * 0301 - B1 * 0302*) (Hermann et al., 2004). One or both of these haplotypes were found in more than 95% of people with T1DM younger than 30 years but also in approximately 40–50% of the general population (Notkins and Lernmark, 2001).

The CTLA-4 polymorphisms were linked to T1DM susceptibility in several studies, but not in all populations nor in studies that included pooled datasets from multiple countries (Marron et al., 1997). CTLA-4 is expressed by $CD4^+$ and $CD8^+$ T cells and (similar to CD28) binds B7-1 and B7-2 ligands during presentation of antigens bound to major histocompatibility complex (MHC) by antigen-presenting cells. Upon binding of B7, CTLA4 down-regulates T-cell proliferation and cytokine production, whereas binding of B7 to CD28 results in a co-stimulatory response.

It is thought that the CTLA4 function is critical for regulating peripheral self tolerance and prevention of auto immunity and it has therefore long been considered as a candidate gene for T1DM (Gough et al., 2005).

The *PTPN22* gene codes for the tyrosine phosphatase non-receptor type 22, or Lyp, a negative regulator of T cell receptor (TCR) signals (Cohen et al., 1999). Susceptibility maps to a missense mutation resulting in an arginine to tryptophan change at position 620 (R620W) (Onengut-Gumuscu et al., 2004). *In vitro*, T cells from patients carrying the R620W mutation secrete less IL-2 and show reduced phosphorylation of TCR signals compared with patients carrying the wild-type allele (Vang et al., 2005). Thus, the disease-predisposing R620W mutation is a gain-of-function variant that may predispose to autoimmunity by suppressing TCR signaling more potently. The mutation may also affect T cell function in the periphery, as well as the function of regulatory T cells and lymphocytes (Rieck et al., 2007).

The IL2RA gene codes for the α-chain of the IL-2 receptor (IL-2Rα, or CD25). Two single nucleotide polymorphisms (SNPs) in the IL2RA intron 1 and 5' region were initially associated with T1DM (Smyth et al., 2004). It promotes T cell proliferation and expansion and maintains the homeostasis of $CD4^+$ $CD25^+$ regulatory T cells. Clinical studies have provided initial evidence for a functional correlation, since patients homozygous for predisposing IL2RA alleles have lower levels of soluble IL-2 receptor, which correlate with the number of circulating activated T cells (Pugliese, 2010).

The insulin gene (*INS*) was one of the obvious candidate genes for T1DM, in part because of the existence of *INS*-specific autoantibodies (Pugliese et al., 1997). The region surrounding *INS* on chromosome 11p15 has been consistently linked to T1DM for more than two decades (the IDDM2 locus) (Bell et al., 1984). The main association was found around the insulin gene variable number tandem repeat (INS-VNTR) polymorphism in a 4.1 kb region encompassing the *INS* gene (Barratt et al., 2004). Homozygosity for class I VNTR alleles is found in approximately 75–85% of patients compared with 50–60% in the general population. It predisposes to T1DM and increases the probability that identical twins will be concordant for disease development (Metcalfe et al., 2001).

There is increasing evidence that some loci are subject to epigenetic regulation, which adds another layer of complexity, as it modulates transcription of inherited genes.

1.4.2 TYPE 2 DIABETES

The T2DM is largely known as a genetically determined disease. A large body of evidence on the high prevalence of T2DM in certain ethnic groups, the high concordance rate in monozygotic twins, familial transmission and familial aggregation patterns suggest that the genetic component plays a strong etiological role in the development of T2DM (Doria et al., 2008; Lawrence et al, 2009).

Studies showed a strong association with a region on chromosome 10q25 located in the *TCF7L2* gene. Clinically, carriers of the high-risk *TCF7L2* genotype have reduced insulin secretion (Florez et al, 2006), suggesting a possible role for TCF7L2 in the β cell dysfunction of T2DM. Over expression studies in β cells, showing a blunting of glucose-stimulated insulin secretion (Lyssenko et al, 2007) and in another a beneficial effect to protect islets from glucose- and cytokine-induced apoptosis and impaired function (Shu et al., 2008). Other studies suggest roles for TCF7L2 in T2DM *via* control of the incretin axis, HGP, and adipocyte function (Cauchi et al, 2006).

Another strongest association was found within the coding region of SLC30A8, a zinc membrane transporter (Zn-T8) that is highly expressed in pancreatic islets (Chimienti et al, 2004). This gene first emerged as a T2DM locus in the McGill/Imperial study (Sladek et al, 2007). The SLC30A8-overexpressing cells display enhanced glucose-stimulated insulin secretion (Chimienti et al, 2006), suggesting that the risk allele might act by impairing transporter function, thereby decreasing the amount of zinc available for cocrystallization with insulin in the secretory vesicles of β cells. Reduced pancreatic and islet zinc levels have been observed in some animal models of T2DM (Taylor, 2005), and zinc supplementation has been shown to improve glucose tolerance.

Mutations in hepatocyte nuclear factor-4 alpha (*HNF4A*) and insulin promoter factor-1 (*IPF1*) genes were also identified in a number of families with late- onset T2DM (Hani et al., 1999). The IPF-1/Pdx-1 has a dose- dependent regulatory effect on the expression of β-cell specific genes and therefore assists in the maintenance of euglycemia. As a consequence, frequent variations in the regulatory sequences controlling IPF- 1/ Pdx-1 expression in the β- cell, or in genes coding for transcription factors known to regulate IPF-1, could contribute to common T2DM susceptibility (Holmkvist et al., 2006).

Another well-replicated association was observed in the *CDKAL1* gene coding for cyclin-dependent kinase 5 (CDK5) regulatory subunit-associated protein 1- like 1, with the strongest association observed in the DeCODE study (Steinthorsdottir et al., 2007). The *CDKAL1* gene encodes a 65 kD protein that is expressed in a broad range of tissues and is believed to be an inhibitor of CDK5. The CDK5 itself has been shown to blunt insulin secretion in response to glucose and to play a permissive role in the decrease of insulin gene expression that results from glucotoxicity (Ubeda et al., 2006).Thus, it can speculate that reduced expression of CDKAL1 would result in enhanced activity of CDK5 in β cells, and this would lead to decreased insulin secretion; in agreement, this locus was significantly associated with small decreases in insulin response to a glucose load (Saxena et al, 2007).

The association with the *KCNJ11* gene concerns a common glutamate to lysine substitution at position 23 (E23K). A common variant, E23K, of *KCNJ11* /K IR 6.2 has now been convincingly associated with an increased risk of T2DM and decreased insulin secretion in glucose-tolerant subjects (Doria, et al., 2008). The lysine allele has been shown to reduce the sensitivity of β cell ATP-sensitive K^+ channels toward inhibitory $ATP4^-$, thereby increasing the threshold for insulin release (Schwanstecher et al., 2002). Consistent with this, this polymorphism has been associated with an insulin secretory defect in multiple studies (Nielsen et al, 2003). Thus, the *KCNJ11* polymorphisms could contribute to loss of glucose sensing in the β cell, leading to impairment in insulin secretion and action.

Another candidate gene that was extensively studied is the *PPAR-γ* gene. A common amino-acid polymorphism (Pro12Ala) in *PPAR* has been associated with the risk of T2DM. There is also evidence for interaction between this polymorphism and the insulin secretion in response to fatty acids, and body mass index (BMI) (Altshuler et al., 2000; Stefan et al.,

2001). The identified polymorphism in PPAR; PPAR-γ, which appears to modify susceptibility to T2DM and obesity, was identified a decade ago and produces a Pro12-to-Ala (P12A) change in the PPAR (Beamer et al, 1998).

The knowledge of the genetics of T2DM has come a long way since the days of a few candidate genes studied by means of one or two haphazardly chosen restriction fragment length polymorphisms. Also, the current analyses have only considered the effects of individual SNPs in isolation from the effect of other genes or environmental factors. As the effect of these variants becomes increasingly established, attention needs to be focused on gene and gene-environment interactions.

1.4.3 LINKAGE DISEQUILIBRIUM (LD) ANALYSIS REVEALS THE GENOMICS OF DIABETES

The availability of cost-efficient genotyping technologies and the development of very dense maps of polymorphic loci within the human genome have paved the way for large-scale genetic studies. Studies, which include genome wide association (GWA) studies, exploit LD relationships between variations at marker loci genotyped on a large number of subjects and variations at loci that reside in the vicinity of these marker loci. The LD is a statistical association between alleles at separate but linked loci, commonly resulting from a special ancestral haplotype, being common in the population studied (Doria et al., 2008). Haplotype analysis employing LD has been significant in deciphering the genetic bases of diabetes.

The GWA screen identified dozens of potential candidates; at least 15 loci emerged as been most consistently associated with risk of T2DM across multiple studies. The strongest association in all of the studies is with a region on chromosome 10q25 located in a 92 kb LD block in the *TCF7L2* gene (Grant et al., 2006), the association of the *TCF7L2* locus with T2DM is by far the strongest and most consistent signal across the GWA studies. Individuals homozygous for the high-risk allele have about a doubling of diabetes risk or about 12% of them will have T2DM versus 9% of heterozygotes and 6% of non-carriers (Watanabe et al., 2007).

The HHEX/IDE/KIF11 (10q23) is a locus on 10q23 ranked for association with T2DM in the McGill scan, and many other independent studies. The association signal lies in a 295 Kb block of LD that includes at least three potential T2DM genes— *HHEX* (a homeobox transcription factor), *KIF11* (a kinesin interacting factor), and *IDE* (insulin degrading enzyme) genes. Each of these genes show rather broad tissue expression (Farris et al., 2003), IDE would be considered as the strongest biological candidate gene at this locus.

The *KCNJ11* gene identified through the candidate gene approach ranked high for association with T2DM in the GWA studies. Both were found to be associated with T2DM in the WTCCC, Fusion, and DGI studies (Zeggini et al, 2007; Saxena et al, 2007), and both involve non-synonymous polymorphisms.

1.4.4 PROTEIN KINASE B (PKB) AND ITS ROLE IN DIABETES

In addition to a number of deleterious effects on cellular integrity and functions, diabetic pathogenesis milieu has been implicated in a rapidly growing number of alterations in signal transduction. The serine-threonine kinase Akt also known as PkB is one of the most studied molecules. It is a serine/threonine kinase with the pleckstrin homology domain (PH) in its NH_2 terminal region and catalytic domain closely related to protein kinase C (PKC) and protein kinase A (PKA) family members (Staal, 1987). Three *Akt* genes are present in the mammalian genomes; *Akt1*, *Akt2*, and *Akt3* that code for three widely expressed isoforms of Akt kinase (Woodgett, 2005). The Akt is an important mediator of biological functions of insulin. One of the major effects of this hormone is the enhancement of glucose uptake in muscle, adipocytes, liver, and other tissues (Zdychova and Komers, 2005). Therefore, it is not surprising that Akt signaling has major impact on glucose metabolism. Earlier studies recognized that PI3K is mainly responsible for the insulin mediated stimulation of glucose transporter type 4 (GLUT4), the crucial insulin-regulated glucose transporter, which transports glucose from intracellular vesicles to the plasma membrane in insulin-sensitive cells (Okada et al. 1994). Upon insulin stimulation Akt associates with GLUT4 transporters and glucose uptake is mediated by

Akt-induced translocation of vesicles containing GLUT4 from intracellular stores to the plasma membrane (Kohn et al. 1996). In this cellular location, GLUT4 mediate glucose uptake. Furthermore, in response to insulin, Akt promotes glycogen synthesis *via* serine phosphorylation and inactivation of glycogen-synthase kinase-3 (GSK-3) (Lawrence and Roach, 1997).

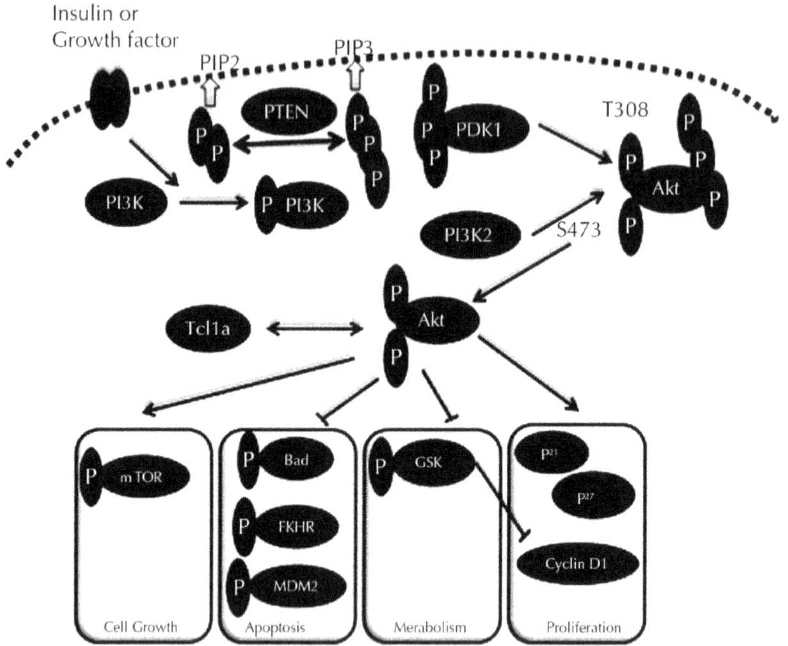

FIGURE 2 Schematic representation of phosphatidylinositol 3-kinase (PI3-K)/Akt pathway.

The Akt can be activated by a wide variety of growth stimuli such as growth factors and cytokines. The role of Akt kinase, its alterations in DM, and its importance in the pathophysiology of diabetic microvascular complications have been widely studied. A schematic diagram of Akt pathway is given in Figure 2. There is convincing evidence suggesting defective Akt signaling in the development of insulin resistance (Krook et al., 1997). An accumulating body of evidence indicates that abnormal regulation of the PI3-K/Akt pathway may be one of several factors contributing to vascular dysfunction in diabetes. The PI3-K pathway activates Akt, the serine/threonine protein kinase enhances nitric oxide (NO) synthase phosphorylation and NO production (Elghazi et al., 2006). The several studies suggest that in diabetes the relative ineffectiveness of insulin and the hyperglycemia act together to reduce activity in the insulin-receptor substrates such as (IRS)/PI3-K/Akt pathway, caused impairments of both IRS/PI3-K/Akt-mediated endothelial function and NO production (Fulton et al., 1999). Similar defects have been reported in endothelium of T2DM models, probably contributing to the development of endothelial dysfunction under these conditions (Mcveigh et al., 1992). Other factors such as glucosamine, a product of hexosamine pathway, intensively studied in the pathophysiology of diabetic complications (Schleicher and Weigert, 2000), has also been shown to diminish Akt activation in endothelial cells (Du et al., 2001). Another factor implicated in impaired Akt activation in diabetic tissues is oxidative stress (Tirosh et al., 1999). Overproduction of hydrogen peroxide (H_2O_2) in adipocytes leads to 90% reduction of Akt phosphorylation.

Macro and microvascular disease states currently represent the principal causes of morbidity and mortality in patients with T1DM or T2DM. Therefore, pharmacological modulation of Akt activity is one of possible targets in future treatment of early stages of T1DM that may prevent or delay the destruction of β-cells.

1.4.5 VASCULAR ENDOTHELIAL GROWTH FACTOR (VEGF) MODULATES VASCULAR COMPLICATIONS IN DIABETES

The VEGF is implicated in the pathogenesis of many diabetic complications including nephropathy, retinopathy, neuropathy, and CVD (Duh and Aiello, 1999). The VEGF is an angiogenic factor with endothelial cell-selective mitogenic activity that plays a critically important role in vasculogenesis (Olsson et al., 2006). The VEGF is a highly conserved homodimeric glycoprotein composed of four isoforms resulting from alternative messenger ribonucleic acid (mRNA) splicing in humans (Ferrara et al., 1991). The VEGF mediates its action predominately through two known VEGF receptors referred to as Flt-1 (*VEGFR1*) and Flk-1/KDR (*VEGFR2*) (Neufeld et al., 1999). These receptors are expressed predominantly in endothelial cells although they have been identified in renal mesangial cells, monocytes, hematopoietic cells, and the retina (Aiello and Wong, 2000).

Recently, much research has focused on VEGF because this potent biogenic permeability factor plays an important role in the pathogenesis of vascular complications in diabetes and is one of the major factors promoting diabetic retinopathy. Elevated VEGF in the vitreous of people with diabetic retinopathy and in animal models of diabetes is sufficient to increase both vascular proliferation and permeability (Adamis et al., 1993). Accumulated evidence has suggested that molecular processes involved in vascular growth and vascular hyper permeability are based on the inappropriate regulation of VEGF (Lorenzi and Cagliero, 1991).

The evidence that VEGF is involved in diabetic renal disease is less extensive than the evidence for its involvement in retinopathy, but several investigations suggest such an association. Increased VEGF mRNA and protein levels have been observed in models of diabetic kidney disease (Schrijvers et al., 2004). There is increasing evidence that the VEGF-A/VEGF receptor and the angiopoietins/Tie-2 (tyrosine kinase with Ig and EGF homology domain 2) receptor systems are involved in the maintenance of the integrity of the glomerular filtration barrier in the kidney in both physiology and diseases (Cas and Gnudi, 2012). VEGF-A is the predominant VEGF isoform found in the glomerulus. The VEGF-A is highly expressed during glomerular development, and plays a central role in vasculogenesis and neoangiogenesis by promoting the migration, survival and proliferation of endothelial cells, and in regulating vessels' permeability and in vascular repair by recruiting inflammatory and endothelial precursor cells (Baelde et al., 2007). However, the precise role of VEGF in diabetic nephropathy is uncertain.

Although, not currently directly implicated in the development of diabetes-related atherosclerotic disease, VEGF may serve a salutary role in the hypoxic myocardial tissues of coronary artery disease by promoting development of collateral circulation (Woodfield et al., 1996). Overall, VEGF appears to play a central role in mediating diabetic vasculopathy in many organs. Further investigations to understand molecular mechanisms underlying these processes have permitted development of novel therapeutic approaches, several of which are now in human clinical trials.

1.4.6 CYTOKINE SNPS ASSOCIATED WITH T2DM

Cytokines are protein mediators of intercellular stress communication with multiple modes of action. Virtually all nucleated cells produce and respond to cytokines under defined conditions, mostly in response to stress factors and in parallel to their differentiated functions. Deficiency in expression or over expression of cytokine molecules leads to diseases such as, heart disease, cancer, and diabetes (Hotamisligil, 2006). The cytokine group of molecules encompasses several hundred individual proteins including 37 interleukins (ILs) and a multitude of chemokines (King, 2008). Such variations manifesting as SNPs may also be directly responsible for causality of disease acting either as a non-synonymous or synonymous SNP. Several GWA studies have identified and confirmed cytokine SNPs being associated with diseases in a particular population (Mandrup-Poulsen, 2005).

In accordance with this, several studies have demonstrated associations between SNPs in cytokine genes and T2DM (Rabinovitch and Suarez-Pinzon, 2003). The T2DM is characterized by the failure of the β-cells to compensate for peripheral insulin resistance (Shoelson et al., 2006). A vast number of epidemiological, genetic studies have investigated the putative role of action/lack of action of IL-6 in the pathogenesis underlying insulin resistance, β-cell destruction, and T2DM (Hu et al., 2004). These studies suggest both protective and pathogenic actions of IL-6 in diabetes. Several genetic studies of *IL6* in relation to T1DM and T2DM and studies of *IL6R* in relation to T2DM have been reported. Elevated levels of IL-6 predict future risk of T2DM (Pradhan et al., 2001).

The TNF-α is a potent cytokine that was originally identified as a factor with a wide range of pro-inflammatory activities (Hotamisligil et al., 1995). However, later on, an important role of TNF-α in the pathogenesis of insulin resistance was also indicated, as many human studies showed a relationship between serum TNF-α levels and insulin resistance (Moller, 2000). Therefore, TNF-α seems to impair insulin action, and, thus lead to the development of T2DM (DM). The association of the *TNF-α* gene polymorphisms with DM and its related conditions, such as insulin resistance and obesity, has been extensively examined (Kroeger et al., 1997). Among them, two SNPs, G-308A and G-238A, of the promoter region of the *TNF*-α gene were the well-annotated SNPs shown to be associated with DM in many populations (Walston et al., 1999). Furthermore, these SNPs were shown to be probably functional: The A allele of the SNP G-308A was shown by *in vitro* analysis to have increased transcriptional activity over the G allele, and the SNP G-238A was shown to be located in a repressor site of the gene (Rasmussen et al., 2000).

The proinflammatory cytokine IL-1β is known for its cytokine- meditated β-cell destruction in T1DM (Mandrup-Poulsen, 1996) but more recently, it has received attention for its role in the pathogenesis of T2DM. At low concentrations, IL-1β enhances human β-cell proliferation and decreases its apoptosis, whereas at higher concentration it impairs β-cell insulin release and increases its apoptosis (Maedler et al., 2006). The IL-1β up regulates Fas expression within β-cells, ultimately enabling Fas-induced apoptosis (Maedler et al., 2001).

The IL-4, mainly secreted by activated T cells, $Fc\varepsilon R1^+$ cells, and eosinophils, is an important anti-inflammatory cytokine that can inhibit the secretion of the proinflammatory cytokines from macrophages (Paul, 1997). An association between homologous IL-4, -589 C/C genotype and lower high-density lipoprotein cholesterol (HDL-C) level is observed, suggesting that polymorphisms of the IL-4 promoter may contribute to the HDL-C metabolism, T2DM predisposition, and diabetic complications (Hoa et al., 2010). A variant of IL8 to be associated with higher risk of diabetic nephropathy. The IL8 T-251A variant lies in the regulatory region and increases the gene expression (Tashiro et al., 2002), suggesting that this genotype could regulate *IL8* gene expression. This variant has been associated with inflammatory renal injury (Rovin et al, 2002) showing an association of this allele with increased risk of diabetic nephropathy.

The causal association of SNP to disease can be important in understanding the genetic basis of disease at a single nucleotide level, and hence be a better source for a drug target since allele specific drugs can be improved drugs with high specificity and high sensitivity.

1.5 PERSONALIZED TREATMENT-PROSPECTS

The different pathogenic mechanisms are involved in the development of various forms of diabetes, including genetic and environmental alterations in the action and secretion of insulin (Chaturvedi, 2007). Within this spectrum of diabetes pathophysiology and subtypes there is established heterogeneity in the determinants of diabetes and the risk of diabetes complications (Malandrino and Smith, 2011). Understanding the basis of this heterogeneity provides an opportunity for personalizing prevention and treatment strategies according to individual patient clinical and molecular characteristics.

Personalized medicine represents an approach for defining disease subtypes and defining biomarkers that can identify patients who are most likely to benefit from a specific treatment and other patients who are unlikely to respond or likely to experience side events (Malandrino and Smith, 2011). Not every patient with diabetes with the same age, disease duration, body mass index, and hemoglobin A1c (HbA1c) will respond the same way to a given treatment. The reason may be a genetic propensity to respond or not respond to a drug (Woodcock, 2007). Given the remarkable progress over the past few years in characterization of human gene sequences, there now is particular interest in the potential for using individual molecular biomarkers to direct patient specific decisions on the management of diabetes.

Both T1DM and T2DM are thought to be complex diseases that develop through the interplay of numerous susceptibility and protective genes, results in action in concert with negative and positive environmental factors (Pearson et al., 2003). Multiple genetic factors have been associated with T1DM, which may ultimately define individualized strategies for preventing β-cell destruction. While knowledge of these specific genes and loci does not yet have practical application in individualizing T1DM management, it can be assumed that such genetic markers ultimately may have utility in defining personalized approaches to both prevention and treatment of T1DM (Bozkurt et al., 2007). Candidate gene and GWA studies thus far have identified at least 23 genes with sequence variations associated with T2DM across multiple populations (Klonoff, 2008). Patients who are identified by genetic testing to be at high risk for diabetes can be directed to preventative strategies, such as lifestyle modifications to delay or prevent the disease (Pearson, 2009). Personalized medicine allows for personalized drug prescribing with less trial and error and less time wasted with an inadequate response or with side effects (McCarthy and Hattersley, 2008).

Much of the mortality of T1DM and T2DM results from long-term microvascular complications (diabetic retinopathy, nephropathy, and neuropathy) and macrovascular complications (peripheral vascular disease, and stroke) (Golubnitschaja, 2010). The onset and progression of diabetes complications correlate substantially with glycemic control. Just as the choice of specific drugs for management of glycemia in diabetes. There is a similar potential for individualizing decisions on treatment and drug choice for management of nonglycemic risk factors for diabetes complications on the basis of individual characteristics.

1.6 CAUSES AND RISK FACTORS OF DIABETES

1.6.1 DIET

The excessive caloric intake is a major driving force behind escalating obesity and T2DM epidemic globally, but diet quality also plays a significant role (Hu, 2011). The Nurses' Health Study (NHS), found that the quality of fats and carbohydrates play an important role in diabetes development, independent of BMI and other risk factors (Hu et al., 2001). In particular, higher dietary glycemic load (GL) and trans fat are associated with increased diabetes risk, meanwhile higher consumption of polyunsaturated fat and cereal fiber is associated with low risk. In epidemiological studies, a high saturated fat intake has been associated with higher risk of IGT and higher fasting glucose and insulin levels (Feskens et al., 1995; Parker et al., 1993; Bo et al., 2001). Higher proportions of saturated fatty acids in serum lipids/muscle phospholipids have been associated with higher fasting insulin levels, lower insulin sensitivity and higher risk of developing T2DM (Schuster, 2010). Many developing nations experience rapid economic and social development with concomitant shifts in lifestyle habits and dietary structure. Data from the 1992–2002 Chinese National Nutrition Survey show that the proportion of energy from animal foods increased from 9.3 to 13.7%, while the proportion of fat rose from 22 to 29.8% (Wang et al., 2007). This nutritional shift typically involves increased consumption of energy dense foods, animal fat, decreased fibre, and more frequent intake of fast foods. At the same time, the common diets of many Asian countries, which are mainly based on polished white rice and refined wheat, have a high glycemic index (GI) (Yoon et al., 2006). Trans fat intake is associated with adverse cardio metabolic risk profiles and increased risk of cardiac diseases, and it may also play a role in the development of insulin resistance and chronic inflammation (Lopez-Garcia et al., 2005). Evidence also indicates that higher consumption of sugar-sweetened beverages (SSBs) increases the risk of T2DM even after taking into account the effects of body weight. The recent meta analysis found that individuals in the highest quantity of SSB intake (most often 1–2 servings/day) had a 26% greater risk of developing the disease than those in the lowest (Malik et al., 2010).

1.6.2 SMOKING

Cigarette smoking is an independent risk factor for T2DM. According to a meta-analysis found that current smokers had a 45% increased risk of developing diabetes compared with non-smokers (Willi et al., 2007). Cigarette smoking may increase risk of diabetes in many ways. Smoking has been shown to cause elevations in blood glucose concentration and may increase insulin resistance (Facchini et al., 1992). Current smokers also tend to have higher blood concentrations of glycosylated hemoglobin (HbA1c) than do non-smokers (Nilsson et al., 1995). Smoking has been associated with increased risk of central obesity or abdominal fat (Barrett-Connor and Khaw, 1989), an established risk factor for insulin resistance and diabetes.

1.6.3 PHYSICAL INACTIVITY

The numerous studies have indicated the importance of physical inactivity in the development of T2DM (Manson et al., 1991, Burchfiel et al., 1995). Prolonged television watching as a surrogate marker of sedentary lifestyle was reported to be positively associated with diabetes risk in both men and women (Hu et al., 2003). The deleterious effect of low levels of physical activity is seen particularly among those subjects who have other risk factors such as high BMI, HTN, or parental diabetes. But for equivalent degrees of obesity, physically active subjects have a lower incidence of diabetes (Manson et al., 1992).

1.6.4 OBESITY

The overweight and obesity are driving the global diabetes epidemic. They are the major factors that affect the majority of adults in most developed countries and are increasing rapidly in developing countries (Bouchard et al., 1990). Obesity has increased rapidly in many populations in recent years because of an interaction between genetic and environmental factors. These factors include: Metabolic characteristics, physical inactivity, habitual energy intake in relation to expenditure, and macronutrient composition of the diet (Grundy et al., 1992). Overweight or obesity is the single most important predictors of T2DM, and the effect of obesity on lifetime risk of T2DM is stronger in younger adults. The data from the NHS suggest that the lowest risk of diabetes occurs in individuals who have a BMI, with increasing prevalence seen as obesity levels increase (Kuczmarski et al., 1994). The several studies indicate that waist circumference or waist-to-hip ratio may be a better indicator of the risk of developing diabetes than BMI (Chan et al., 1994; Despres, 2001). Such data suggest that the distribution of body fat is an important determinant of risk as these measures reflect abdominal or visceral obesity. Results of a 5 yr prospective study of insulin resistance in Pima Indians showed a clear relationship between IGT and the subsequent development of T2DM (Lillioja et al., 1993).

1.6.5 ETHNICITY

The prevalence of type 2 varies considerably among populations of different ethnic origins living in apparently similar environments. High prevalence rates of diabetes have also been found among Asian Indians compared with the indigenous populations in Fiji, the United Kingdom, South Africa, and in the Caribbean (Mather et al., 1998; Omar et al., 1993). Considerable differences in the prevalence of diabetes have also been described among the multi-ethnic populations of New Zealand and Hawaii, where the Maori populations and Native Hawaiians, both of Polynesian origin, have higher prevalences than other ethnic groups (Simmons et al., 1996; Steyn et al., 2004). While environmental factors undoubtedly account for some of these variations, also they are more likely to reflect inherent ethnic differences in susceptibility to the disease.

The SEARCH study reviewed five major races and ethnic groups in the U.S., non-Hispanic white, Asian and Pacific Islander, African American, Hispanic, and Navajo populations (Mayer-Davis et al., 2009; Lawrence et al, 2009). In the non-Hispanic white population the prevalence rate of T1DM was 2 out of 1,000 and the incidence was 23.6/100,000 (Bell et al., 2009). The study concludes that these rates of T1DM among non-Hispanic white youth are among the highest in the world. These youth had higher cardio metabolic risk profiles (>40% with elevated low-density lipoprotein (LDL)) which put them at risk for future health complications related to diabetes (Maahs et al., 2011).

1.6.6 GENETIC SUSCEPTIBILITY

Although, the majority of T1DM cases occurs in individuals without a family history of the disease, T1DM is highly influenced by genetic factors. Of the multiple genes implicated in susceptibility to T1DM, the major one is the HLA complex on chromosome 6, mainly the HLA class II. Two susceptibility haplotypes present in the HLA class II region are now considered the principal susceptibility markers for T1DM (Ng et al., 2008). Although, 90–95% of young children with T1DM carry either or both susceptibility haplotypes, approximately 5% or fewer persons with HLA-conferred genetic susceptibility actually develop clinical disease (Wu et al., 2008). Genetic susceptibility for T1DM ranges from marked in childhood-onset T1DM to a more modest effect in adult-onset T1DM, in which children having a higher identical twin concordance rate and a greater frequency of HLA genetic susceptibility are more prone to develop

T1DM (Southam et al., 2009). Siblings of children with onset of T1DM before the age of 5 yrs have a three- to five-fold greater cumulative risk of diabetes by age 20 compared to siblings of children diagnosed between 5 and 15 yrs of age (Hales et al., 2001). Common variants of the TCF7L2 gene that are significantly associated with diabetes risk represent in 20–30% of Caucasian populations but only 3–5% of Asians (Ng et al., 2008). Conversely, a variant in the *KCNQ1* gene associated with a 20–30% increased risk of diabetes in several Asian populations is common in East Asians, but rare in Caucasians (Yasuda et al., 2008).

1.7 FREE RADICALS AND OXIDATIVE STRESS IN DIABETES

The balance between the rate of free radical generation and elimination is important. Excessive generation of free radical can be harmful, increased oxidative stress is a widely accepted participant in the development and progression of diabetes and its complications (Baynes and Thorpe, 1999). There is convincing experimental and clinical evidence that the generation of reactive oxygen species (ROS) increases in both types of diabetes and that the onset of diabetes is closely associated with oxidative stress (Rains and Jain, 2011). Many studies have shown that increased lipid peroxides and/or oxidative stress are present in diabetic subjects (Maritim and Sanders, 2003). Oxidative stress can be increased before clinical signs of diabetic complications. In diabetes, oxidative stress seems caused by both increased production of free radicals, considerable reduction in antioxidant defences and altered cellular redox status.

During diabetes, persistent hyperglycemia causes increased production of free radicals, from glucose auto-oxidation and protein glycosylation (Tsai et al., 1994; Hori et al., 1996). The aetiology of oxidative stress in diabetes arises from a variety of mechanisms such as auto-oxidation of glucose, non enzymatic protein glycosylation, shifts in redox balances, decreased tissue concentrations of low molecular weight antioxidants including reduced glutathione (GSH) and vitamin E, impaired activities of antioxidant defence enzymes such as superoxide dismutase (SOD), catalase (CAT) and decreased ascorbic acid levels. As the development of DM is characterized by high serum glucose levels, can be an origin of ROS over production. High glucose levels can initiate the production of H_2O_2 and superoxide, precursors of reactive free radicals, which are capable of disrupting the antioxidant systems, damage cellular biomolecules, and increase the level of lipid peroxidation in diabetes (Saxena et al., 1993; Halliwell and Gutteridge, 1996).

The oxidative stress is currently the unifying factor in the development of diabetes complications. There are mainly four mechanisms by which chronic hyperglycemia cause diabetes complications: Activation of the polyol pathway, increased formation of advanced glycosylation end products, activation of PKC, involved in many molecular signaling pathways, and activation of the hexsosamine pathway (Baynes, 1991; McLennan et al., 1991). The disorders of the physiological signaling functions of ROS (superoxide and H_2O_2) and reactive nitrogen species (NO and peroxynitrite (ONOO)) are important features of diabetes (Oberly, 1988). Enhanced oxidative stress in T2DM has further a variety of important effects in atherogenesis, particulary LDL oxidation (Leiter L. 1999).

The enhanced oxidative stress may directly induce endothelial dysfunction by the decreased synthesis or release of NO by endothelial cells and by inactivating NO with superoxide in sub endothelial space (Stocker, 1999). The decreased NO release or inactivation of NO by ROS may be responsible for these impaired endothelium-dependent vasodilator responses. The majority of human studies suggest abnormal endothelium dependent vasodilatation in T1DM (Gazis et al., 1999). In inflammatory conditions, such as obesity, the immune system generates both superoxide and NO, that may react together to produce significant amounts of ONOO- anion (Li and Forstermann, 2000). The ONOO is a potent oxidizing agent that can cause deoxyribonucleic acid (DNA) fragmentation and lipid peroxidation. There are multiple lines of evidence demonstrating the formation of ONOO in diabetic vasculature, both in experimental models and in humans (Bergendi et al., 1999). The mechanisms that underlie ONOO-induced diabetic complications and vascular alterations are multiple. One of the important pathways of ONOO-mediated vascular dysfunction in diabetes involves activation of the nuclear enzyme poly (ADP-ribose) polymerases (PARP enzymes).

1.8 PHYSICAL STRESS AND DIABETES

While, stress has long been considered an important factor in diabetes, there has been very little experimental evidence to show how it might affect the development of the disease. In people who have diabetes, stress can alter blood sugar levels.

The effects of stress on glucose metabolism are mediated by a variety of counter-regulatory hormones that are released in response to stress and that result in elevated blood glucose levels and decreased insulin action (Mitra, 2008). However, in diabetes, because of a relative or absolute deficiency of insulin, stress-related increases in blood glucose cannot be adequately metabolized. The stressful stimuli can also result in elevated blood glucose levels via several different hypothalamic pituitary pathways (Surwit et al., 2002). The cortisol causes enhanced glucose production by the liver and diminished cellular glucose uptake. This mechanism may lead to both central obesity and a predisposition to diabetes if individuals are exposed to chronic stress (Bjorntorp, 1991). The stress-induced release of growth hormone and beta-endorphin can also decrease glucose uptake, suppress insulin secretion, and elevate glucose levels (Guillemin, 1978). Furthermore, in people diagnosed with T2DM, hormones that include adrenaline and cortisol results in the mobilization of stored energy including glucose and fatty acids. The direct effects of stress on the nerves controlling the pancreas can also inhibit insulin release. Energy mobilization is part of the 'fight or flight' response and is useful to prepare individuals to deal with stressors. In people who have diabetes, the fight-or-flight response does not work well. In this condition insulin is not always able to let the extra energy into the cells, so glucose piles up in the blood (Surwit and Williams, 1996). Stress increases the release of mediators of inflammations, leading to insulin resistance and hyperglycemia (McMahon et al., 1995). Inflammatory cytokines such as IL-6 and TNF-α may directly or indirectly enhance both hepatic gluconeogenesis and glycogenolysis.

Physical stress, including illness or injury, increase blood glucose levels in people with either type of diabetes. The stress blocks the body from insulin release in people with T2DM (Mitra, 2008). For some people with diabetes, limiting stress with relaxation therapy seems to help. It is more helpful for people with T2DM than people with T1DM. The T1DM patients do not make insulin, so stress controlling does not have this effect. Simple stress management techniques can have a significant impact on long-term blood glucose control and can constitute a useful tool in the management of this common condition (Gilbert et al., 1989).

Therapeutic approaches aimed at reducing the stress response and its metabolic effects in diabetic patients have included intensive family therapy, and long term beta blockade (Kashiwagi et al., 1986).

1.9 ROLE OF DIETARY SUGARS IN INSULIN RESISTANCE

The wide distribution of fructose and other individual sugars in foods and limitations in the available data describing its content in the majority of food items, it is not easy to accurately calculate fructose and other sugar intakes for an individual. For added sugar intake, U.S. Department of Agriculture (USDA) provides the added sugar content in foods, which can be used to calculate an individual's total added sugar intake (Sun et al., 2011). Added sugars mainly include dietary sugar/molasses from beet or cane, corn sweeteners (including high fructose corn syrup such as HFCS-55, HFCS-42, and corn syrup), honey, maple sugar/syrup, and sorghum syrup (Stanhope and Havel, 2010).

From the early 1970s through the mid-1990s, HFCS gradually replaced sugar in many manufactured products, and almost entirely replaced sugar in soft drinks manufactured in the USA. In 1970, individual consumption of fructose was only 0.5 lb/yr. The last 25 yrs have witnessed a marked increase in total per capita fructose intake as a sweetener in the food industry, firstly in the form of sucrose (a disaccharide containing of 50% fructose) and high-fructose corn syrup (HFCS; 55–90% fructose content) (Bray et al, 2004). The disturbing fact is fructose consumption (excluding that which occurs naturally in fruits and vegetables) increased from 0.5 g/day in 1970 to more than 40 g/day in 1997 (more than an 80-fold increase) (Gaby, 2005). Several studies have concluded that intakes of fructose or high fructose corn syrup (HFCS) were associated with increased risk of obesity or metabolic syndrome (Hu and Malik, 2010; Stanhope and Havel, 2008). In addition, excessive fructose consumption may be responsible in part for the increasing prevalence of DM and CVDs (Jurgens et al., 2005).

The high flux of fructose to the liver disturbs glucose metabolism and uptake pathways and leads to metabolic disturbances that underlie the induction of insulin resistance, a hallmark of T2DM (Bezerra et al., 2001). The relationship between sugar consumption and indicators of metabolic syndrome in individuals is a current debate among health professionals.

1.10 OBESITY AND DIABETES

The epidemic of obesity is worldwide – the WHO statistics from 2005 demonstrated that 400 million people were obese in the world, with a prospective increase to 700 million by 2015 (Schuster, 2010).This increase in obesity is a prelude to multiple obesity-associated health problems including CVD, T2DM (DM), and HTN, and often these occur together (Stunkard et al., 1986). The aetiology for the increasing incidence of obesity is primarily lifestyle-related reduced physical activity and over nutrition but susceptibility to obesity is complex and involves environment influenced by genetics (Must et al., 1992). According to twin studies the heritability of obesity is high, ranging between 0.6 and 0.9, with only slightly lower values in twins raised apart compared with those raised together (Bougneres, 2002). Obese adults demonstrate reduced glucose disposal, initially at the skeletal muscle (peripheral insulin resistance), as well as deterioration in insulin action on nonesterified fatty acid oxidation leading to insulin resistance and abnormal lipolysis (Goodpaster, 1997).

The obesity is obviously associated with an increased number and/or size of adipose tissue cells. These cells overproduce hormones, such as leptin, and cytokines, such as TNF-α, some of which appear to cause cellular resistance to insulin (Shoelson et al., 2006; Lumeng et al., 2007; Margetic et al., 2002). Retinol-binding protein-4, produced by the adipose tissue, induces insulin resistance through reduced phosphatidylinosital-3-OH kinase signaling in the muscle and increase expression of phosphenolpyruvate carboxykinase in the liver, along with diminished adiponectin and PPAR-γ activity typical for obesity (Sprangler et al., 2003; Yang et al., 2005; Adams et al., 1997; Kahn and Hull, 2006). One striking clinical feature of overweight individuals is a marked elevation of serum levels of NEFAs, cholesterol, and triacylglycerols irrespective of the dietary intake of fat. The insulin resistance in adipose tissue results in increased activity of the hormone-sensitive lipase, which would explain the increase in circulating NEFAs (Iozzo, 2009). The high circulating levels of NEFAs may also contribute to insulin resistance in the muscle and liver.

It is widely accepted that the current worldwide epidemic of obesity is largely a consequence of dramatic changes in lifestyle and environment which emerged over the past 30–50 years. A rather novel phenomenon is the expansion of the fast food culture characterized by high-fat, low-starch foods together with a high intake of sugar-sweetened beverages (Olsen and Heitmann, 2008). Another aspect in the context of high fast food consumption which may further explain the elevated risk of obesity is the energy density of modern foods (Prentice and Jebb, 2003; Rosenheck, 2008).

The cornerstones of a weight reduction program for obese patients with diabetes include a moderately hypocaloric diet, an increase in physical activity and behavior modification (Hauner, 2004). At present, only two compounds are available that has demonstrated efficacy and safety in obese subjects with and without T2DM. Orlistat is a gastric and pancreatic lipase inhibitor that impairs the intestinal absorption of ingested fat. Sibutramine is a selective serotonin and noradrenaline reuptake inhibitor that enhances satiety and slightly increases thermogenesis (Lloret et al., 2008).

1.11 DIAGNOSIS OF DIABETES

Blood glucose values are normally maintained in a narrow range usually 70 to 120mg/dL. The search for diabetes in an individual is often driven by the presence of characteristic symptoms such as polyuria, recurrent infections and weight loss in more severe cases, pre-coma. Individuals' belonging to this class, a single elevated casual plasma glucose value is sufficient to confirm the diagnosis. The diagnosis of diabetes established by any one of the following criteria, serum glucose-based tests and glycated proteins (Barr et al., 2002). Serum glucose-based tests include fasting plasma glucose (FPG), random plasma glucose (RPG), and the oral glucose tolerance test (OGTT). The most thoroughly studied and useful glycated protein is A1C (HbA1c) (ADA, 2003). The ADA has established criteria for testing undiagnosed people (Cox and Edelman, 2009). An FPG greater than 126 mg/dL is diagnostic for diabetes. If the FPG is 110 to 126 mg/dL, then an OGTT, should be performed to determine the degree of glucose intolerance. If the FPG score is less than 110 mg/dL, the test should be repeated at 3 yr intervals. In each instance, positive findings must be confirmed by repeat testing on a subsequent day. The commonly used diagnostic tests for diabetes are given as follows.

1.11.1 FASTING PLASMA GLUCOSE TEST (FPG)

The FPG test is a simple plasma glucose measurement obtained after at least 8 hours of fasting (usually an overnight fast) (Sacks et al., 2002). In a comparative analysis, FPG show better intra-individual reproducibility than 2 hr post-load plasma glucose, with intra-individual coefficients versus 14.3–16.7% for 2 hr plasma glucose with intra-individual coefficients of variation of 6.4–11.4% for FPG versus 14.3–16.7% for 2 hr plasma glucose (Cheng et al., 2006). A FPG level 126mg/dL (7.0 mmol/L) meets the threshold for the diagnosis of diabetes.

1.11.2 RANDOM PLASMA GLUCOSE TEST (RPG)

Advantages of the RPG measurement are that it is easily obtained and does not require fasting (Saudek et al., 2008). The commonly held RPG threshold is ≥ 200 mg/dL, along with symptoms such as polyuria, polydipsia, and unusual weight loss to indicate a second test for confirmation of diagnosis. An RPG of 140–199 mg/dL is suggestive of pre-diabetes (Edelman et al., 2004). Based on diagnosis by OGTT, an RPG ≥ 200 mg/dL is insensitive but has a specificity approaching 100%, which, in the background of symptoms, is unlikely to lead to a false-positive diagnosis.

1.11.3 THE ORAL GLUCOSE TOLERANCE TEST (OGTT)

The OGTT was introduced in 1922 and has been one of the diagnostic tests of choice for the past 80 yrs (Ko et al., 1998). In symptomatic individuals with RPG values >200 mg/dL, the OGTT is not required for a diagnosis of diabetes. Nevertheless in asymptomatic subjects and to establish a diagnosis of IGT, the OGTT is necessary (Engelgau et al., 2000). The test should be performed in the morning on subjects who have had at least 3 days of unrestricted diet. The individual should have fasted overnight for 10–16 hrs and remain seated and not smoke throughout the analysis. Primarily a fasting blood sample should be collected, after that the subject should drink 75 g of glucose in a concentration no greater than 25 g per 100 mL. It was originally suggested that blood samples be taken at mid test (1–2 hr, 1 hr, or 11–2 hrs) and at 2 hrs.

1.11.4 GLYCATED HAEMOGLOBIN (HbA_{1c})

The introduction of HbA_{1c} as a means to test glycemic control has had an enormous impact on patient care (Kim et al., 2008). It has been proposed many times that it could prove a useful means of diagnosing diabetes as it requires neither fasting nor an OGTT. The A1C test is a blood test that provides information about a person's average levels of blood glucose or blood sugar for the last 3 months. International Expert Committee of ADA released the formal recommendation of an A1C level ≥ 6.5% for diabetes diagnosis (Edelman et al., 2004).

1.11.5 DIAGNOSIS OF GESTATIONAL DIABETES

Gestational diabetes mellitus (GDM) is defined as a form of diabetes first diagnosed during pregnancy (Mottola, 2008).The screening and diagnosis of GDM is the subject of intense debate and controversy worldwide (Holt et al., 2011). Early detection and management of GDM improves outcomes for both mother and child. The GDM is diagnosed if two or more plasma glucose levels meet or exceed the following thresholds: Fasting glucose level of 95 mg/dL, 1 hr glucose level of 180 mg/dL, 2 hr glucose level of 155 mg/dL, or 3 hr glucose level of 140 mg/dL (ADA, 2004). The WHO recommends screening high-risk women with a 75g OGTT in the first trimester of pregnancy and all other women at 24–28 weeks, with fasting glucose measurements of 126 mg/dL and 2 hr glucose levels of 140 mg/dL being considered abnormal (Lindsay, 2009).

1.11.6 PREDIABETES TESTS

Pre-diabetes represents an elevation of plasma glucose above the normal range but below that of clinical diabetes. It is a characterized by perturbations in glucose homeostasis that significantly increase the chance for progression to T2DM. Prediabetes can be diagnosed on the basis of either impaired fasting glucose (IFG) or IGT, according to the revised ADA criteria (Genuth et al., 2003). The IFG is defined as a fasting plasma glucose concentration of 100 mg/dL but <126 mg/dL. The IGT is defined as a 2 hr response to a 75 g OGTT of 140 mg/dL and < 200 mg/dL. Both IFG and IGT are risk factors for T2DM, and risk increased when IFG and IGT occur together. The pathophysiology of prediabetes includes alterations in insulin sensitivity and pancreatic β-cell function, normally on a background of elevated adiposity (Abdul-Ghani et al., 2006).

1.11.7 CONTINUOUS GLUCOSE MONITORING (CGM)

The self-monitoring of blood glucose is a fundamental part of diabetes management. It is important to obtain good metabolic control, as better glycemic control will help to adjust the insulin doses and plan the schedule of administration. The continuous monitoring can provide information include quantifying the response in a trial of a diabetes therapy, assessing the consequences of lifestyle modifications on glycemic control, diagnosing and then preventing hypoglycemia (e.g., during sleep, with hypoglycemia unawareness) and diagnosing and preventing postprandial hypoglycaemia

(Pickup et al., 2011). The most important use of continuous blood glucose monitoring is to facilitate adjustments in therapy to improve control.

The CGM is a developing technology in the field of diabetes treatment. Over the last years, CGM Systems have become a very useful tool for the treatment of T1DM and several studies have shown their utility in lowering HbA1c and reducing glycemic variability (Klonoff, 2005). The CGM provides information about the direction, magnitude, frequency, duration and causes of fluctuations in blood glucose levels. The emergence of CGM followed in the 1990s, with the first reports on CGM by micro dialysis in 1992 (Feldman et al., 2003). Retrospective needle-type CGM systems were introduced just before the turn of the century (Chase et al., 2001). Currently, there are five subcutaneous CGM systems are approved by the U.S. Food and Drug Administration (FDA) for use in the U.S. (Vazeou, 2011). These have real-time glucose values on display every 1–5 min and feature an alarm function for hypo and hyperglycemia. Monitoring System Gold (CGM System Gold; Medtronic MiniMed, Northridge, CA), the GlucoWatch G2 Biographer (GW2B; Cygnus, Redwood City, CA), the Guardian Telemetered Glucose Monitoring System (Medtronic MiniMed), the GlucoDay (A. Menarini Diagnostics, Florence, Italy), and the Pendra (Pendragon Medical, Zurich, Switzerland). All of these measure glucose via the glucose-oxidase reaction.

The GlucoWatch (Cygnus Inc., Redwood City, CA, USA) is a widely used CGM in the form of a wrist-worn device intended for detecting trends and tracking patterns in glucose levels in adults with diabetes (Girardin et al.,2009). The glucose measurement was done by reverse iontophoresis based extraction of interstitial fluid (ISF) through the skin. This was done by directing 300 μA electric current between two electrodes contacting the skin on the backside of the device (Potts et al., 2000). It enables the taking out of ISF into two collection disks that act as anode and cathode. The glucose molecules are extracted through the epidermis to the iontophoretic cathode along with Na^+ ions by electro-osmosis. The biographer uses the calibration value previously entered by the patient to convert the signal into a glucose measurement. The glucose measurement is then displayed on the biographer and stored in memory.

The currently available CGMs measure blood glucose either with minimal invasiveness through continuous measurement of ISF or with the non invasive method of applying electromagnetic radiation through the skin to blood vessels in the body (Girardin et al., 2009). The technologies for bringing a sensor into contact with ISF include inserting an indwelling sensor subcutaneously (into the abdominal wall or arm) to measure ISF in situ or harvesting this fluid by various mechanisms that compromise the skin barrier and delivering the fluid to an external sensor.

The CGM devices display blood glucose concentrations measured in near real-time at the subcutaneous tissue. The system has many advantages. The devices display up and down arrows indicating the rate of blood glucose change and the trend of blood glucose variability and alarms for low and high blood glucose levels. Data are stored and can be reviewed later for detection of glucose trends which can be of great benefit in improving glycemic control. The CGM System data can be sent to health care professionals through the internet system allowing treatment adjustments in a more convenient way and can serve as a powerful means of patient education, allowing the patient to further understand blood glucose changes (Vashist, 2012).

1.11.8 GLUCOSE BIOSENSORS

The development of biosensor technique started being aimed at the continuous measurement of the circulating blood glucose concentration. As a first step bedside devices had been developed and applied which were able to estimate blood glucose concentration transiently under clinical conditions (Albisser et al, 1977). In principle, many transducers could be used in a biosensor for the measurement of glucose, but in practice, electrochemistry has dominated. The most commonly used enzymes in the design of glucose biosensors contain redox groups that change redox state during the biochemical reaction. Major enzymes belongs to this type are glucose oxidase (GOx) and glucose dehydrogenase (GDH) (Wang, 2008). In nature, oxidase enzymes such as GOx act by oxidation of their substrates by accepting electrons and thereby changing to an inactivated reduced state (Clark and Lyons, 1962). These enzymes are normally returned to their active oxidised state by transferring these electrons to molecular oxygen, ensuing the production of H_2O_2:

$$\text{Glucose} + O_2 \rightarrow \text{gluconolactone} + H_2O_2$$

Glucose may also be oxidised by GDH. One mechanism relies on nicotinamide adenine dinucleotide (NAD^+) acting as a cofactor, rather than oxygen as a co-substrate (Clark and Duggan, 1982). In this case NADH is produced:

$$\text{Glucose} + NAD^+ \rightarrow \text{gluconolactone} + NADH$$

A third mechanism involves the use of quinoprotein GDH, which requires no oxygen or NAD^+. Quinoproteins are a class of enzymes, which require orthoquinone cofactors to oxidise a wide variety of alcohols and amines to their corresponding aldehydes and ketones (Newman et al., 2005). The soluble quinoprotein GDH uses pyrroloquinoline quinine (PQQ) as a cofactor.

$$\text{Glucose} + \text{PQQ (ox)} \rightarrow \text{gluconolactone} + \text{PQQ (red)}$$

Most of the current blood glucose biosensors measure the glucose in a small sample of capillary blood. Early work involved abrasion of the skin, but a more recent approach is based on electro osmosis and electrochemical measurement of ISF (Wang, 2001).

SpectRx Inc. at Norcross, Georgia, USA developed a biophotonics based noninvasive glucose monitor (NGM) device, which employs a handheld Altea MicroPor™ laser to create micropores in the stratum corneum i.e. the outermost layer of skin through which the ISF comes out and gets collected in an external patch on the skin containing glucose sensor (Vashist, 2012). It has a wireless transmitter and a handheld display. The glucose measurements in the ISF by this device correlated well with the blood glucose measurements done with a commercial analyzer and glucose meters. It can detect glucose in the ISF in the range of 60–400 mg/dL.

There are methods for the measurement of glucose non-invasively. The Bayer Microlet® Vaculance is suitable for non-finger use (Vashist, 2012). The Vaculance is pressed against the puncture site and the lancet fired when the plunger is completely pushed down. Then an airtight seal is formed by slowly releasing the plunger which creates a vacuum. This causes the skin to bulge into the end cap, dilating the puncture and increasing the flow of blood. The transparent end cap enables the operator to see when sufficient blood has been collected, at that point the vacuum is dispensed by partially depressing the plunger. Blood is then applied to a glucose test strip in the usual way.

GlucoTrack™ was a handheld real-time continuous NGM device developed by Integrity Applications Ltd., Israel. It determines the glucose concentration in the blood by employing three NGM techniques i.e. ultrasonic, electromagnetic and heat capacity (Weiss et al., 2007). The device measures glucose concentration in the earlobe by attaching personal ear clip (PEC) equipped with sensors and calibration electronics.

OrSense NBM-200G is a CE approved device from OrSense Ltd, Israel that allows non-invasive measurement of glucose as well as haemoglobin and oxygen saturation with very high sensitivity (Vashist, 2012). It employs red near-infrared radiation (NIR) occlusion spectroscopy, which is based on detecting the red NIR optical signal of blood due to changes in the glucose concentration in blood vessels of finger. The device is portable, easy-to-use, and measures glucose in less than a minute.

IMPLANTABLE DEVICES

The miniaturized implantable biosensors form a highly desirable proposition for diabetes management which at present relies on data obtained from test strips using blood drawn from finger pricking, a procedure that is not only painful but also is incapable of reflecting the overall direction, trends, and patterns associated with daily habits (Reach and Wilson, 1992).

A major historical advance in the *in vivo* application of glucose biosensors was the needle-type enzyme electrode for subcutaneous implantation (Shichiri et al, 1982). In early 2000, after a long research program, MiniMed (Sylmar, CA, USA) began human testing of an implantable subcutaneous blood glucose sensor, which led to its successful launch in 2002.

Therasense (Alameda CA, USA) has also developed a miniaturised subcutaneous sensor designed for insertion into the skin by the user to continuously monitor glucose levels and provide immediate results while also storing the results for future analysis (Newman and Turner, 2005). Therasense designed their system to measure ISF, which requires a needle only long enough to cross the outer dermis and makes the needle essentially pain-free.

A different approach is being adopted by Animas (Frazer, PA, USA), with the intention of developing a long-term (more than 5 yr) implantable sensor, which will provide accurate and continuous monitoring of blood glucose levels (Newman and Turner, 2005). This device will be equipped with alarms to give warnings of impending hypoglycaemia and hyperglycaemia. The ultimate aim is to link the sensor to an insulin infusion pump to provide closed-loop control of blood glucose levels. The Animas sensor measures the near-infrared absorption of blood, and it can be implanted across a vein with readings transmitted *via* radio wave (RF) telemetry to a small display unit worn on the wrist.

1.11. 9 NANOTECHNOLOGY IN GLUCOSE MONITORING

Globally, diabetes is a rapidly growing problem that is managed at the individual level by monitoring and controlling blood glucose levels to minimize the negative effects of the disease. Due to the limitations in diagnostic methods, considerable research efforts focus on developing improved methods to measure glucose. The use of nanotechnology in the development of glucose sensors is also a prominent focus on non-invasive glucose monitoring systems. Nanotechnology can now offer implantable devices of wearable sensing technologies that provide continuous and accurate medical information (Cash and Clark, 2010). Although, there is no cure for diabetes, patients can cut down the disease-associated complications through the tight control of blood glucose levels. To attain optimal control, patients must monitor their blood glucose levels. The most common application of nanotechnology for sensors in diabetes is the use of nanomaterials to assist the standard enzymatic electrochemical detection of glucose. The incorporation of nanomaterials into these sensors offers a variety of advantages including increased surface area, more effective electron transfer from enzyme to electrode and the ability to include additional catalytic steps (Chopra et al, 2007). Carbon nanotube (CNT) incorporation is a heavily investigated modification to the enzymatic electrode detection of glucose, mainly because of the electron transfer capabilities of CNTs as well as their large surface areas. The electrode can be replaced with a highly porous nanofiber onto which GOx is immobilized (Qiu et al, 2009). The CNTs can be coupled with other nanomaterials or polymers to form nanocomposites for glucose detection. The commonly used magnetic nanoparticles made from iron oxide were also used for glucose sensors. These nanoparticles can be combined with other systems such as CNTs. The magnetic nature of these nanoparticles simplifies the assembly of GOx-labeled nanoparticles onto the electrode as well as enabling the formation of nanoparticle conductive wires on the surface of the electrode (Li et al., 2009). Nanostructured polymers can improve the development of glucose sensors. Hollow spheres of conductive polymers can be used to transfer electrons from GOx to the electrode (Santhosh et al., 2009) Conductive polymer electrodes can be used in a method similar to other nanostructured surfaces, on which GOx is immobilized directly on the modified electrode.

For *in vivo* continuous monitoring, the use fluorescence-based sensors offer several advantages. The most important among them is the ability to optically interrogate the sensors through the skin rather than having an electrode system implanted.

This approach often involves a 'smart tattoo' for the patient, because sensors would be implanted into the skin of the patient similar to regular tattoos (Rahiman and Tantry, 2010). The sensors would change fluorescence properties in response to blood glucose, and this variation could be read out using optical interrogation through the skin. This strategy would avoid or reduce the need for patients to take blood samples while allowing data to be collected in a more continuous manner.

Quantum dots (QDs) can be used for biomedical purposes as a diagnostic as well as therapeutic tool. These are nanosized (2–10 nm) semiconductor crystals, including cadmium selenide coated with a shell, such as zinc sulphide (Michalet et al., 2005). Semiconductor QDs have excellent optical properties, such as narrow fluorescence peaks and minimal photo bleaching so that they can use in sensors. Several research groups have coupled cadmium telluride (CdTe) QDs with GOx to fabricate sensing systems (Li et al., 2009).

The luminescence of these QDs is quenched by the H_2O_2 generated by the enzyme in the presence of glucose. Adhering the enzyme directly to a CdTe QD or using layer-by-layer assembly to form a nanofilm of CdTe QDs covered by a nanofilm of GOx (Barone and Strano, 2009) allows the rapid optical detection of glucose. However, the QDs themselves do not interact with glucose, and thereby have no inherent recognition ability and must be coupled to a recognition element for successful implementation.

The use of polyethylene glycol beads coated with fluorescent molecules to monitor diabetes blood sugar levels is very effective in this method the beads are injected under the skin and stay in the ISF. When there is a considerable drop in glucose levels in the ISF, glucose displaces the fluorescent molecules and glow is created. This glow is seen on a tattoo placed on the arm (Burge et al., 2008).

So, far nanomedicine in the treatment of diabetes aims mainly to improve the life-quality of patients by providing a non-invasive insulin administration and glucose control. While, the novel glucose detection systems promise a better opportunity to control the glucose level more frequently and hence allow a better insulin management.

1.12 DIABETES PREVENTION AND MANAGEMENT

The DM is a major health problem worldwide with its prevalence increasing, thus becoming a pandemic (Hjelm et al., 2003). In the past decade, major advances have been made in our understanding of the prevention of diabetes.

Though, both forms of diabetes are believed to be the products of complex interplay between genetic susceptibility and environmental factors, regarding T1DM there are limited known modifiable environmental risk factors (Nathan et al., 2005). The goal of primary prevention is to help those who are at risk of developing the disease and hence prevent or postpone the onset of disease by establishing more active lifestyles and healthier eating habits.

Primary prevention of T2DM has been performed in two different approaches, pharmacological intervention and lifestyle modification both of which are aiming to decrease insulin resistance and to promote and sustain pancreatic β-cell function. Lifestyle modification applied management of weight, altered diet composition and exercise (Ahmad and Crandall, 2010). Diabetes prevention trials using lifestyle modification have been proven effective in reducing the risk of developing T2DM, and have shown to be even more effective than pharmacological interventions (Li et al., 2008). Large scaled prospective prevention studies–Diabetes Prevention Program (DPP) and the Finnish diabetes prevention study (FDPS), demonstrated that lifestyle intervention is effective in preventing development of DM from IGT (Ahmad and Crandall, 2010). For these patients and those who progress despite successful weight loss, supplementary therapeutic options are needed. A large number of pharmacological agents have been studied in clinical diabetes prevention trials. Several trials have evaluated the efficacy of drugs in the prevention or delay of T2DM (Yang et al., 2001; Kahn et al., 2006). Therefore, lifestyle interventions coupled with some medications, are likely to enhance both insulin sensitivity and secretion (Kosaka et al., 2005).

The T1DM is a clearly heritable disease with multiple genetic and environmental risk factors. Lifestyle modification, although different, is an equally integral part of T1DM management (Haller et al., 2005). Patients with T1DM, because of their worldly need for insulin, should learn to calculate or at least closely estimate the amount of carbohydrate they consume to help regulate their blood glucose levels and adjust their insulin doses (Skyler et al., 2008). Obviously, earlier intervention, before the autoimmune reaction has begun or in advance enough to prevent significant islet loss, holds the assurance of true diabetes prevention. Antigen-specific interventions currently in development include the use of a GAD vaccine and the isolation and expansion of regulatory T-cells that are able to suppress islet-reactive lymphocytes in an antigen-specific manner (Tang et al., 2004). In addition, systemic anti-inflammatory agents such as IL-1 receptor antagonists and agents that stimulate β-cell proliferation are being studied as potential components of a multidrug prevention of β-cell destruction (Hu et al., 2007; Larsen et al., 2007).

It is difficult to overstate the importance of the relationship between lifestyle and the risk of developing T2DM. It is crucial, therefore, to properly educate obese patients and patients with glucose intolerance or IFG about the significance of exercise and weight loss and a healthful diet in individuals already diagnosed with diabetes.

1.12.1 DIET CONTROL

CARBOHYDRATE

Large observational studies have provided conflicting results, showing both positive and negative associations of total carbohydrate intake with diabetes risk (Schulze et al., 2008). Instead, the quality of carbohydrates ingested may be of extreme importance in determining the ability to raise glucose levels, which depends to a great extent on its influence on gastro-intestinal transit and the velocity of nutrient absorption, and the long-term risk of diabetes. Since 1994, the ADA has instructed that, for individuals with T1DM, 60–70% of total calories come from carbohydrate and mono-unsaturated fat (ADA, 2010). Not only the amount of carbohydrate, but also the quality of carbohydrate is important for individuals with diabetes (Toeller, 2010).

Four important qualitative features of dietary carbohydrates relevant to diabetes are fibre, wholegrain seeds, GI, and simple sugars in beverages (Rizkalla et al., 2004). Dietary fibre is the indigestible component of complex carbohydrates. Observational studies almost unanimously suggest that high intakes of fibre or fibre-rich whole grain foods are independently associated with a reduced risk of obesity and diabetes (Schulze et al., 2007). Soluble viscous fibre plays an important role in controlling postprandial glycemic and insulin responses and satiety, which is attributable to its effect of slowing gastric emptying and intestinal nutrient absorption (Slavin et al., 1999). Most prospective studies have found that insoluble fibre, but not soluble fibre, relates inversely to incident diabetes (Salmeron et al., 1997).

The GI of a carbohydrate containing food describes its post-prandial blood glucose response over 2 hr in the area under the blood glucose curve compared with a reference food with the same amount of carbohydrate, usually 50 g glucose (Rizkalla et al., 2004). Different carbohydrates have different glycemic effects. Besides the amount of carbohydrate, other factors including the nature of starch, the amount of dietary fibre and the type of sugar influence the glycemic response to carbohydrate - containing foods (Jarvi et al., 1999). Therefore, foods with known low GI (e.g. legumes, pasta, parboiled rice, wholegrain breads, oats and certain raw fruits) should be substituted when possible for those with a high GI (Gilbertson et al., 2001).

Moderate intake of sucrose (10% total energy) or other added sugars may be included in the diet of people with diabetes without worsening glycemic control (Tariq et al., 2001). The Federal Drug Administration (FDA) has approved several sugar alcohols such a sorbitol for use as sweeteners. Despite a lower risk of cavities, they have not been demonstrated to facilitate weight loss or improve glycemic control (Heilbronn et al., 1999).

Several non-nutritive sweeteners are also available and do not affect blood glucose levels. These include saccharin, aspartame and sucralose (Toeller, 2010). These sweeteners have not been shown to facilitate weight loss or improve glycemic control. Approved non-nutritive sweeteners may also be used by people with diabetes although a special long-erm benefit in metabolic control has not been proven. They are safe when acceptable daily intakes (acceptable daily intake (ADI) values) are followed. But recent observational studies have consistently shown that their consumption relates to an increased risk of diabetes after adjustment for various confounders (Schulze et al., 2004; Odegaard et al., 2010).

PROTEIN

Although,the majority of clinical focus on the management of diabetes is on carbohydrate metabolism, metabolism of proteins in the state of diabetes is also abnormal. Protein degradation appears to be exacerbated by hyperglycemia and improved by controlling glucose levels with insulin therapy (Gougeon et al., 1998). Studies suggest that the protein requirements for people with T2DM may be slightly greater than those for non-diabetic individuals (Gougeon et al., 2000; Fowler, 2010). Patients with T1DM can and do convert amino acids into glucose depending on the level of insulinization; so that protein consumption may cause hyperglycemia (Gannon et al., 2001).

Several studies have focused on protein restriction as a means to reverse or retard the progression of proteinuria in people with diabetes (Pijls et al., 2002). Progression of diabetes complications may be modified by improving glycemic control, reducing blood pressure and potentially lowering protein intake. There may also be an association between high-protein diets and the risk of developing diabetic nephropathy (Meloni et al., 2002). In some studies of subjects, particularly with T1DM and macroalbuminuria, urinary albumin excretion rates and decline in glomerular filtration were favorably influenced by a reduction of protein intake; however, there is insufficient evidence to make recommendations about the preferred type of dietary protein (Hansen et al., 2002). Studies of patients with T2DM, nevertheless, have shown that protein consumption does not increase plasma glucose concentrations and that endogenous insulin release is, in fact, fostered by protein consumption (Toeller, 2010).

FAT

The recommendations regarding fat in the diet of people with diabetes are similar to those for patients with coronary artery disease (Fowler, 2010). Because saturated fats are the major dietary determinants of serum LDL cholesterol levels, individuals with diabetes should directed to keep saturated fat consumption to < 7% of total daily calories and to minimize consumption of trans-fatty acids. Cholesterol intake should be limited to < 200 mg/day. The primary goal concerning dietary fat intake is to restrict the consumption of saturated fatty acids, trans-fats and dietary cholesterol to reduce the risk of vascular disease (Tanasescu et al., 2004). Compared with the non-diabetic population, people with diabetes have an increased risk of developing vascular disease. Fat modification in people with diabetes is an established principle to assist in achieving desirable serum lipid concentrations and to avoid vascular lesions in high-risk groups. Monounsaturated or polyunsaturated fats appear to have beneficial effects on insulin action, whereas food with high amount of saturated fats and diets with high total-fat content appear to decrease insulin sensitivity in animal studies (Toeller and Mann, 2008). The effects of trans-fats are similarly adverse as those of saturated fatty acids in raising LDL cholesterol. Therefore, their intake should be minimized. Plant sterols are plant esters that decrease intestinal absorption of both dietary and hepatobiliary cholesterol (Lee et al., 2003). They have been shown in prospective studies of diabetic patients to decrease LDL cholesterol.

MICRONUTRIENTS

There has been a great deal of interest in using micronutrients including zinc, chromium, antioxidants, and herbal supplements to improve diabetes control. Currently, there are no large convincing studies that prove benefit of micronutrients in the management of diabetes. Vegetables, legumes, fresh fruit, whole grain foods, and low fat milk products should be part of a healthy diet (Toeller, 2010). These foods provide also a range of micronutrients and fibre. Regular consumption of a variety of vegetables, fresh fruit, legumes, low fat milk products, vegetable oils, nuts, whole grain breads, and oily fish should be encouraged to ensure that recommended vitamin and mineral requirements are met (Hasanain and Mooradian, 2002).

1.12.2 EXERCISE/PHYSICAL ACTIVITY

Several lines of evidence support the concept that physical activity contributes to the prevention of diabetes. Increases in physical activity have been demonstrated to reduce the risk of developing diabetes (Myers et al., 2003). The convincing epidemiologic data support the role of physical activity in preventing diabetes. Physical activity is considered as a cornerstone of weight management. The practising aerobic exercise by obese and overweight adults results in modest weight loss independent of the effect of caloric reduction through dieting. In people with diabetes, the advantages of regular physical activity have been well documented: improved glycemic control and insulin sensitivity, reduced visceral and total fat and improved physical functioning. Studies have shown that many beneficial effects can be achieved with activities of moderate intensity such as walking (Waden et al., 2008; Hu et al., 1999; Sigal et al., 2006). In patients in whom the metabolic regulation is well maintained, exercise promotes the use of glucose and FFA in the muscles. Therefore, physical exercise combined with dietary restriction has beneficial effects for prevention and treatment of metabolic syndrome/obesity (Guelfi et al., 2007). And exercise after meals by diabetic patients with relatively good glucose control may lead to better control of diabetes by suppressing the rapid postprandial elevation of blood glucose (Wei et al., 2000).

Higher amounts of habitual physical activity are associated with decreased incidence of diabetes related complications and reduced mortality in individuals with T1DM (Moy et al., 1993). In large prospective cohort studies, higher levels of physical activity and/or cardio respiratory fitness have consistently been associated with reduced risk of developing T2DM (Krause et al., 2007). The T2DM is linked to adult onset weight gain and a sedentary lifestyle. Regular physical activity has been recommended for patients with T2DM (Marliss and Vranic et al., 2002). In addition, physically active societies have a lower incidence of diabetes than less active societies, and cross sectional studies have indicated an inverse association between the predominance of T2DM and physical activity. This inverse correlation has been mainly attributed to the fact that exercise elevates insulin sensitivity, improves glucose tolerance, and supports weight loss. Comparable magnitudes of risk reduction are seen by walking compared to more vigorous activity when total energy expenditures are similar (Hu et al., 1999). Several clinical trials have demonstrated that supervised structured physical activity programs, with or without concomitant dietary interventions, reduce the risk of developing T2DM in individuals with IGT (Pan et al., 1997). Sedentary male patients were three times more likely to die than the active ones after adjusting for age, body mass index, smoking and diabetic complications.

Physical exercise is a key component of lifestyle modification that can help individuals. Although, diet is probably more important in the initial phases of weight loss, including exercise as part of a weight-reduction regimen helps maintain weight loss and prevent weight regain. Mild to moderate activity levels have been associated with a lower risk of developing diabetes or pre-diabetes.

1.12.3 DIABETIC FOOT CARE: ORTHOTICS AND FOOT WEAR

The diabetic foot is at particular risk of developing pressure-related injury when the architecture of the foot changes, resulting in a reduction in the surface area and elevated pressure being exerted through the load-bearing areas (Reiber et al, 1999). This is often further complicated by peripheral vascular disease that affects healing by lowering the oxygen concentration of the localised tissue (Apelqvist et al., 1990). Foot disorders are a major source of morbidity and a leading cause of hospitalization for persons with diabetes. Infection, ulceration, gangrene, and amputation are serious complications of this disease, with a cost estimated to billions of dollars each year. Current guidelines recommend annual screening for the high risk foot and those so identified should receive enhanced foot care and education additional to that given to all people with diabetes (Clayton and Elasy, 2009). Low risk patients should be instructed about foot hygiene, nail care, footwear, avoidance of trauma, smoking cessation and actions to take if problems develop. Inappropriate footwear is a common cause of foot ulceration in insensitive feet, whereas good footwear can reduce ulcer occurrence.

The use of orthotic devices that are custom built for each patient's requirements has been advocated as a strategy to prevent and treat diabetic foot ulcers (DFU) (Kato et al., 1996; Armstrong et al., 2001). The off-loading of pressure from the affected areas is an established treatment option for diabetic ulcers. It heals by reducing mechanical stresses and repetitive trauma. The custom-moulded orthotics is recognized and recommended as an adjunctive measure in the management of the diabetic foot (Myerson et al., 1992). Custom-moulded orthotics decrease plantar pressures, particularly over bony prominences, to block the reocurrence of ulcers and possibly treat ulcers in a fashion similar to the total contact cast (TCC) (Edmonds et al., 1986). The TCC has been shown to heal a higher proportion of diabetic foot wounds than other therapeutic interventions as it leads to optimal weight off-loading, reduced edema, decreased patient movement, foot protection and it cannot be detached, thus ensuring compliance. Custom-made insoles function to their highest efficiency in proper fitting footwear.

The materials used to make the custom-moulded orthotics need to be sufficiently firm to support the foot and off-load the problem area, able to endure cyclic compression, for force distribution of plantar pressure throughout the material (Uccioli et al., 1995). The materials used for the base of the orthotic must be carefully selected to ensure that they should be lightweight, strong, resilient, flexible, and sustain their shape despite compressive forces. The material which comes in contact with the foot is usually made of an expanded rubber or a polyurethane foam (e.g., PPTTM) and ethylene vinyl acetate (EVA) as they provide cushioning and decrease friction and shear forces (Hogge et al., 2000).

Clinical recommendations for people with diabetes include provision of special footwear to individuals with diabetes and foot risk factors (Litzelman et al., 1997; Knowles et al., 1996). Footwear benefits have been widely promoted and accepted in the clinical community despite limited experimental evidence on the effectiveness of therapeutic footwear in preventing foot reulceration (Calhoun et al., 2002). Therapeutic shoes with pressure-relieving insoles and high toe boxes are important adjunctive treatments that can reduce the occurrence of ulceration and resultant amputation in high-risk patients. Patients with severely deformed feet require custom molded shoes (Slavens and Slavens, 1995), and patients with minor foot deformities may benefit from using athletic shoes (Soulier, 1988). Nevertheless, patients with foot deformities that cannot be accommodated by standard therapeutic footwear should have custom shoes that provide appropriate fit, depth, and a rocker insole (Boulton et al., 1999). Therapeutic footwear is often prescribed to interrupt ulceration, especially for patients who have suffered prior ulceration. The footwear's primary intention is to redistribute pressure on the plantar foot surface to relieve pressure at locations that are at risk for (re)ulceration.

1.13 COMPLICATIONS ASSOCIATED WITH DIABETES

1.13.1 FOOT ULCERS AND WOUNDS

One of the most common complications of diabetes in the lower extremity is the DFU. Approximately 15% of patients with diabetes will develop a lower extremity ulcer during the course of their disease (Reiber, 2001). Several population-based studies indicate a 0.5% to 3% annual cumulative incidence of DFUs (Moss et al., 1992). Foot ulcers cause substantial morbidity, diminish quality of life, create high treatment costs (Kumar et al., 1994; Ramsey et al., 1999) and are the most important risk factor for lower-extremity amputation (Margolis et al., 2005).

The multifactorial nature of diabetic foot ulceration has been elucidated by numerous observational studies (Blumberg et al., 2012; Frykberg et al., 1998). Risk factors identified include vascular diseases, peripheral neuropathy, foot deformities, minor trauma, a history of ulceration or amputation, and impaired visual acuity (Boulton et al., 2004). Peripheral sensory neuropathy is identified as the primary factor leading to diabetic foot ulcerations (Edmonds et al., 1999; Levin, 1994).Other forms of neuropathy may also play a role in foot ulceration. Ulceration is the most common single reason to lower extremity amputations among persons with diabetes (Larsson et al., 1998).

Wound healing is a complex process involving three sequential and overlapping phases, proliferation, inflammation, and remodelling (Martin, 1997). In individuals with DM, wounds remain in a chronic inflammatory state and fail to heal in a timely and orderly manner. Continual influx of inflammatory cells and sustained production of their inflammatory mediators cause imbalances in wound proteases and their inhibitors, preventing extracellular matrix (ECM) synthesis and remodelling that are essential for normal wound healing (Parks, 1999; Mast and Schultz, 1996). Diabetes impairs the functions of neutrophils and macrophages, including cell adherence, chemotaxis, phagocytosis, and cytokine production and secretion (Marhoffer, 1992). Keratinocytes and fibroblasts from diabetic wounds show reduced migratory capability, diminished response to growth factors, and increased apoptosis (Brem, 2007). The complexity of DFU pathophysiology is multifactorial and evidently necessitates intervention at multiple levels to accelerate healing.

A number of newer approaches to promote more rapid healing in diabetic foot lesions have been described over the last two decades (Wu et al., 2007) Growth factor treatment may be a promising approach to diabetic foot wounds. A number of growth factors and other agents designed to modify abnormalities of the biochemistry of the wound bed or surrounding tissues have been described, but there is still no consensus as their place in day-to-day clinical practice (Lin et al., 2008). One example is platelet-derived growth factor (PDGF) which is available for clinical use in a number of countries.

Stem cell therapy has emerged as a promising treatment modality aiming to address the underlying pathophysiology of DFUs. Stem cells have been shown to mobilize and home to ischemic and wounded tissue where they secrete chemokines and growth factors that promote angiogenesis and ECM remodelling, creating a local environment conducive to wound healing (Li et al., 2006). Several types of stem cells have been used to promote healing in DFUs. These can be grossly categorized into allogenic and autologous stem cells, based on their source of procurement.

1.13.2 MACRO AND MICROVASCULAR COMPLICATIONS

Diabetes is a group of chronic diseases characterized by hyperglycemia. Generally, the injurious effects of hyperglycemia are separated into macrovascular complications (stroke and peripheral arterial disease (PAD)) and microvascular complications (diabetic nephropathy, neuropathy, and retinopathy). Macro and microvascular complications can result in significant morbidity and mortality in people with diabetes. Hence these conditions posit an enormous challenge to the healthcare system.

PERIPHERAL ARTERIAL DISEASE (PAD)

Peripheral vascular diseases includes diseases to arteries and veins outside the thoracic region. The most common arterial disease is the PAD. The PAD occurs when arteries become narrowed or blocked by fatty deposits and injury to the wall of the artery (ADA, 2003). While PAD is a major risk factor for lower-extremity amputation, it is also associated with a high prospect for symptomatic cardiovascular and cerebrovascular disease (Sillesen, 2010). The PAD is a manifestation of atherosclerosis characterized by atherosclerotic occlusive disease of the lower extremities and is a marker for atherothrombotic disease in other vascular beds.

The PAD is usually characterized by occlusive arterial disease of the lower extremities. The most common symptom of PAD is intermittent claudication, characterized by pain, cramping, or aching in the thighs, calves or buttocks that appears intolerable with walking exercise and is relieved by rest (Murabito et al., 1997). More extreme presentations of PAD include rest pain, gangrene or tissue loss; these devastating manifestations of PAD are collectively termed critical limb ischemia (CLI). The reduced walking speed and distance associated with intermittent claudication may result in progressive loss of function and long-term disability (McDermott et al., 2004). As the disease becomes severe, CLI may develop, leading to ischemic ulceration of the foot and risk of limb loss (Hiatt, 2002). Importantly, PAD is associated with a substantial increase in the risk of fatal and non-fatal cardiovascular and cerebrovascular events, including myocardial infarction (MI) and stroke (Weitz et al., 1996).

Inflammation has been established as both a risk marker and perhaps a risk factor for atherothrombotic disease states, including PAD. Elevated levels of C-reactive protein (CRP) are strongly associated with the development of PAD (Ridker et al., 1998). In addition, levels of CRP are abnormally elevated in patients with impaired glucose regulation syndromes, involving IGT and diabetes. In addition to being a marker of disease presence, increase in CRP level may also be a culprit in the causation or exacerbation of PAD (Cermak et al., 1998). The CRP has been found to bind to endothelial cell receptors promoting apoptosis and has been shown to co-localize with oxidized LDL in atherosclerotic plaques. Moreover CRP also enhances endothelial production of procoagulant tissue factor, leukocyte adhesion molecules and chemotactic substances and inhibits endothelial cell NO synthase, resulting in abnormalities in the regulation of vascular tone (Williams et al., 1996). The CRP may also increase the local production of compounds impairing fibrinolysis that includes plasminogen activator inhibitor (PAI)-1. Most patients with diabetes, including those with PAD, demonstrate abnormalities of endothelial function and vascular regulation (De Vriese et al., 2000).

A thorough medical history and physical examination are of primary importance in evaluating a diabetic individual for the presence of PAD. Knowledge about the onset and duration of symptoms, pain features, and any mitigating factors is helpful. Currently exercise rehabilitation is suggested as the key therapy, as well as the potential use of pharmacologic agents.

STROKE

Patients with DM are more prone to develop macrovascular diseases, including strokes. In addition to being a deadly disorder in diabetics, stroke is a disabling disorder. The DM not only significantly increases the chance of stroke, but also is a predictor of reduced survival following stroke. Stroke is the second most frequent cause of death worldwide and the most frequent cause of permanent disability (Sander et al., 2008; Sacco et al., 1997). An initial diagnosis of DM is often made at the time of acute hospitalization for stroke. Case control studies of stroke patients and prospective epidemiologic studies have confirmed an independent effect of diabetes on ischemic stroke in both men and women, with an increased relative risk in diabetics ranging from 1.8 to nearly 6-fold (Folsom et al., 1999). Since diabetics have an increased susceptibility to developing atherosclerosis, it is very likely that DM is a risk factor that plays an essential role in producing the vascular pathology underlying ischemic stroke.

A FPG level over 5.5 mmol/L is strongly linked with ischaemic cerebrovascular events in patients with pre-existing atherothrombotic disease and stress hyperglycaemia following a primary stroke increases the probability of a poor outcome (Tanne et al., 2004; Selvin et al., 2004). Chronic hyperglycaemia, as manifested by elevated HbA1c levels, is associated with a 17% increase in the risk of stroke with each 1% rise of HbA1c (Capes et al., 2001). The DM is estimated to have a population accountable risk of approximately 35%. This figure for DM is greater than the estimates of the population attributable risk for cigarette smoking (12.3%) and atrial fibrillation (9.4%) (Kissela et al., 2005).

Prevention of stroke in the patient with diabetes is best served through aggressive management of concurrent HTN and hyperlipidemia (Sander et al., 2008). Careful glycemic control likely reduces the risk of stroke as well, but the risk reduction is not nearly as robust. Preventing stroke in people with diabetes is feasible through identifying and treating risk factors, especially HTN, cigarette smoking, and high LDL cholesterol. Antiplatelet therapy also has important role; a single antithrombotic agent is sufficient for the prevention of ischemic stroke (Idris et al., 2006; Biller et al., 1993).

MICROVASCULAR COMPLICATIONS

DIABETIC RETINOPATHY

Diabetic retinopathy is a complication of diabetes that results from damage to the blood vessels of the retina in the back of the eye (Moore et al., 2009). The risk of related visual loss in people with diabetes is up to 25 times higher than the population not affected by diabetes. Twenty years after the onset of diabetes almost all patients with T1DM and over 60% of patients with T2DM will have some degree of retinopathy, and even at the time of diagnosis of T2DM, approximately one-quarter of patients already have established background retinopathy (Fowler, 2008; Watkins, 2003).

The risk of developing diabetic retinopathy or other microvascular complications of diabetes depends on both the duration and the severity of hyperglycemia. There are several proposed pathological mechanisms by which diabetes may lead to development of retinopathy. There are two major stages of diabetic retinopathy: an early stage non-proliferative diabetic retinopathy and a later stage proliferative diabetic retinopathy. The latter is characterized by the formation of new blood vessels on the surface of the retina and can lead to vitreous hemorrhage (Fong and Aiello, 2004; Wilkinson et al., 2003). White areas on the retina (cotton wool spots) can be a sign of impending proliferative retinopathy. If proliferation progresses, blindness can occur through vitreous hemorrhage and traction retinal detachment. Without any intervention, visual loss may occur (Scanlon et al., 2010). Laser photocoagulation can often prevent proliferative retinopathy from progressing to blindness, therefore, close surveillance for the presence or progression of retinopathy in patients with diabetes is crucial (Watkins, 2003). Background retinopathy includes such features as small haemorrhages in the middle layers of the retina. Diabetic retinopathy is due to microangiopathy affecting the retinal precapillary arterioles, venules and capillaries. Damage is caused by both microvascular leakages due to break down of the inner blood-retinal barrier and microvascular occlusion (Kunisaki et al., 1995). It has long been appreciated that persons with diabetes are at substantial risk for tissue injury in organs supplied by an end arterial system due to microangiopathy.

Aldose reductase may participate in the development of diabetes complications. It is the initial enzyme in the intracellular polyol pathway (Aiello, 2003). This pathway involves the conversion of glucose into glucose alcohol (sorbitol). Elevated glucose levels increase the flux of sugar molecules through the polyol pathway, which causes sorbitol agglomeration in cells. Osmotic stress results from sorbitol accumulation have been postulated as an underlying mechanism in the development of diabetic retinopathy (Gabbay, 2004). Cells are also thought to be injured by glycoproteins. Increased glucose concentrations can promote the nonenzymatic formation of AGEs (Fong et al., 2004). In animal models, these substances have also been associated with formation of microaneurysms and pericyte loss (Stitt et al., 1995). Oxidative stress may also play an important role in cellular injury from hyperglycemia. High glucose levels can promote free radical generation and ROS formation.

Growth factors, including VEGF, transforming growth factor β and growth hormone, have also been hypothesized to play important roles in the development of diabetic retinopathy (Aiello et al., 1995). The VEGF production is augmented in diabetic retinopathy, probably in response to hypoxia.

As treatment is now available to prevent blindness in the majority of cases, it is essential to identify patients with retinopathy before their vision is affected. Investigative techniques to assess diabetic retinopathy include Fundus fluorescein angiography, retinal photography, ultrasound B scan examination, optical coherence tomography and perimetry (Scanlon et al., 2010).

DIABETIC NEPHROPATHY

Diabetic nephropathy is a microvascular complication of diabetes characterized by persistent proteinuria, decreased glomerular filtration rate, and increased blood pressure (McKnighta et al., 2007). It is defined by proteinuria > 500 mg in 24 hr in the setting of diabetes, but this is anticipated by lower degrees of proteinuria or microalbuminuria. Microalbuminuria is explained as albumin excretion of 30–299 mg/24 hr (Gross et al., 2005). Without proper interference, diabetic patients with microalbuminuria typically progress to proteinuria and overt diabetic nephropathy. This progression occurs in both T1DM and T2DM. As many as 7% of patients with T2DM may already have microalbuminuria at the time they are diagnosed with diabetes (Fowler, 2008; Forsblom et al., 1998).

The main potentially modifiable diabetic nephropathy initiation and progression factors in susceptible individuals are sustained hyperglycemia and HTN (Gall et al., 1997). Other putative risk factors are glomerular hyperfiltration (Caramori et al., 1999), smoking (Hovind et al., 2003), proteinuria levels, dyslipidemia, and dietary factors, such as the source and amount of protein and fat in the diet (Ruggenenti et al., 1998; Toeller et al., 1997).

Diabetic nephropathy is characterized by the development of proteinuria followed by decreased glomerular filtration in association with glomerulosclerosis (Brito et al., 1998). Development of proteinuria is mainly due to injury of the glomerular filtration barrier, which consists of the glomerular basement membrane, glomerular endothelium and podocytes placed outside of the capillary (Nelson et al., 1997). The pathological changes to the kidney include elevated glomerular basement membrane thickness, mesangial nodule formation and microaneurysm formation and other changes (White and Bilous, 2000). Diabetes causes unique changes in kidney structure. Although, diabetic nephropathy is traditionally considered a non immune disease, accumulating evidence now indicates that immunologic and inflammatory mechanisms play a significant role in its development and progression (Fioretto et al., 1996).

The screening for diabetic nephropathy may be accomplished by either a 24 hr urine collection or a spot urine measurement of microalbumin (Forsblom et al., 1998). Measurement of the microalbumin-to-creatinine ratio may help account for concentration or dilution of urine, and spot determinations are more comfortable for patients than 24 hr urine collections.

Initial treatment of diabetic nephropathy is prevention. Similar to other microvascular complications of diabetes, there are strong correlation between glucose control (as measured by HbA1c) and the risk of developing diabetic nephropathy (Chaturvedi et al., 2001; Gross et al., 2005). Patients should be treated to the lowest safe glucose level that can be obtained to prevent or control diabetic nephropathy. In addition to aggressive treatment of elevated blood glucose, patients having diabetic nephropathy benefit from treatment with antihypertensive drugs. Hyperglycaemia leads to the overproduction of the hormones renin, angiotensin and aldosterone which is the key cascade in diabetic nephropathy (Figure 3). Blockade of renin-angiotensin system has additional benefits beyond the simple blood pressure-lowering effect in patients with diabetic nephropathy (Kelly et al., 2003). Several studies have demonstrated renoprotective effects of treatment with angiotensin receptor blockers (ARBs) and angiotensin converting enzyme (ACE) inhibitors, which appear to be present independent of their blood pressure-lowering effects, probably because of decreasing intraglomerular pressure (Rossing et al., 2003). Both ACE inhibitors and ARBs have been shown to decrease the risk of progression to macroalbuminuria in patients with microalbuminuria by as much as 60–70%. These drugs are recommended as the first-line pharmacological treatment of microalbuminuria, even in patients without HTN (Weinberg et al., 2003). Similarly, patients with macroalbuminuria benefit from control of HTN.

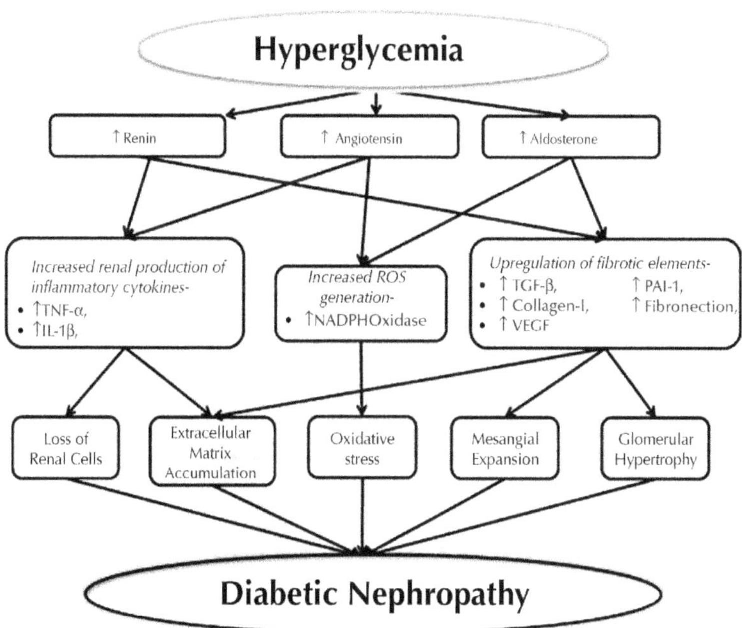

FIGURE 3 Role of hyperglycemia in diabetic nephropathy.

1.13.3 DIABETIC PERIPHERAL NEUROPATHY

Diabetic neuropathies constitute a diverse group of conditions. Diabetic neuropathy is recognized by the ADA as 'the presence of symptoms and/or signs of peripheral nerve dysfunction in people with diabetes after the exclusion of other causes' (Boulton et al., 1998). Diabetic neuropathy is the nerve damage caused by diabetes. Numerous classifications of the variety of syndromes affecting the peripheral nervous system in diabetes have been proposed in recent years. The classification shown in Figure 4 is based on that originally proposed by Thomas (Thomas, 1997). Diabetic neuropathy is the result of slowed motor and sensory nerve conduction that most commonly develops between 5 and 10 yr after onset of disease (Vinik et al., 2003; Boulton et al., 1998). More than 80% of amputations occur after foot ulceration, which can result from diabetic neuropathy (McCabe et al., 1998). As with other microvascular difficulties, risk of developing diabetic neuropathy is proportional to both the degree and duration of hyperglycemia, and some patients may have genetic attributes that affect their predisposition to developing such complexities (Fowler, 2008).

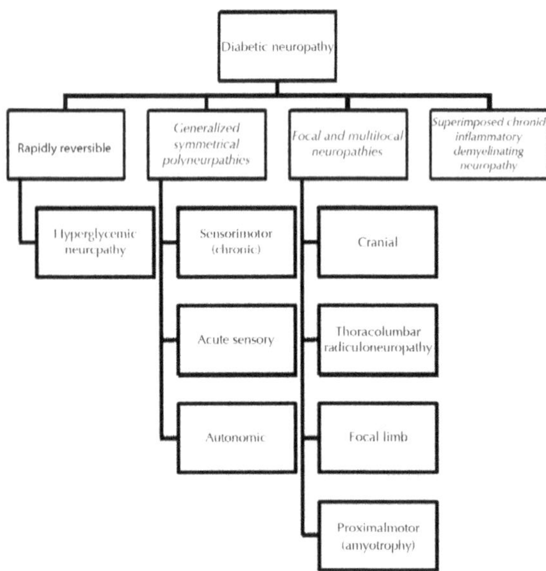

FIGURE 4 Classification of diabetic neuropathy.

The type of neuropathy affecting the hands, arms, legs and feet is known as diabetic peripheral neuropathy (Boulton, 1998b). Three different groups of nerves can be affected by diabetic neuropathy. Peripheral neuropathy in diabetes may manifest in several different forms, including focal/multifocal, sensory and autonomic neuropathies. The peripheral sensorimotor neuropathy is symmetric and mostly affects the feet, leading to decreased sensation and paresthesia (Boulton, 1999; Mendell and Sahenk, 2003). Diminished sensation can cause altered perception of foot pressures and altered foot architecture. Commonly, patients experience burning, tingling, but sometimes they may experience simple numbness.

Diabetic autonomic neuropathy (DAN) is among the least recognized and understood complications of diabetes. A subtype of the peripheral polyneuropathies that follow diabetes, DAN can incorporate the entire autonomic nervous system (ANS) (Vinik and Erbas, 2001; Spruce et al., 2003). It is manifested by dysfunction of one or more organ systems (e.g., cardiovascular, gastrointestinal etc). Major clinical manifestations of DAN include exercise intolerance, resting tachycardia, orthostatic hypotension, gastroparesis constipation, impaired neurovascular function, and hypoglycemic autonomic failure (Maser et al., 2003; Pfeifer et al., 1984).

Hypotheses concerning the multiple aetiologies of diabetic neuropathy include a metabolic insult to nerve fibers, autoimmune damage, neurovascular insufficiency and neurohormonal growth factor deficiency (Vinik, 1999). Several different factors have been implicated in this pathogenic process. Hyperglycemia induced activation of the polyol pathway leading to accumulation of sorbitol and potential changes in the NAD: NADH ratio may cause direct neuronal damage and/or decreased nerve blood flow (Sundkvist et al., 2000; Oates, 2002; Dyck et al., 1988, King, 2001). Activation of PKC induces vasoconstriction and diminishes neuronal blood flow (Cameron and Cotter, 2002). Increased oxidative stress, with elevated free radical production, results in vascular endothelium damage and reduces NO bioavailability (Low et al., 1997). Alternately, excess NO production may result in development of ONOO and deteriorate endothelium and neurons, a process known as nitrosative stress (Hoeldtke et al., 2002; Cameron and Cotter, 1997). In a subpopulation of individuals with neuropathy, immune mechanisms may also be involved (Sundkvist et al., 1991).

There is no specific treatment of diabetic neuropathy, albeit several drugs are available to treat its symptoms. The primary intention of therapy is to restrict symptoms and prevent worsening of neuropathy through improved glycemic control. Conventional treatments include antidepressants (tricyclics-TCAs and serotonin selective reuptake inhibitors- SSRIs), antiarrhythmics (sodium-channel blockers; mexiletine), anticonvulsants, opioid and non-opioid analgesics, N-methyl-D aspartate (NMDA) receptor antagonists and aldose reductase inhibitors (Boulton et al., 1998).

1.14 THERAPEUTIC STRATEGIES

Physicians can use a wide range of therapeutic agents, singly and in combination, to help lower and stabilise blood sugar levels. The major therapeutic strategies used in the treatment of diabetes are given in Figure 5.

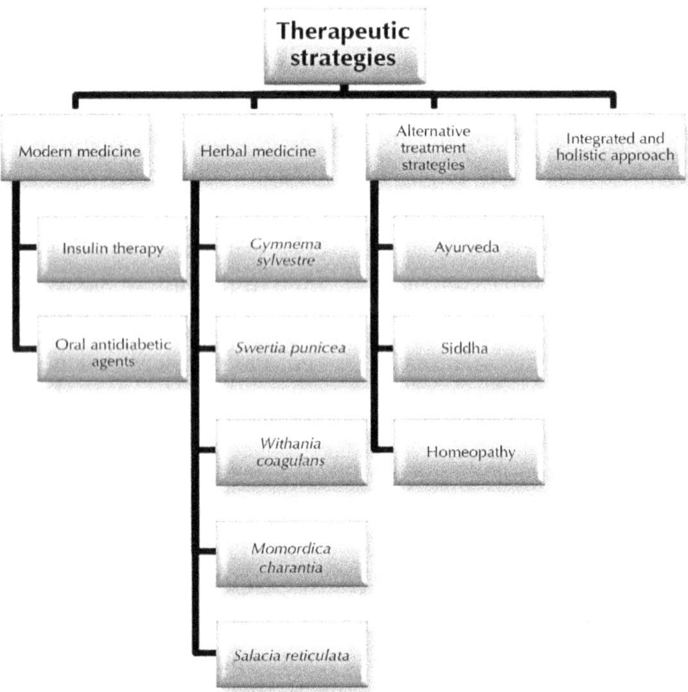

FIGURE 5 Major therapeutic strategies used in the treatment of diabetes.

1.14.1 MODERN MEDICINE

INSULIN THERAPY

The purification of insulin by Banting, Best, Collip, and Macleod in 1921 was one of the most important scientific achievements of the 20th Century (Banting et al., 1991). It gave hope to thousands of patients with T1DM, prolonged their life span by decades, and allowed them to lead a highly improved quality of life. Human insulin produced biosynthetically was first introduced commercially in 1982 (Howey et al., 1994). Commonly available conventional insulin is derived from animal sources (bovine, porcine), while human insulin is manufactured by recombinant DNA technology. Since the advent of recombinant human insulin this has become the preferred method for commercial production (Heinemann and Richter, 1993). The principle of intensive insulin therapy is to provide an adequate amount of basal insulin and also provide insulin to prevent the anticipated hyperglycemia following meals; thus mimicking the physiologic insulin profile.

In order to achieve better control of diabetes, efforts have been made to modify the insulin molecule leading to the development of insulin analogs. The pharmacologic characteristics of the insulin analogs allow clinicians to use them in specific situations to achieve better control of diabetes. Currently available insulin analogs can be divided into three categories based on their duration of action, short acting, intermediate acting and long acting insulins (Gossain, 2003).

Short acting insulin analogs, made through genetic modification of human insulin, were introduced to the public in the mid-1990s (Hirsch, 2005). The three products currently available (lispro, aspart, and glulisine) are absorbed rapidly with general onset in 5–15 min, reaches peak in 1–2 hr, with a duration averaging 3–5 hr, though there may be slight differences among the products (Koivisto, 1998; Bolli et al., 1999). The rapid onset of these insulin products allows for optimal mealtime flexibility, conceiving them ideal for individuals with varying or unpredictable meal schedules.

Intermediate acting insulin consists of regular insulin modified by adding zinc (lente) or basic protein (neutral protamine hagedorn (NPH)) (Owens et al., 2001). These are used primarily to provide basal insulin replacement. This insulin has duration of action of 12–14 hr and usually need to be given twice in a day to provide cover for the entire 24 hr (Francis et al., 1983). The long-acting insulin analogs currently available are glargine and detemir (Heinemann et al., 2000). The onset of insulin glargine occurs in 4–6 hr with no appreciable peak and duration of 24 hr in most patients. Insulin detemir is newer long acting insulin with onset similar to glargine at 3–4 hr. Anyhow, detemir has a potential peak at 3–4 hr and a prolongation that is dose dependent ranging from 5.7 hr and 23.2 hr at lower and higher doses respectively (Bloomgarden, 2006).

Although, intensive exogenous insulin therapy can closely mimic the physiological management of glucose, and delay or restrict the onset of chronic complications, multiple daily injections or regular subcutaneous infusion of insulin is cumbersome and sometimes causes hypoglycemia. Therefore, more-efficient methods are needed for the constant delivery of physiological levels of insulin and the tight control of blood glucose level in a safe and cost-effective manner. The lasting cure of T1DM has long been sought using several different approaches, including insulin gene therapy (Levine and Leibowitz, 1999; Felgner, 1997). As T1DM is caused by insulin deficiency, it is a good candidate for gene therapy to rectify the insulin deficiency. The intramuscular injection of plasmid DNA has been shown to result in local expression of the gene for a considerable length of time (Bartlett et al., 1998). The delivery of the insulin gene by direct injection into the skeletal muscle led to the production of physiological concentrations of proinsulin for over 30 weeks.

Before starting insulin therapy, the patient should be well acquainted with the techniques of home glucose monitoring (HGM), proper insulin application, and self-management of the insulin dose, if appropriate, as well as conscious about dietary and exercise strategies (Mooradian et al., 2006). The HGM using any of the commercially available glucose monitors is an essential component of any insulin therapy regimen and is useful both to monitor glycemic control and to adjust insulin doses.

ORAL ANTIDIABETIC AGENTS

Today's clinicians are presented with an extensive range of oral antidiabetic drugs for diabetes. The number of approved diabetes drug therapies has grown significantly in the past two decades. There are seven distinct classes of hypoglycaemic agents are available in the market which includes biguanides, sulfonylureas, meglitinides, thiazolidinediones, α-glucosidase inhibitors, incretin mimetics and DPP-4 inhibitors (Rotenstein et al., 2012) (Table 2).

TABLE 2 Oral antidiabetic agents

Class	Examples
Biguanides	Metformin
Sulfonylureas	Glimepiride, gliclazide, glibenclamide, glipizide
Meglitinides	Repaglinide, nateglinide
DPP-4 inhibitors	Sitagliptin, vildagliptin,saxagliptin
Thiazolidinediones	Pioglitazone, rosiglitazone
α - Glucosidase inhibitors	Acarbose, miglitol, voglibose
GLP-1 receptor agonists	Exenatide, Albiglutide

Sulfonylureas are insulin secretagogues are well studied and, like metformin, lower A1C by ~1.5%. It is generic and inexpensive. Sulfonylureas potentiate insulin action and variably increase insulin secretion following a meal, decreasing blood glucose concentrations (Lebovitz et al., 1983). The drugs in this class, including glyburide, tolbutamide, glibenclamide, glimepiride, and glipizide are generally used as second-line therapy after metformin (Bailey and Krentz, 2010). Sulfonylureas act directly on the β-cells of the islets of Langerhans to stimulate insulin secretion. They enter the β-cell and bind to the cytosolic surface of the sulfonylurea receptor 1(SUR1), which forms part of a transmembrane complex with ATP-sensitive Kir6.2 potassium channels (K^+ ATP channels) (Ashcroft and Gribble, 1999). The binding of a sulfonylurea closes the K^+ ATP channel, reducing the efflux of potassium and enabling membrane depolarization. Localized membrane depolarization opens adjacent voltage-dependent L-type calcium channels, increasing calcium influx and raising the cytosolic free calcium concentration. This activates calcium-dependent signaling proteins that control the contractility of microtubules and microfilaments that mediate the exocytotic release of insulin (Gribble and Reimann, 2002).

Biguanides act chiefly by reducing HGP. They also stimulate peripheral glucose uptake, and to some extent decrease carbohydrate absorption. Metformin is the most widely used only biguanide (Bailey and Krentz, 2010). Metformin increases insulin sensitivity and thus decreases the insulin resistance in T2DM. Metformin lowers glucose levels by decreasing gluconeogenesis, although the exact mechanism by which it does this is not well understood (Bosi, 2009; Bailey, 1996).

The meglitinides, are short-acting glucose-lowering drugs for therapy of patients with T2DM alone or in combination with metformin (Dornhorst, 2001). The pharmacokinetic properties of these compounds favoured a rapid but short-lived insulin secretory effect that suited administration with meals to promote prandial insulin release. They are structurally different than sulfonylureas but their mechanism of action closely resembles that of sulfonylureas, (they act by regulating ATP-dependent potassium channels in pancreatic beta cells), because they stimulate the release of insulin from the pancreatic beta cells through a different binding site on the "sulfonylurea receptor" (Fuhlendorff et al., 1998). Moreover, meglitinides have different half-life compared to sulfonylureas. Two agents, the meglitinide derivative repaglinide and the structurally related phenylalanine derivative nateglinide are the important drugs belong to this category.

The hypoglycaemic activity of a thiazolidinedione (including rosiglitazone and pioglitazone) was reported in the early 1980s (Stafford and Elasy, 2007). In the early 1990s the PPAR family was identified as part of the nuclear receptor superfamily 1, and it became evident that thiazolidinediones were potent agonists of PPAR-α (Staels and Fruchart, 2005; Semple et al., 2006). Most of the antidiabetic efficacy of thiazolidinediones appears to be achieved through stimulation of PPAR–α leading to increased insulin sensitivity (Day, 1999). When activated it forms a heterodimeric complex with the retinoid X receptor and binds to a nucleotide sequence termed the peroxisome proliferator response element (PPRE) located in the promoter regions of PPAR- responsive genes. In conjunction with co-activators such as PGC-1, this alters the transcriptional activity of a range of insulin-sensitive and other genes. Many of these genes participate in lipid and carbohydrate metabolism. Thiazolidinediones also increase glucose uptake into adipose tissue and skeletal muscle *via* increased availability of GLUT 4 glucose transporters (Bailey, 2005).

The α-glucosidase inhibitors competitively inhibit the activity of α-glucosidase enzymes in the brush border of enterocytes lining the intestinal villi (Scheen, 2003). They bind to the enzymes with high affinity, preventing the enzymes from cleaving disaccharides and oligosaccharides into monosaccharides. This delays completion of carbohydrate digestion and can defer the process distally along the intestinal tract, leading to a delay in glucose absorption (Lebovitz, 1998). Acarbose acts in this way and can be used alone or in combination with other oral hypoglycaemic agents.

Dipeptidyl peptidase-4 (DPP-4) inhibitors act by competitively inhibiting the enzyme DPP-4 (Pratley and Salsali; 2007). The DPP-4 inhibitors act to prevent the aminopeptidase activity of DPP-4, an enzyme found free in the circulation and tethered to endothelia and other epithelial cells in most tissues, especially in the intestinal mucosa which breaks down GLP-1 and GIP, thus increasing the concentrations of these incretins (Herman et al., 2007). The GLP-1 and GIP suppress the release of glucagon after a meal, increase the secretion of insulin and increase satiety, effectively decreasing blood glucose (Green et al., 2006). The DPP-4 inhibitors have been shown to improve glycemic control in both fasting and postprandial states and increase β-cell function (Weber, 2004). They have also been shown to decrease HbA1C by reducing postprandial glucose and FPG (Pratley and Gilbert, 2008).

A novel category of antihyperglycemic therapy based on modulation of the incretin system has recently appeared. Incretins are gut-derived peptides secreted in response to meals, precisely the presence and absorption of nutrients in the intestinal lumen (Silvio, 2008). The major incretins are GLP-1 and GIP. The GLP-1 and GIP stimulate insulin output from pancreatic β-cells in a glucose-dependent fashion (enhancement of secretion linked to the presence of hyperglycemia) (Chee et al., 2009). In addition, GLP-1 reduces pancreatic β-cell secretion of glucagon that augments HGP. GLP-1 also decreases gastric emptying and likely has a direct suppressive effect on central appetite centers (Baggio and Drucker, 2007). Exenatide is a synthetic version of exendin-4, a peptide identified in the salivary secretions of the reptile *Heloderma suspectum* (the Gila monster) (DeFronzo et al., 2005). Exenatide shares partial homology with human GLP-1 and activates human GLP-1 receptors. Pivotal trials have assessed its efficacy at lowering glucose in patients with T2DM in combination with sulfonylureas and/or metformin (Buse et al., 2004).

INSULIN DELIVERY SYSTEMS

The advent of insulin revolutionised the treatment of diabetes and must be one of the most outstanding achievements of twentieth century medicine. The administration of insulin in the form of a bolus subcutaneous injection has remained the basis of insulin therapy since its introduction. Efforts to develop alternative routes and delivery systems for administering insulin began soon after the introduction of insulin therapy in the 1920s (Owens, 2002). Since then, almost every conceivable route has been tried, but with only limited success. Strategies for enhancing the flux of insulin across the various epithelia include chemical strategies (enzyme (protease) inhibitors, permeation enhancers and insulin modifications and formulations), physical methods (Iontophoresis and Sonopheresis), pH sensitive systems and different combinations of these (Marschutz, 2000). Recently, however, attention has focused on the delivery of inhaled insulin by the pulmonary route.

ORAL DELIVERY SYSTEMS

Success in the oral delivery of therapeutic insulin can significantly improve the quality of life of diabetic patients who must routinely receive injections of this drug. Nevertheless, oral absorption of insulin is constrained by various physiological barriers and remains a major scientific challenge. Several technological solutions have been developed to augment the oral bioavailability of insulin. Enhancing the chemical stability of insulin, shielding against proteolytic enzymes, fusing insulin into liposomes and using surfactants or emulsions to increase the permeability of the intestinal mucosa have achieved only variable success in improving absorption (Carino and Mathiowitz,1999). Entrapment of insulin into conventional 'liposomes' has been extensively investigated (Damge, 1991) and more recently, liposomes that are made resistant to the gastrointestinal environment by polymerization have been developed (Langer, 1998). Considerable effort has also been made in the encapsulation of insulin, with or without the addition of inhibitors of proteases, into pH-dependent and enteric-coated biodegradable-polymer microspheres (Mathiowitz et al., 1997), some of which also show strong adhesive interactions with the intestinal mucosa. Diverse polymer-based systems include insulin that is incorporated with an absorption enhancer coated with an enteric polymer, or insulin is microencapsulated in systems in which polymers are administered with absorption promoters (Yadav et al., 2009). Non-degradable and degradable polymers have been used to produce microspheres in the nanometre size range that can be absorbed intact by the intestinal epithelium.

BUCCAL/SUBLINGUAL DELIVERY SYSTEMS

The administering insulin through the mucosa of the mouth is a potentially attractive option. Sublingual delivery is achieved through the mucosal membranes lining the floor of the mouth (Varshosaz, 2007). The route is easily accessible, protease activity is minimal and the lining of the mouth is greatly vascularised. Nevertheless, the buccal and sublingual mucosae present special problems for insulin delivery due to the associated effects of the comparatively thick, multilayered buccal barrier and the constant flow of saliva. More recently, a liquid-insulin aerosol formulation known as Oralin has been introduced, which is being assessed in healthy and diabetic subjects (Schwartz and Modi, 2000). Future progress in this area might involve the use of combination strategies to improve absorption.

INTRANASAL DELIVERY SYSTEMS

The nasal mucosa is another potentially interesting route. It is easily accessible, contributes a relatively large surface area for absorption (~150 cm^2), and has a rich, vascular sub epithelium and lymphatic system (Gizurarson and Bechgaard, 1991). Since the 1980s, absorption enhancers, such as bile salts (1–4% sodium glycocholate and deoxycholate spray or drops, and 1% taurodihydrofusidate spray), surfactants (Laureth-9 spray) and phospholipids (2% didecanoyl-phosphatidylcholine spray), as well as variety of formulation methods, have been used to enhance absorption and bioavailability (Hinchcliffe and Illum,1999).

PULMONARY DELIVERY

Over the years, certain drugs have been sold in compositions suitable for forming drug dispersion for oral inhalation (pulmonary delivery) to treat various conditions in humans. These pulmonary drug delivery formulations are designed to be delivered by inhalation by the patient of a drug dispersion so that the active drug within the dispersion can reach the lung The respiratory tree has a surface area of ~140 m^2, and offers the largest available surface area for drug delivery, Early attempts to deliver insulin as an inhaled aerosol began in the 1920s, and hence patient technique, and are subject to large inter and intra subject variability (Corne et al., 1997). Pulmonary drug delivery can itself be achieved by different strategies, including aerosol based metered dose inhalers (MDIs), liquid nebulizers, and dry powder dispersion devices (Hitzman et al., 2006). Current aerosol devices include pressurized metered-dose inhalers (pMDIs) and dry-powder inhalers (DPIs). The DPI devices are further limited by powder hygroscopicity, which reduces the respirable fraction (Borgstom et al., 2000).

ARTIFICIAL PANCREAS

An artificial pancreas system is an automated, closed-loop system which integrates a continuous glucose monitor and insulin pump, together with an automated algorithm to control insulin delivery, the patient would be removed from the decision loop, and the system would essentially function as an artificial pancreas (Steil et al., 2006). Development of the first generations of an artificial pancreas is underway and several studies have already demonstrated that glycemic control can be achieved with an automated closed loop system in investigational and controlled hospital settings. Medtronic MiniMed has developed an external physiologic insulin delivery system that combines an external insulin pump and continuous glucose sensor with a variable insulin infusion rate algorithm designed to emulate the physiologic characteristics of the β-cell (Weinzimer et al., 2008).

pH-SENSITIVE SYSTEMS

The main hurdles in developing oral insulin delivery devices are attributed to poor intrinsic insulin permeability across the biological membrane (Mundargi et al., 2011). Insulin has high molecular weight, and is easily degraded by proteolytic enzymes of the stomach or small intestine (Jain et al., 2006). Therefore, to protect insulin in acidic conditions, efforts have been made to develop pH-sensitive polymers or hydrogels for an effective oral formulation of insulin. In pH-sensitive systems insulin has to be delivered in response to pH in the body. Hydrogels are three-dimensional hydrophilic cross linked polymer networks, due to their high swollen nature and permeability to hydrophilic agents, hydrogels have also been proposed as controlled drug delivery system for insulin delivery (Rasool et al., 2010). Poly (glycolic acid, poly (acrylic acid) and poly (methacrylic acid) are commonly used for the preparation of hydrogels.

1.14.2 HERBAL MEDICINE

The plant kingdom is a good potential source for the discovery of novel medicines to treat numerous diseases including DM. Presently; about 400 plants included more than 700 recipes and compounds which have been evaluated extensively for the treatment of diabetes throughout the world (Bailey and Day, 1989). A multitude of spices, herbs and other plant materials have been assigned for the treatment of diabetes throughout the world. Indeed, in many parts of the world, particularly undeveloped countries, this may be the only form of therapy available to treat diabetic patients (Coman et al., 2012). Renewed attention to alternative medicines and natural therapies has stimulated a new wave of research interest in traditional practice.

Traditional antidiabetic plants might provide a useful source of new oral hypoglycemic compounds for development as pharmacological entities, or as simple dietary adjuncts to existing therapies. In many cases, very little is known about the mechanism of action of traditionally used antidiabetic plants, thus preventing them from being used in standard diabetes care (Singh et al., 2011). Recently, more research is being focused on elucidating the action of these plants and their active constituents.

MEDICINAL PLANTS USED FOR DIABETES

Several plants have been tested for their anti-diabetic potential. For most of them, the findings have been based on the ethno-botanical claims. The present non-exhaustive list gives an overview of some plants with well-known profiles of anti-diabetic claims. Table 3 presents a number of plants that are currently used for their antidiabetic properties, together with their active biomolecules, on the basis of recent studies.

TABLE 3 Some herbal plants with proven antidiabetic properties

Plant	Family	Parts used	Active compounds
Azadirachta indica	Meliaceae	Leaves, seed	Azadirachtin and nimbin
Tinospora cordifolia	Menisperma-ceae	Root	Tinosporone, tino-sporic acid
Momordica charan-tia	Cucurbitaceae	leaves	Charantin, sterol
Aloe vera	Asphodelaceae	Leaf,	Lophenol, Lectins
Syzygium cumini	Myrtaceae.	seeds, leaves,	Mycaminose
Morus alba	Moraceae	leaves	Chalcomoracin, mora-cin C
Liriope spicata	Liliaceae	root	Beta-sitosterol
Salacia oblonga	Celastraceae	Root, stem	Salacinol, kotalanol
Curcuma longa	Zingiberaceae	rhizome	Curcumin

TABLE 3 *(Continued)*

Picea mariana	Pinaceae	fruit	Quercetin
Nigella sativa	Apiaceae	seeds	Chlorogenic acid, apigenin
Pinus pinaster	Pinaceae	bark	Catechin, epicatechin
Gallega officinalis	Faboideae	leaves, seeds	Galegine
Phyllanthus amarus	Phyllanthaceae	whole plant	Phyllanthin
Beta vulgaris	Amaranthaceae	Root	Phenolics, betacyanins
Annona squamosa	Annonaceae	Fruits	Liriodenine, moupin-amide
Camellia sinensis	Theaceae	Leaves	Caffeine and catechins
Lantana camara	Verbenaceae	Leaves	Lantanoside, lantanone
Ricinus communis	Euphorbiaceae	Root	Ricinolic acid
Prunus amygdalus	Rosaceae	Seeds	Amygdalin

GYMNEMA SYLVESTRE

Gymnema sylvestre (Asclepiadaceae) is emerging as a potential treatment for the management of diabetes, the leaves of this plant is used in herbal medicine preparations. The main constituent of gymnema is gymnemic acid, a complex mixture of at least nine closely related acidic glycosides, the main ones being gymnemic acid A-D. The drug acts indirectly through stimulation in insulin secretion of the pancreas on the carbohydrate metabolism (Sahu et al., 1996). This hypoglycaemic effect was due to the ability of gymnemic acids to delay the glucose absorption in the blood. Gymnemic acid molecules incorporate the receptor location in the absorptive external layers of the intestine thereby preventing the sugar molecules absorption by the intestine, which results in low blood sugar level (Daisy et al., 2009).

SWERTIA PUNICEA

The hypoglycemic activity of this plant is due to the presence of two important constituents which are *Methylswertianin* and *Bellidifolin.* These active ingredients significantly reduced Fasting Blood Glucose after 1 week of administration, and the Fasting Blood Glucose levels were stable within 4 weeks (Tian et al., 2010). The mechanism of action of hypoglycemic effect of *Swertia Punicea* was found that is, by the improvement of insulin resistance.

WITHANIA COAGULANS DUNAL

Withania coagulans Dunal commonly known as Indian cheese maker, belongs to the family Solanaceae. *Withania coagulans* is rich in steroidal lactones, which are known as withanolides. From ethyl acetate extract of its fruits a steroidal lactone (withanolide) and sitosterol β-D glucosides were isolated. Steroidal lactones isolated from fruits are responsible for its hypoglycaemic effect (Yasir et al., 2012).

MOMORDICA CHARANTIA

Momordica charantia commonly known as bitter or bitter gourd belongs to the family Cucurbetaceae. The plant has many different chemical ingredients, which help medicinally either alone or when combined. One of the major hypoglycemic components is a steroid saponin called momocharin (charantin) with insulin-like chemical effect (Singh et al., 2011). Charantin has a molecular weight of 9.7 kDa and it is assumed that charantin is the active agent of *M.charantia.*

SALACIA RETICULATA

Salacia reticulata has been traditionally used for the treatment of T2DM in countries such as Sri Lanka, India, and Thailand. The plant contains α-glucosidase inhibitors, such as salacinol, kotalanol, de-*O*-sulphated-salacinol, and de-I-sulphated-kotalanol (Muraoka et al., 2008). The α-glucosidase the decomposition of disaccharides to glucose. Any inhibitory of α-glucosidases leads to the retardation of their action, consequently becoming an effective approach for the treatment of T2DM (Goldstein and Muller-Wieland, 2008).

IMPORTANT PHYTOCONSTITUENTS/ACTIVE AGENTS

Plants have evolved secondary biochemical pathways allowing them to synthesize a raft of chemicals called secondary metabolites, often in response to specific environmental stimuli, including pathogen attacks, herbivore-induced damage, or nutrient depravation (Hermsmeier et al, 2001, Coman et al., 2012). These chemicals also help humans to protect themselves against diseases and are called Phytochemicals. Synthetic drugs currently in use for diabetes treatment sometimes have side effects (Stumvoll et al., 2005). Table 4 shows the different classes of plant compounds with antihyperglycaemic activity, together with few examples from each class.

TABLE 4 List of phytoconstituents with antidiabetic properties

Compounds	Class of compounds
Catechins, epicatechins	Flavan-3-ols
Vanillic acid, gallic acid	Organic acids
Coumarin	Phenylpropanoids
Enhydrin	Sesquiterpenes
Mangiferin,bellidifolin	Xanthones
Gensenoside	Steroid glycoside
Genistein	Isoflavones
Quercetin, kaempferol, myricetin	Flavones
Cyanidin, delphynidin	Anthocyanidins

TABLE 4 *(Continued)*

Caffeic acid, ferulic acid	Cinamic acid derivatives
Salacinol, kotalanol,	Sugars
Curcumin, demethoxycurcumin	Curcuminoids
Phytoestrogens	Isoflavonoids
Cyanidin 3-galactoside	Anthocyanins
Davidigenin ,gallotannins	Chalcones
Ellagitannins, mallotinic acid	Tannins
Piperine, pipernonaline, dehydropiper-nonaline	Alkaloids

PHENOLIC COMPOUNDS

Polyphenolic compounds are among the classes of compounds that have received the most attention with regard to their antidiabetic properties (Marles and Farnsworth, 1995). The two main types of polyphenols are flavonoids and phenolic acids. Flavonoids are themselves distributed among several classes: Flavones, flavonols, flavanols, flavanones, isoflavones, proanthocyanidins, and anthocyanins. Dietary intake of flavonoids might prove to be important for alternative diabetes treatments or reduction of the risk of the disease. Attempts have been made to determine their potential in preventing β-cell apoptosis, promoting β-cell proliferation and insulin secretion (Pinent et al., 2008), and enhancing insulin activity (Ahmed et al., 2010). Structure of some of the phytoconstituents with antidiabetic property are given in Figure 6.

Rutin the flavonoid from *Ruta graveolens* decreased glycaemia, lipidaemia, serum insulin concentrations, liver glycogen content, and hexokinase activities (Coman et al.., 2010). Rutin was also effective in increasing the expression of the receptor PPAR-γ, leading to improved muscle insulin sensitivity and insulin signaling by increasing insulin-stimulated GLUT4 receptor activity (Petersen et al., 2006).

Genistein, an isoflavone found in soy products, increased glucose-stimulated insulin secretion in cell lines and mouse pancreatic islets (Liu et al., 2006). The mechanism of their action involved the activation of the cyclic adenosine monophosphate/protein kinase A (cAMP/PKA) signaling cascade, which led to an increase in intracellular Ca^{2+}, leading to the stimulation of insulin secretion.

Cyanidin 3-glucoside, an anthocyanin from black rice, exhibited a protective effect on insulin sensitivity in experiments on insulin-resistant adipose tissue cells induced by H_2O_2 or TNF-α (Guo et al., 2008). It is known that both H_2O_2 and the inflammatory TNF-α molecule inhibit the process of insulin signaling (Sesti, 2006). The exposure to H_2O_2 or TNF-α leads to insulin receptor substrate (IRS) serine phosphorylation concurrent with a decrease in insulin-stimulated IRS tyrosine phosphorylation and a decrease of cellular glucose uptake.

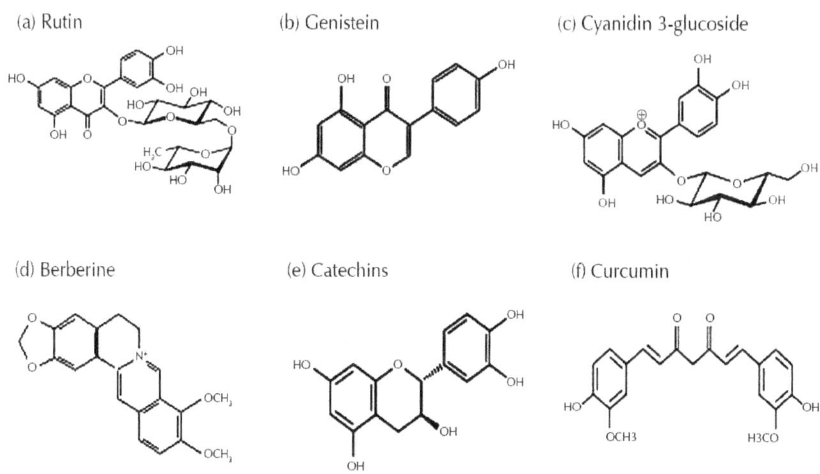

FIGURE 6 Structure of some phytoconstituents with antidiabetic potential.

ALKALOIDS

Another group of compounds are the alkaloids. In the plant they may exist in the free state, as salts or as *N*-oxides. Conophylline, an alkaloid compound extracted from the leaves of the tropical plant *Ervatamia microphylla*, was effective in stimulating the differentiation of progenitor cells into β-cells (Kojima and Umezawa, 2006). Other alkaloid compounds isolated from *Piper retrofractum*, such as piperine, pipernonaline, and dehydropipernonaline, activated AMP-activated protein kinase (AMPK) signalling and the PPAR-γ protein (Kim et al., 2011) in 3T3-L1 adipocytes and L6 myocytes, suggesting potential antidiabetic effects.

Berberine a quaternary ammonium salt from the protoberberine group of isoquinoline alkaloids is used successfully in experimental (Wang et al., 2010) and clinical DM (Gu et al., 2010). It is found in such plants as *Berberis aquifolium* (Oregon grape), *Berberis vulgaris* (Barberry). Berberine has been shown to lower elevated blood glucose as effectively as metformin (Yin et al., 2008). The mechanisms of action include inhibition of aldose reductase, inducing glycolysis, hindering insulin resistance through increasing insulin receptor expression.

Natural products such as plant extracts, phytochemicals are attracting more and more attention for their potential uses in the treatment and prevention of T2DM. Some of them show very promising effects, which demonstrated that the dietary intake of phytochemicals could be a promising strategy for diabetes prevention. Additionally, therapies based on phytochemicals could constitute a novel pharmacological approach for treatment or an approach that would reinforce existing treatments.

1.14.3 ALTERNATIVE TREATMENT STRATEGIES

AYURVEDA

Ayurveda which means "Science of life is derived from the Sanskrit words *Ayur* meaning life and *Veda* meaning knowledge (Sharma et al., 2007). Ayurveda is perhaps, the most ancient of all medical traditions is considered to be the origin of systematic medicine. It is really a practical and holistic set of guidelines to maintain balance and harmony in the system. Illness is the consequence of imbalance between the various elements and it is the goal of the treatment to restore his balance. Ayurveda was first referred to in the *Vedas* (*Rigveda* and *Atharva Veda* 1500 BC). The DM (*Madhumeha*) was known to ancient Indian physicians and an elaborate description of its clinical features and management appears in Ayurvedic texts (Modak et al., 2007).

Ayurveda treat diabetes with a multi-pronged approach, using diet modification, *Panchkarma* to cleanse the system, herbal preparations, yoga and breathing exercises (Manyam, 2004). First, it addresses diet modification, excluding sugar and simple carbohydrates, and affirming complex carbohydrates. Protein is restricted, since large intake can damage the kidneys. Fat is also reduced because there is often a deficiency of pancreatic enzymes, resulting fat digestion tough. Since several diabetics have autoantibodies, a cleansing program is established. *Panchakarma* is usually used for this purpose. This starts with herbal massages and an herbal steam bath, followed by fasting to cleanse the body. This is succeeded by a herbal purge for the pancreas, liver and spleen (Sharma, 2011). Ayurveda use several herbal preparations for diabetics. The herbs which are used to treat diabetes include famous Ayurvedic medicinal plants include *Azadirachta indica* (Neem), *Centella asiatica* (Gotu Kola), *Cinnamomum camphora* (Camphor), *Elettaria cardamomum* (ela or cardamomum), *Santalum album* (Sandalwood), *Terminalia* species (Myrobolan) and *Withania somnifera* (Aswargandha), *Rauwolfia serpentina* (Indian snake root), *Curcuma longa* (turmeric), (Saxena 2004; Sharma et al., 2007). Decoctions of triphala, fenugreek, and shilajit are commonly used. Powders (*Churana*) used include *Amalaki Churna*, *Haldi* powder (Turmeric powder) and *Naag Bhasma* (Modak et al., 2007).

It is postulated that Ayurvedic medications may act through potential pancreatic as well as extra pancreatic effects. The probable mechanisms of action include: delaying gastric emptying, slowing carbohydrate absorption, inhibition of glucose transport, increasing the erythrocyte insulin receptors and peripheral glucose utilization, increasing glycogen synthesis, modulating insulin secretion, decreasing blood glucose synthesis through depression of the enzymes fructose-1,6-bisphosphatase, glucose-6-phosphatase, and enhanced glucose oxidation by the enzyme glucose-6-phosphatase-dehydrogenase pathway (McWhorter 2001).

SIDDHA

Siddha is one of the oldest medical systems in India in which pulse is used to diagnose the diseases (Thiyagarajan, 2006). It was developed and practiced widely not only in India, but also in other countries like Egypt, China, and Greece. It is a non invasive pulse diagnosis method. Physicians mostly use the pulse to determine the heart rate. There are three *doshas* which govern the function of entire human body. They are *vata, pitta, and kapha*, called as *Tridosha. Siddha* practitioners locate three different pulses in single artery on each wrist, corresponding to each of the three *doshas*. *Siddha* system of medicine practiced in India describes number of preparations using herbals, metals, minerals, animals and the mixture of above for the management of DM (Sathish et al., 2012).

Siddha literature describes the DM as *madhumegam or neeazhivu*, which means sweet urine. It emphasizes to use herbo-mineral preparations if herbals alone could not provide relief in DM (Shankar and Singhal, 1995). *Siddha* literature describe different preparations/formulations of *abraga chendhooram*.

Eventhough, biotite or mica is the common mineral constituent, each preparations varies by different herbal ingredients. *Sesbania grandiflora, Calotropis gigantea* flower and *Momordica charantia* (bitter melon) are three herbal ingredients in *abraga chendhooram*. A 45 day clinical trial by *abraga chendooram* in NIDDM has shown statistically significant fall in both fasting as well as post prandial blood glucose level without toxic report (Shankar and Singhal, 1995). *Abraga chendhooram* exhibited a dose dependent α-glucosidase inhibitory activity. Unlike other α-glucosidase inhibitors, *abraga chendhooram* did not produce any gastrointestinal adverse effects (Boonmee et al., 2007).

HOMEOPATHY

Homeopathic treatment with drugs can improve the general well being of the person with diabetes. In peoples with poor general health it can be very burdensome to accomplish good control of diabetes. Improvement of general health enhances the general sense of well-being; decreases the dose and number of drugs needed to control blood glucose and improve blood glucose control. Remedies such as uranium nitricum, Syzygium, phloridzin (obtained from the root of the apple and other fruit trees) are given to augment the general health of the patient. The metals are used for treatment of patients with diabetic nephropathy, HTN arteriosclerosis, physically and mentally exhausted and many other symptoms. The vegetables, minerals and animal products are used to manage symptoms such as gangrene, weakness and prostration, impotence, diabetes complicated with digestive troubles, ocular troubles and other complications of diabetes (Witt et al., 2008). The homeopathic remedy prescribed to a patient depends on his/her symptoms. Hence, two patients may have diabetes but their medications may be totally different. The homeopathy drug treatment used in diabetes can be classified in to six groups namely metals, other minerals, acids, vegetables, drugs from animals, and organo therapy remedies (Adler, 2011). Acids are often used in patients with debility or persistent weakness. The acids used for treatment of diabetes are acetic acid, lactic acid and phosphoric acid. Vegetables (such as *Cephalandra indica, Helleborus niger*), and products from Animal kingdom are prescribed based on the individual characteristics and symptoms of the patients.

1.14.4 INTEGRATED AND HOLISTIC APPROACH IN DIABETES MANAGEMENT

Integrated care for people with diabetes refers to the need to provide care for conditions coexisting with diabetes within the same primary health care service. Within most high income countries, primary health care has been developed to provide a range of services covering most of the needs with people with diabetes, and indeed with other chronic conditions.

People with diabetes come into contact with all parts of the health care systems. As they incur complications and culminating disability, their care may also need involvement from social services in the community. Thus diabetes care should be integrated over all of these services (Rovira, 2002). The choice of the person with diabetes must always be appreciated, such that care planning is a joint activity regularly undertaken between the physician or care provider (e.g. diabetic nurse) and the patient with involvement of his family as appropriate (Funnell and Anderson,2003). Care planning and management must also be seen as dynamic processes that evolve around the changing needs of the patient and events that trigger the need for targeted interventions.

The present day life style contributes to the alarming rise in the occurrence of this disease. Lifestyle modifications inclusive of dietary alterations, weight reduction and regular physical activity are indicated for prevention of diabetes. Accordingly, a holistic health care approach (instead of a conventional drug-based approach alone) for the treatment is highly warranted. Chronic diseases such as diabetes are associated with diminished quality of life and psychological depression and anxiety (Kutty and Raju, 2010). Mind-body therapies have behavioral and psychological effects that may help patients cope with disease and improve mood and quality of life (Astin et al., 2003). Medical Nutrition Therapy (MNT) is a component of diabetes management and of diabetes self-management education. The MNT is the preferred term and should replace other terms, such as dietary management and diet therapy. The MNT for people with diabetes should be individualized with consideration given to each individual's metabolic profile, usual food and eating habits, treatment goals, and prospected outcomes. The monitoring of metabolic parameters such as HbA1c, glucose, blood pressure, lipids, body weight, and renal function, as well as quality of life is essential to assess the need for changes in therapy and ensure successful outcomes (Tinker et al., 1994).

1.15 CONCLUSION

The present day life style contributes to the alarming rise in the occurrence of diabetes and the ailments associated with it. Lifestyle modifications inclusive of dietary alterations, weight reduction and regular physical activity are indicated for prevention of diabetes. Accordingly, a holistic health care approach (instead of a conventional drug-based approach alone) for the treatment is highly warranted. Chronic diseases such as diabetes are associated with diminished quality of life and psychological depression and anxiety. Mind-body therapies have behavioural and psychological effects that may help patients cope with disease and improve mood and quality of life. The MNT is a component of diabetes management and of diabetes self-management education. The MNT is the preferred term and should replace other terms, such as dietary management and diet therapy. The MNT for people with diabetes should be individualized with consideration given to each individual's metabolic profile, usual food and eating habits, treatment goals, and prospected outcomes. Monitoring of metabolic parameters such as HbA1c, glucose, blood pressure, lipids, body weight, and renal function, as well as quality of life is essential to assess the need for changes in therapy and ensure successful outcomes.

KEYWORDS

- **Diabetes mellitus**
- **Epodermiology**
- **Classification**
- **Pathophysiology**
- **Diagnosis**
- **Treatment**

REFERENCES

1. Abdul-Ghani, M. A.,Tripathy, D., and DeFronzo, R. A. Contributions of beta-cell dysfunction and insulin resistance to the pathogenesis of impaired glucose tolerance and impaired fasting glucose. *Diab Care,* **29**, 1130–113 (2006).
2. Adamis, A. P. Shima, D. T.,Yeo, K. T., Yeo, T. K., Brown, L. F., Berse, B., D'Amore, P. A. and Folkman, J. Synthesis and secretion of vascular permeability factor/vascular endothelial growth factor by human retinal pigment epithelial cells. *Biochem. Biophys. Res. Commun.* **193**, 631–638 (1993).
3. Adams, M., Montague, C. T., Prins, J. B. et al. Activators of peroxisome proliferator-activated receptor gamma have depot-specific effects on human preadipocyte differentiation. *J. Clin. Invest.*, **100**, 3149–3153 (1997).
4. Adler, U. C. Low-grade inflammation in chronic diseases: An integrative pathophysiology anticipated by homeopathy? *Med. Hypotheses*, **76**, 622–626 (2011).

5. Ahmad, L. A. and Crandall, J. P. Type 2 Diabetes Prevention: A Review. *Clin Diab.*, **28**(2), 53–59 (2010).
6. Ahmed, O. M., Moneim, A. A., Yazid, I. A., and Mahmoud, A. M. Antihyperglicemic antihyperlipidemic and antioxidant effects and the probable mechanisms of action of Ruta graveolens infusion and rutin in nicotinamide-streptozotocin-induced diabetic rats. *Diabetol. Croatica*, **39**, 15–35 (2010).
7. Ahren, B., Larsson, H., and Holst, J. J. Effects of glucagon-like peptide-1 on islet function and insulin sensitivity in noninsulin-dependent diabetes mellitus. *J. Clin. Endocrinol. Metab.*, **82**, 473–8 (1997).
8. Aiello, .L. P., Pierce, E. A., Foley, E. D., Takagi, H., Chen, H., Riddle, L., Ferrara, N., King, G. L., and Smith, L. E. Suppression of retinal neovascularization in vivoby inhibition of vascular endothelial growth factor (VEGF) using soluble VEGF-receptor chimeric proteins. *Proc. Natl. Acad. Sci.*, **92**, 10457–10461 (1995).
9. Aiello, L. M. Perspectives on diabetic retinopathy. *Am. J. Ophthalmol.*,**136**, 122–135 (2003).
10. Aiello, L. P. and Wong, J. S. Role of vascular endothelial growth factor in diabetic vascular complications. Kidney Int., **58**(77), S113–S119 (2000).
11. Albisser, A. M., Leibel, B. S., Zingg, W., Botz, C. K., Marliss, E. B., Denoga, A., and Zinman, B. The development of an artificial endocrine pancreas and its application in research and clinical investigation. *Horm. Metab. Res.* (Suppl.) **7**, 87–94 (1977).
12. Aljasem, L. I., Peyrot, M., Wissow, L., and Rubin, R. R. The impact of barriers and self efficacy on self-care behaviors in type 2 diabetes. *Diab Educator*, **27**(3), 393–404 (2001).
13. Altshuler, D., Hirschhorn, J. N., Klannemark, M., Lindgren, C. M., Vohl, M. C., Nemesh, J., Lane, C. R., Schaffner, S. F., Bolk, S., Brewer, C., Tuomi, T., Gaudet, D., Hudson, T. J., Daly, M., Groop, L., and Lander, E. S. J. The common PPAR γ Pro12Ala polymorphism is associated with decreased risk of T2D. *Nat. Genet.*, **26,** 76–80 (2000).
14. American Diabetes Association, Report of the Expert Committee on the diagnosis and classification of diabetes mellitus, *Diab. Care*, **20**, 1183–1197 (1997).
15. American Diabetes Association. Diagnosis and Classification of Diabetes Mellitus. *Diab.Care*, **33**(1), S62–S69n (2010),
16. American Diabetes Association. Diagnosis and Classification of Diabetes Mellitus. *Diab. Care,* **27**(1), S5-S10 (2004).
17. American Diabetes Association. Diagnosis and Classification of Diabetes Mellitus. *Diab. Care*, **30**(1), S42–S47 (2007).
18. American Diabetes Association. Diagnosis and Classification of Diabetes Mellitus. *Diab care*, **32**(1), S62–S67 (2009).
19. American Diabetes Association. Peripheral arterial disease in people with diabetes. *Diab. Care*, **26**, 3333–3341 (2003).
20. American Diabetes Association. Tests of glycemia in diabetes. *Diab. Care*, **26**(1), S106–S108 (2003).
21. American Diabetes Association: Nutrition recommendations and interventions for diabetes. *Diab. Care*, **30**(1), S48–S65 (2007).
22. Amoah, A. G., Owusu, S. K., and Adjei, S. Diabetes in Ghana: acommunity based prevalence study in Greater Accra. *Diab. Res. Clin. Pract.*, **56**(3), 197–205 (2002).

23. Apelqvist, J., Larsson, J., and Agardh, C. D. Theinfluence of external precipitating factors and peripheral neuropathy on the development and outcome of diabetic foot ulcers. *J Diabetes Complications*, **4**, 21–25 (1990).
24. Armstrong, D. G., Nguyen, H. C., Lavery, L. A., van Schie, C. H., Boulton, A. J., and Harkless, L. B. Off-loading the diabetic foot wound:a randomized clinical trial. *Diab. Care*, **24**(6), 1019–22 (2001).
25. Ashcroft, F. M. and Gribble, F. M. ATP- sensitive K^+ channels and insulin secretion: their role in health and disease. *Diabetologia*, **42,** 903–919 (1999).
26. Astin, J. A., Shapiro, S. L., Eisenberg, D. M., and Forys, K. L. Mind-body medicine: state of the science, implications for practice. *J. Ann. Board. Farm. Med.*, **16**, 131–47 (2003).
27. Atkinson, M. A. and Eisenbarth, G. S. Type 1 diabetes: new perspectives on disease pathogenesis and treatment. *Lancet*, **358**, 221–229 (2001).
28. Bach, J. F. Insulin-dependent diabetes mellitus as an autoimmune disease, *Endocrine Rev.*, **15**, 516–542 (1994).
29. Baelde, H. J., Eikmans, M., Lappin, D. W., Doran, P. P., Hohenadel, D., Brinkkoetter, P. T., van der Woude, F. J., Waldherr, R., Rabelink, T. J, de Heer, E, and Bruijn, J. A. Reduction of VEGF-A and CTGF expression in diabetic nephropathy is associated with podocyte loss. *Kidney Int.*, **71**, 637–45 (2007).
30. Baggio, L. L. and Drucker, D. J. *Biology of incretins: GLP-1 and GIP. Gastroenterol.* **132**, 2131–2157 (2007).
31. Bailey, C. J. Treating insulin resistance in type 2 diabetes with metformin and thiazolidinedione. *Diab. Obes. Metab.*, **7,** 675–691 (2005).
32. Bailey, C. J. and Day, C. Hypoglycemic agents from traditional plant treatments for diabetes. *Diab. Care*, **12**(8), 553–564 (1989).
33. Bailey, C. J. and Krentz, A. J. Oral Antidiabetic Agents. In Textbook of Diabetes, 4th edition., R. Holt, C. Cockram, A. Flyvbjerg, and B. Goldstein (Eds.).West Sussex, *Wiley-Blackwell*, pp. 460–462 (2010).
34. Bailey, C. J. and Turner, R. C. Metformin. *N. Engl. J. Med.*, **334**, 574–9 (1996).
35. Banting, F. G., Best, C. H., Collip, J. B., Campbell, W. R., and Fletcher, A. A. Pancreatic extracts in the treatment of diabetes mellitus: preliminary report. 1922. *Can. Med. Asso.c J.*, **145**, 1281–6 (1991).
36. Barone, P. W. and Strano, M. S. Single walled carbon nanotubes as reporters for the optical detection of glucose. *J. Diabetes. Sci.Technol.*, **3**, 242–252 (2009).
37. Barr, R. G., Nathan, D. M., Meigs, J. B., and Singer, D. E. Tests of glycemia for the diagnosis of diabetes mellitus. *Ann. Intern. Med.*, **137**, 263–272 (2002).
38. Barratt, B. J., Payne, F., Lowe, C. E., et al. Remapping the insulin gene/IDDM2 locus in type 1 diabetes. *Diabetes*, **53**, 1884–9 (2004).
39. Barrett-Connor, E. and Khaw, K. T. Cigarette smoking and increased central adiposity. *Ann. Intern. Med.*, **111**, 783–787 (1989).
40. Bartlett, R. J., Denis, M., Secore, S. L., Alejandro, R., and Ricordi, C. Toward engineering skeletal muscle to release peptide hormone from the human pre-proinsulin gene. *Transplant.Proc.*, **30**, 451 (1998).
41. Basta, G., Schmidt, A. M., and De Caterina, R. Advanced glycation end products and vascular inflammation: implications for accelerated atherosclerosis in diabetes, *Cardiovasc. Res.*, **63**, 582–592 (2004).

42. Baynes, J. W. Role of oxidative stress in development of complications in diabetes. *Diabetes*, **40**, 405–412 (1991).
43. Baynes, J. W. and Thorpe, S. R. Role of oxidative stress in diabetic complications: A new perspective on an old paradigm. *Diabetes*, **48**, 1–9 (1999).
44. Bays, H., Mandarino, L., and DeFronzo, R. A. Role of the adipocyte, free fatty acids, and ectopic fat in pathogenesis of type 2 diabetes mellitus: peroxisomal proliferator-activated receptor agonists provide a rational therapeutic approach. *J. Clin. Endocrinol. Metab.*, **89**, 463–78 (2004).
45. B. E. Metzger, T. A. Buchanan, D. R.Coustan, A. de Leiva, D. B. Dunger, D. R. Hadden, B. E. Metzger, D. R. Coustan (Eds.). Proceedings of the Fourth International Workshop - conference on gestational diabetes mellitus. *Diab. Care*, **21**, B1–B167 (1998).
46. Beamer, B. A., Yen, C. J., Andersen, R. E., Muller, D., Elahi, D., Cheskin, L. J., Andres, R., Roth, J., and Shuldiner, A. R. Association of the Pro12Ala variant in the peroxisome proliferator-activated receptor g2 gene with obesity in two Caucasian populations. *Diabetes*, **47**, 1806–1808 (1998).
47. Bell, G. and Polonsky, K. Diabetes mellitus and genetically programmed defects in β-cell function. *Nature*, **414**, 788–791 (2001).
48. Bell, G. I., Horita, S., and Karam, J. H. A polymorphic locus near the human insulin gene is associated with insulin-dependent diabetes mellitus. *Diabetes*, **33**, 176–83 (1984).
49. Bell, G. I., Kayano, T., Buse, J. B., Burant, C. F., Takeda, J., Lin, D., Fukumoto, H., and Seino, S. Molecular biology of mammalian glucose transporters. *Diab.* Care, **13**, 198–20 (1990).
50. Bell, R. A., Mayer-Davis, E. J., Beyer, J. W, et al. Diabetes in non-Hispanic white youth: prevalence, incidence, and clinical characteristics: the SEARCH for Diabetes in Youth Study. *Diab. Care*, **32**(2), S102–S111 (2009).
51. Bergendi, L., Benes, L., Durackova, Z., and Ferencik, M. Chemistry, physiology, and pathology of free radicals. *Life Sci.*, **65**, 1865–1874 (1999).
52. Bergman, R. N. and Mittelman, S. D. Central role of the adipocyte in insulin resistance. *J Basic Clin. Physiol. Pharmacol.*, **9**, 205–21 (1998).
53. Bezerra, R. M., Ueno, M., Silva, M. S., Tavares, D. Q.,Carvalho, C. R., Saad, M. J., and Gontijo, J. A. A high-fructose diet induces insulin resistance but not blood pressure changes in normotensive rats. *Braz. J. Med. Biol. Res*, **34**(9), 1155–60 (2001).
54. Biller, J. and Love, B. B. Diabetes and stroke. *Med. Clin. North Am.*, **77**, 95–110 (1993).
55. Bjorntorp, P. Metabolic implications of body fat distribution. *Diab. Care*, **14**, 1132–143 (1991).
56. Bloomgarden, Z. T. Insulin treatment and type 1 diabetes topics. *Diab Care*, **294,** 936–944 (2006).
57. Blumberg, S. N., Berger, A., Hwang, L., Pastar, I., Warren, S. M., and Chen, W. The role of stem cells in the treatment of diabetic foot ulcers. *Diab. Res. Clin. Prac.*, **96**, 1–9 (2012).
58. Bo, S., Menato, G., Lezo, A., Signorile, A., Bardelli, C., De Michieli, F., Massobrio, M., and Pagano, G. Dietary fat and gestational hyperglycemia. *Diabetologia*, **44**, 972–8 (2001).

59. Boddula, R., Yadav, S., Bhatia, V., Genitta, G., Pandey, D., Kumar, A., Singh, H. K., Ramesh, V., Julka, S., Bansal, B., Srikant, K., Bhatia, E., et al. High prevalence of type 2 diabetes mellitus in affluent urban Indians. *Diab. Res. Clin. Pract.*, **81**, 4–7 (2008).
60. Boden, G. Role of fatty acids in the pathogenesis of insulin resistance and NIDDM. *Diabetes*, **46**, 3–10 (1997).
61. Boden, G., Cheung, P.; Stein, T. P., Kresge, K., and Mozzoli, M. FFA cause hepatic insulin resistance by inhibiting insulin suppression of glycogenolysis. *Am. J. Physiol. Endocrinol. Metab.*, **283**, E12–9 (2002).
62. Bolli, G. B., Di Marchi, R. D., Park, G. D., Pramming, S., and Koivisto, V. A. Insulin analogues and their potential in the management of diabetes mellitus. *Diabetologia*, **42**, 1151–67 (1999).
63. Bonifacio, E., Lampasona, V., Genovese, S., Ferrari, M., and Bosi, E. Identification of protein tyrosine phosphatase - like IA2 (islet cell antigen 512) as the insulin - dependent diabetes-related 37/40K autoantigen and a target of islet - cell antibodies. *J. Immunol.*,**155**, 5419–5426 (1995).
64. Boonmee, A., Reynolds, C. D., and Sangvanich, P. Alpha-glucosidase inhibitor proteins from Sesbania grandiflora flowers. *Planta Med.*, **73**, 1197–201 (2007).
67. Borgstom, L., Bengtsson, T., Derom, E., and Pauwels, R. Variability in lung deposition of inhaled drug, within and between asthmatic patients, with a pMDI and dry powder inhaler, Turbuhaler. *Int. J. Pharm.*, **193**, 227–230 (2000).
68. Bosi, E. Metformin. The gold standard in type 2 diabetes: what does the evidence tell us? *Diab. Obes. Metab.*, **11**, 3–8 (2009).
69. Bottini, N., Vang, T., Cucca, F., and Mustelin, T. Role of PTPN22 in type 1 diabetes and other autoimmune diseases. *Semin. Immunol.*, **18**, 207–213 (2006).
70. Bouchard, C., Tremblay, A., Despres, J. P., Nadeau, A., Lupien, P. J., Theriault, G., Dussault, J., Moorjani, S., Pinault, S., and Fournier, G. The response to long-term overfeeding in identical twins. *N. Engl. J. Med.*, **322**, 1477–82 (1990).
71. Bougneres, P. Genetics of obesity and type 2 diabetes tracking pathogenic traits during the predisease period. *Diabetes*, **51**(3), S295–S303 (2002).
72. Boulton, A. J., Kirsner, R. S., and Vileikyte, L. Clinical practice. Neuropathic diabetic foot ulcers. *N. Engl. J. Med.*, **351**, 48–55 (2004).
73. Boulton, A. J., Meneses, P., and Ennis, W. J. Diabetic foot ulcers: a framework for prevention and care. *Wound Repair Regen.*, **7**, 7–16 (1999).
74. Boulton, A. J. M. Neuropathy and diabetes. *Diab. Rev.*, **7**, 235–410 (1999).
75. Boulton, A. J. M., Gries, F. A., and Jervell, J. A. Guidelines for the diagnosis and outpatient management diabetic peripheral neuropathy. *Diabet Med.*, **15**, 508–514 (1998).
76. Boulton, A. J. M. and Malik, R. A. Diabetic neuropathy. *Med. Clin .N .Am.*, **82**, 909–929 (1998).
77. Bozkurt, O., de Boer, A., Grobbee, D. E., Heerdink, E. R., Burger, H., and Klungel, O. H. Pharmacogenetics of glucose-lowering drug treatment: a systematic review. *Mol. Diagn. Ther.*, **11**, 291–302 (2007).
78. Bray, G. A., Nielsen, S. J., and Popkin. B. M. Consumption of high - fructose corn syrup in beverages may play a role in the epidemic of obesity. *Am. J. Clin. Nutr.*, **79** 537–543 (2004).

79. Brem, H., Stojadinovic, O., Diegelmann, R. F., Entero, H., Lee, B., Pastar, I., Golinko, M., Rosenberg, H., and Tomic-Canic, M. Molecular markers in patients with chronic wounds to guide surgical debridement. *Mol. Med.*, **13**(1–2), 30–9 (2007).
80. Brito, P. L., Fioretto, P., Drummond, K., Kim, Y., Steffes, M. W., Basgen, J. M., Sisson-Ross, S., and Mauer, M. Proximal tubular basement membrane width in insulin-dependent diabetes mellitus. *Kidney Int.*, **53**, 754–761 (1998).
81. Burchfiel, C. M., Sharp, D. S., Curb, J. D., Rodriguez, B. L., Hwang, L. J., Marcus, E. B., and Yano, K. Physical activity and incidence of diabetes: The Honolulu Heart Program. *Am. J. Epidemiol.*, **141**, 360–368 (1995).
82. Burge, M. R., Mitchell, S. D. O., Sawyer, A., and Schade, D. S. Continuous glucose monitoring: the future of diabetes management. *Diabetes Spectr.*, **21**, 112–119 (2008).
83. Busch, C. and Hegele, R. Genetic determinants of type 2 diabetes mellitus. *Clin. Genet.*, **60,** 243–254 (2001).
84. Buse, J. B., Henry, R. R., Han, J., Kim, D. D., Fineman, M. S., and Baron, A. D. For the Exenatide- 13 Clinical Study Group. Effects of exenatide (exendin-4) on glycemic control over 30 weeks in sulfonylurea-treated patients with type 2 diabetes. *Diab Care.*, **27**, 2628–2635 (2004).
85. Butler, A. E., Janson, J., Bonner-Weir, S., Ritzel, R., Rizza, R. A., and Butler, P. C. β-cell deficit and increased β-cell apoptosis in humans with type 2 diabetes. *Diabetes*, **52**(1), 102–110 (2003).
86. Calhoun, J. H., Overgaard, K. A., Stevens, M. C., Dowling, J. P. F., and Mader, J. T. Diabetic Foot Ulcers and Infections Current Concepts. *Adv. Skin Wound Care*, **15**, 31–45, (2002).
87. Cameron, N. E. and Cotter, M. A. Effects of protein kinase C beta inhibition on neurovascular dysfunction in diabetic rats: interaction with oxidative stress and essential fatty acid dysmetabolism. *Diab. Metab. Res. Rev.*, **18**, 315–323 (2002).
88. Cameron, N. E. and Cotter, M. A. Metabolic and vascular factors in the pathogenesis of diabetic neuropathy. *Diabetes*, **46**(2), 31S–37S (1997).
89. Capes, S. E., Hunt, D., Malmberg, K., Pathak, P., and Gerstein, H. C. Stress hyperglycemia and prognosis of stroke in nondiabetic and diabetic patients: a systematic overview. *Stroke*, **32**, 2426–32 (2001).
90. Caramori, M. L., Gross, J. L., Pecis, M., and de Azevedo, M. J. Glomerular filtration rate, urinary albumin excretion rate, and blood pressure changes in normoalbuminuric normotensive type 1 diabetic patients:an 8-year follow-up study. *Diab. Care*, **22**, 1512–1516 (1999).
91. Carino, G. P. and Mathiowitz, E. Oral insulin delivery. *Adv. Drug Deliv. Rev.*, **35**, 249–257 (1999).
92. Carpenter, M. W. and Coustan, D. R. Criteria for screening tests for gestational diabetes. *Am. J. Obstet. Gynecol.*, **144**, 768–773 (1982).
93. Carpentier, A., Mittelman, S. D., Bergman, R. N., Giacca, A., and Lewis, G. F. Prolonged elevation of plasma free fatty acids impairs pancreatic beta - cell function in obese nondiabetic humans but not in individuals with type 2 diabetes. *Diabetes*, **49,** 399–408 (2000).
94. Cas, D. A. and Gnudi, L. VEGF and angiopoietins in diabetic glomerulopathy: How far for a new treatment? *Metabol.*, **61**(12), 1666–73 (2012).

95. Cash, K. J. and Clark, H. A. Nanosensors and nanomaterials for monitoring glucose in diabetes. *Trends Mol. Med.*, **16**(12), 584–593 (2010).
96. Castano, L., Ziegler, A. G., Ziegler, R., Shoelson, S., and Eisenbarth, G. S.Characterization of insulin autoantibodies in relatives of patients with type 1 diabetes. *Diabetes*, **42,** 1202–1209 (1993).
97. Cauchi, S., Meyre, D., Dina, C., Choquet, H., Samson C., Gallina, S., Balkau, B., Charpentier, G., Pattou, F., Stetsyuk, V., Scharfmann, R., Staels, B., Frühbeck, G., and Froguel, P. Transcription factor TCF7L2 genetic study in the French population: expression in human beta cells and adipose tissue and strong association with type 2 diabetes. *Diabetes*, **55**, 2903–2908 (2006).
98. Ceriello, A. Oxidative stress and diabetes-associated complications, *Endocr. Pract.*, **12**, 60–62 (2006).
99. Cermak, J., Key, N. S., Bach, R. R., Balla, J., and Jacob, H. S. Vercellotti GM. C-reactive protein induces human peripheral blood monocytes to synthesize tissue factor. *Blood*, **82**, 513–20 (1993).
100. Chan, J. M., Rimm, E. B., Colditz, G. A., Stampfer, M. J. and Willett, W. C. Obesity, fat distribution, and weight gain as risk factors for clinical diabetes in men. *Diab. Care*, **17**, 961 –969 (1994).
101. Chase, H. P., Kim, L. M., Owen, SL., MacKenzie, T. A., Klingensmith, G. J., Murtfeldt, R., and Garg, S. K. Continuous subcutaneous glucose monitoring in children with type 1 diabetes. *Pediatrics*, **107**, 222–226 (2001).
102. Chaturvedi, N. The burden of diabetes and its complications: trends and implications for intervention. *Diab. Res. Clin. Pract.*, **76**, S3-12 (2007).
103. Chaturvedi, N., Bandinelli, S., Mangili, R., Penno, G., Rottiers, R. E., and Fuller, J. H. Microalbuminuria in type 1 diabetes: rates, risk factors and glycemic threshold. *Kidney Int.*, **60**, 219–227 (2001).
104. Chee, W., Egan, C., and Egan, J. M. Incretin-Based Therapies in Type 2 Diabetes Mellitus. *Curr. Protein Pept. Sci.*, **10**, 46–55 (2009).
105. Chen, K. W., Boyko, E. J., Bergstrom, R. W., Leonetti, D. L., Newell-Morris, L., Wahl, P. W., and Fujimoto, W. Y. Earlier appearance of impaired insulin secretion than of visceral adiposity in the pathogenesis of NIDDM. 5-year follow-up of initially nondiabetic Japanese-American men. *Diab. Care*, **18**, 747–53 (1995).
106. Cheng, C., Kushner, H., and Falkner, B. E. The utility of fasting glucose for detection of prediabetes. *Metabol.*, **55**, 434–438 (2006).
107. Chimienti, F., Devergnas, S., Favier, A., and Seve, M. Identification and cloning of a beta cell-specific zinc transporter, ZnT-8, localized into insulin secretory granules. *Diabetes*, **53**, 2330–2337 (2004).
108. Chimienti, F., Devergnas, S., Pattou, F., Schuit, F., Garcia-Cuenca, R., Vandewalle, B., Kerr-Conte, J., Van Lommel, L., Grunwald, D., Favier, A., and Seve, M. In vivo expression and functional characterization of the zinc transporter ZnT8 in glucose-induced insulin secretion. *J. Cell Sci.*, **119**, 4199–4206 (2006).
109. Chopra, N., Gavalas, V. G., Bachas, L. G., Hinds, B. J., and Bachas, L. G. Functional one-dimensional nanomaterials: applications in nanoscale biosensors. *Anal. Lett.*, **40**, 2067–2096 (2007).
110. Clark, L. C Jr. and Duggan ,C. A. Implanted electroenzymatic glucose sensors. *Diab. Care*, **5**, 174–180 (1982).

111. Clark, A. Islet amyloid and type 2 diabetes. *Diabetic Med.*, **6**, 561–567 (1989).
112. Clark, L. C Jr. and Lyons, C. Electrode systems for continuous monitoring in cardiovascular surgery. *Ann. New York Acad. Sci.*, **102**, 29–45 (1962).
113. Clayton, W. Jr. and Elasy, T. A. Review of the Pathophysiology, Classification, and Treatment of Foot Ulcers in Diabetic Patients. *Clin Diab.*, **27**(2), 52–58 (2009).
114. Cockram, C. S. The epidemiology of diabetes mellitus in the Asia-Pacific region. *HKMJ*, **6**, 43–52 (2000).
115. Cohen, S., Dadi, H., Shaoul, E., Sharfe, N., and Roifman, C. M. Cloning and characterization of a lymphoid-specific, inducible human protein tyrosine phosphatase. *Lyp. Blood*, **93**, 2013–24 (1999).
116. Coman, C., Rugina, O. D., and Socaciu, C. Plants and Natural Compounds with Antidiabetic Action. *Not. Bot. Horti. Agrobo.*, **40**(1), 314–325 (2012).
117. Consoli, A., Kennedy, F., Miles, J., and Gerich, J. Determination of Krebs cycle metabolic carbon exchange *in vivo* and its use to estimate the individual contributions of gluconeogenesis and glycogenolysis to overall glucose output in man J. *Clin. Invest.*, **80**, 1301–1310 (1987).
118. Cooper, G. J. S, Willis, A. C, Clark, A., Turner, R. C., Sim, R. B, and Reid, K. B. Purification and characterization of a peptide from amyloid-rich pancreases of type 2 diabetic patients. *Proc. Natl. Acad. Sci.*, **84**, 8628–8632 (1987).
119. Corne, J., Gillespie, D., Roberts, D., and Younes, M. Effect of inspiratory flow rate in intubated ventilated patients. *Am. J. Respir. Crit. Care Med.*, **156**, 304–308 (1997).
120. Coughlan, A., McCarty, D. J., Jorgensen, L. N., and Zimmet, P. The epidemic of NIDDM in Asian and Pacific Island populations: prevalence and risk factors. *Horm. Metab. Res.*, **29**, 323–1 (1997).
121. Cox, M. E. and Edelman, D. Tests for Screening and Diagnosis of Type 2 Diabetes. *Clin. Diab.*, **27**(4), 32–38 (2009).
122. Daisy, P., Eliza, J., and Mohamed Farook, K. A. A novel dihydroxy gymnemic triacetate isolated from Gymnema sylvestre possessing normoglycemic and hypolipidemic activity on STZ-induced diabetic rats. *J. Ethnopharmacol.*, **126**, 39–344 (2009).
123. Damge, C. In Biotechnology of Insulin Therapy. J. Pickup (Ed.) Oxford, *Blackwell Scientific.*, pp.97–112 (1991).
124. Day, C. Thiazolidinediones: a new class of antidiabetic drugs. *Diabet. Med.*, **16,** 1–14 (1999).
125. de Vegt, F., Dekker, J. M., Groeneveld, W. J., Nijpels, G., Stehouwer, C. D., Bouter, L. M., and Heine, R. J. Moderate alcohol consumption is associated with lower risk for incident diabetes and mortality: the Hoorn Study. *Diab. Res. Clin. Pract.*, **57**, 53–60 (2002).
126. De Vriese, A. S., Verbeuren, T. J., Van de Voorde, J., Lameire, N. H., and Vanhoutte, P. M. Endothelial dysfunction in diabetes. *Br. J. Pharmacol.*, **130**, 963–74 (2000).
127. DeFronzo, R. A. Lilly lecture 1987. The triumvirate: beta-cell, muscle, liver. A collusion responsible for NIDDM. *Diabetes*, **37**, 667–87 (1988).
128. DeFronzo, R. A. Pathogenesis of type 2 diabetes: metabolic and molecular implications for identifying diabetes genes. *Diab. Rev.*, **5**(3), 177–269 (1997).
129. DeFronzo, R. A., Ratner, R. E., Han, J., Kim, D. D., Fineman, M. S., and Baron, A. D. Effects of exenatide (exendin-4) on glycemic control and weight over 30 weeks in metformin-treated patients with type 2 diabetes. *Diab. Care.*, **28**, 1092–1100 (2005).

130. Delli, A. J., Larsson, H. E., Ivarsson, S. A., and ke Lernmark, A., Type 1 Diabetes. *In Textbook of Diabetes, 4th edition.* R. Holt, C. Cockram, A. Flyvbjerg, and B. Goldstein, (Eds.), Wiley-Blackwell, West Sussex., pp.142–144 (2010).
131. Deshpande, A. D., Harris-Hayes, M., and Schootman, M. Epidemiology of diabetes and diabetes-related complications. *Phys. Ther.*, **88**, 1254–64 (2008).
132. Despres, J. P. Health consequences of visceral obesity. *Annals Med.*, **33**, 534–41 (2001).
133. Di Lorenzo, T. P., Peakman, M., and Roep, B. O. Translational mini-review series on type 1 diabetes: systematic analysis of T cell epitopes in autoimmune diabetes. *Clin. Exp. Immunol.* **148**, 1–16, (2007).
134. DIAMOND Project Group. *Incidence and trends of childhood type 1 diabetes worldwide 1990–1999. Diabet. Med*, **23,** 857–866 (2006).
135. Donath, M. Y., Storling, J., Berchtold, L. A., Billestrup, N., and Mandrup-Poulsen, T. Cytokines and beta-cell biology: From concept to clinical translation. *Endocr Rev.*, **29**,334–350 (2008).
136. Doria, A., Patti, M. E., and Kahn, C. R. The emerging genetic architecture of type 2 diabetes. *Cell Metab.*, **8,** 186–200 (2008).
137. Dornhorst, A. Insulotropic meglitinide analogues. *Lancet*, **358**, 1709–1715 (2001).
138. Du, X. L., Edelsteinm, D., DImmeler, S., Ju Q, Sui, C., and Brownlee, M. Hyperglycemia inhibits endothelial nitric oxide synthase activity by posttranslational modification at the Akt site. *J Clin Invest*, **108**, 1341–1348 (2001).
139. Duh, E. and Aiello, L. P. Vascular endothelial growth factor and diabetes. The agonist versus antagonist paradox. *Diabetes*, **48**, 1899–1906 (1999).
140. Dyck, P. J., Zimmerman, B. R., Vilen, T. H., Minnerath, S. R., Karnes, J. L., Yao, J. K., and Poduslo, J. F. Nerve glucose, fructose, sorbitol, myo-inositol, and fiber degeneration and regeneration in diabetic neuropathy. *N. Engl. J. Med.*, **319**, 542–548 (1988).
141. Edelman, D., Olsen, M. K., Dudley, T. K., Harris, A. C., and Oddone, E. Z. Utility of haemoglobin A1c in predicting diabetes risk. *J. Gen. Intern. Med.*, **19**, 1175–1180 (2004).
142. Edmonds, M. E.; Blundell, M. P., Morris, M. E., Cotton, L. T., and Watkins, P. J. Improved survival of the diabetic foot: The role of a specialized foot clinic. *Q J Med.*, **60**, 763–71 (1986).
143. Edmonds, M. E. Progress in care of the diabetic foot. *Lancet*, **354**, 270–72 (1999).
144. Elghazi, L., Balcazar, N., and Bernal-Mizrachi, E. Emerging role of protein kinase B/Akt signaling in pancreatic β-cell mass and function. *Int. J. Biochem. Cell Biol.*, **38**(2), 157–63 (2006).
145. Engelau, M. M., Thompson, T. J., Herman, W. H., Boyle, J. P., Aubert, R. E., Kenny, S. J. et al. Comparison of fasting and 2 hour glucose and HbA 1clevels for diagnosing diabetes: diagnostic criteria and performance revisited. *Diab. Care*, **20,** 785–791 (1997).
146. Engelgau, M. E., Narayan, K. M. V., and Herman, W. H. Screening for type 2 diabetes (Technical review). *Diab Care*, **10**, 1563–1580 (2000).
147. Erlich, H. Type 1 Diabetes Genetics Consortium. HLA DR-DQ haplotypes and genotypes and type 1 diabetes risk: analysis of the Type 1 Diabetes Genetics Consortium families. *Diabetes*, **57**, 1084–1092 (2008).

148. Facchini, F. S., Hollenbeck, C. B., Jeppesen, J., Chen, Y. D., and Reaven, G. M. Insulin resistance and cigarette smoking. *Lancet*, **339**, 1128–1130 (1992).
149. Farris, W., Mansourian, S., Chang, Y., Lindsley, L., Eckman, E. A., Frosch, M. P., Eckman, C. B.. Tanzi, R. E., Selkoe, D. J., and Guenette, S. Insulin-degrading enzyme regulates the levels of insulin, amyloid beta -protein, and the beta amyloid precursor protein intracellular domain in vivo. *Proc. Natl. Acad. Sci.*,**100**, 4162–4167 (2003).
150. Feldman, B., Bragz, R., Schwartz, S., and Weinstein, R. A continuous glucose sensor based on wired enzyme technology: Results from 3-day trial in patients with type 1 diabetes. *Diabetes Technol Ther.*, **5**, 769–99 (2003).
151. Felgner, P. L. Nonviral strategies for gene therapy. *Sci. Am.*, **276**, 102–106 (1997).
152. Ferrara, N., Houck, K. A., Jakeman, L. B., Winer, J., and Leung, D. W. The vascular endothelial growth factor family of polypeptides. *J. Cell Biochem.*, **47**, 211–218 (1991).
153. Fery, F. Role of hepatic glucose production and glucose uptake in the pathogenesis of fasting hyperglycemia in type 2 diabetes: normalization of glucose kinetics by short-term fasting. *J. Clin. Endocrinol. Metab.*, **78**(3), 536–42 (1994).
154. Feskens, E. J. M., Virtanen, S. M., Rasanen, L., Tuomilehto, J., Stengard, J., Pekkanen, J., Nissinen, A., and Kromhout, D. Dietary factors determining diabetes and impaired glucose tolerance. A 20-year follow-up of the Finnish and Dutch cohorts of the Seven Countries Study. *Diab. Care*, **18**, 1104–12 (1995).
155. Fioretto, P., Mauer, M., Brocco, E., Velussi, M., Frigato, F., Muollo, B., Sambataro, M., Abaterusso, C., Baggio, B., Crepaldi G., and Nosadini, R. Patterns of renal injury in NIDDM patients with microalbuminuria. *Diabetologia*, **39**, 1569–1576 (1996).
156. Florez, J. C., Jablonski, K. A., Bayley, N., Pollin, T. I., de Bakker, P. I., Shuldiner, A. R., Knowler, W. C., Nathan, D. M., and Altshuler, D. TCF7L2 polymorphisms and progression to diabetes in the Diabetes Prevention Program. *N. Engl. J. Med.*, **355**, 241 (2006).
157. Folsom, A. R., Ma, J., McGovern, P. G., and Eckfeldt, H. Relation between plasma phospholipid saturated fatty acids and hyperinsulinemia. *Metabol.*, **45**, 223–8 (1996).
158. Folsom, A. R., Rasmussen, M. L., Chambless, L. E. et al. Prospective associations of fasting insulin, body fat distribution, and diabetes with risk of ischemic stroke. The Atherosclerosis Risk in Communities (ARIC) Study Investigators. *Diab. Care*, **22**, 1077–83 (1999).
159. Fong, D. S, Aiello, L. P., Ferris, F. L.3rd, and Klein, R. Diabetic retinopathy. *Diab Care*, **27**, 2540–2553 (2004).
160. Forsblom, C. M., Groop, P. H., Ekstrand, A.,Totterman, K. J., Sane, T., Saloranta, C., and Groop, L. Predictors of progression from normoalbuminuria to microalbuminuria in NIDDM. *Diab. Care*, **21**, 1932–1938 (1998).
161. Fowler, M. J. Microvascular and macrovascular complications of diabetes. *Clin. Diab.*, **26**(2), 77–82 (2008).
162. Francis, A. J., Home, P. D., Hanning, I., Alberti, K. G., and Tunbridge, W. M. Intermediate acting insulin given at bedtime: effect on blood glucose concentrations before and after breakfast. *Br. Med. J.*, **286**, 1173–76 (1983).

163. Frank, J. W., Camilleri, M., Thomforde, G. M., Dinneen, S. F., and Rizza, R. A. Effects of glucagon on postprandial carbohydrate metabolism in nondiabetic humans. Metabolism., **47,** 7–12 (1998).
164. Frykberg, R. G., Lavery, L. A., Pham, H., Harvey, C., Harkless, L., and Veves, A. Role of neuropathy and high foot pressures in diabetic foot ulceration. *Diab. Care*, **21**, 1714–719 (1998).
165. Fuhlendorff, J., Rorsman, P., Kofod, H., Brand, C. L, Rolin, B., MacKay, P., Shymko, R., and Carr, R. D. Stimulation of insulin release by repaglinide and glibenclamide involves both common and distinct processes. *Diabetes*, **47**, 345–351 (1998).
166. Fulton, D., Gratton, J. P., MCcabe, T. J., Fontana, J., Fujio, Y., Walsh, K., Franke, T. F., Papapetropoulos, A., and Sessa, W. C. Regulation of endothelium-derived nitric oxide production by the protein kinase Akt. *Nature*, **399**, 597–601 (1999).
167. Funnell, M. M. and Anderson, R. M. Patient empowerment: a look back, a look ahead. *Diab. Educator*, **29**(3), 454–464 (2003).
168. Gabbay, K. H. Aldose reductase inhibition in the treatment of diabetic neuropathy: where are we in 2004? *Curr. Diab, Rep.*, **4**, 405–408 (2004).
169. Gaby, A. R. Adverse effects of dietary fructose. *Altern. Med. Rev.*, **10**(4), 294–306 (2005).
170. Gale, E. A. The rise of childhood type 1 diabetes in the 20th century. *Diabetes*, **51**, 3353–3361 (2002).
171. Gall, M. A., Hougaard, P., Borch-Johnsen, K., and Parving, H. H. Risk factors for development of incipient and overt diabetic nephropathy in patients with non-insulin dependent diabetes mellitus: prospective, observational study. *BMJ*, **314**, 783–788 (1997).
172. Gannon, M. C., Nuttall, J. A., Damberg, G., Gupta, V., and Nuttall, F. Q. Effect of protein ingestion on the glucose appearance rate in people with type 2 diabetes. *J. Clin. Endocrinol. Metab.*, **86**, 1040–1047 (2001).
173. Gastaldelli, A. Role of beta-cell dysfunction, ectopic fat accumulation and insulin resistance in the pathogenesis of type 2 diabetes mellitus. *Diab. Res.Clin. Prac.*, **93**, S60–S65 (2011).
174. Gastaldelli, A., Baldi, S., Pettiti, M., Toschi, E., Camastra, S., Natali, A., Landau, B. R., and Ferrannini, E. Influence of obesity and type 2 diabetes on gluconeogenesis and glucose output in humans: a quantitative study. *Diabetes*, **49**, 1367–73 (2000).
175. Gastaldelli, A., Cusi, K., Pettiti, M., Hardies, J., Miyazaki, Y., Berria, R., Buzzigoli, E., Sironi, A. M., Cersosimo, E., Ferrannini, E., and Defronzo, R. A. Relationship between hepatic/visceral fat and hepatic insulin resistance in nondiabetic and type 2 diabetic subjects. *Gastroenterol.*, **133**, 496–506 (2007).
176. Gastaldelli, A., Toschi, E., Pettiti, M., Frascerra, S., Quinones-Galvan, A., Sironi, A. M., Natali, A., and Ferrannini, E. Effect of physiological hyperinsulinemia on gluconeogenesis in nondiabetic subjects and in type 2 diabetic patients. *Diabetes*, **50**, 1807–12 (2001).
177. Gazis, A., White, D. J., Page, S. R., and Cockcroft, J. R. Effect of oral vitamin E (α-tocopherol) supplementation on vascular endothelial function in type 2 diabetes mellitus. *Diabet. Med.*, **16**, 304–11 (1999).

178. Genuth, S., Alberti, K. G., Bennett, P., Buse, J., Defronzo, R., Kahn, R., Kitzmiller, J., Knowler, W. C. et al.. Follow-up report on the diagnosis of diabetes mellitus. *Diab Care.*, **26**(11), 3160–7 (2003).
179. George, K. and Alberti, M. M. The Classification and Diagnosis of Diabetes Mellitus. *In Textbook of Diabetes, 4th edition.,* R. Holt, C. Cockram, A. Flyvbjerg, B. Goldstein (Eds.) Wiley-Blackwell., West Sussex., pp. 25–26 (2010).
180. Gilbert, B. O., Johnson, S. B., Silverstein, J., and Malone, J. Psychological and physiological responses to acute laboratory stressors in insulin-dependent diabetes mellitus adolescents and nondiabetic controls. *J. Pediatr. Psychol.*, **14**, 577–91 (1989).
181. Gilbertson, H., Brand-Miller, J., Thorburn, A., Evans, S., Chondros, P., and Werther, G. The effect of fl exible low glycemic index dietary advice versus measured carbohydrate exchange diets on glycemic control in children with type 1 diabetes. *Diab. Care*, **24,** 1137–1143 (2001).
182. Girardin, C. M., Huot, C., Gonthier, M., and Delvin, E. Continuous glucose monitoring: A review of biochemical perspectives and clinical use in type 1 diabetes. *Clin Biochem.*, **42** 136–42 (2009).
183. Gizurarson, S. and Bechgaard, E. Intranasal administration of insulin to humans. *Diabetes Res. Clin. Pract.*, **12**, 71–84 (1991).
184. Goldstein, B. J. and Muller-Wieland, D. Type 2 Diabetes: *Principles and Practice, 2nd Ed*, Informa Healthcare, London, New York (2008).
185. Golubnitschaja, O. Advanced Diabetes Care: Three Levels of Prediction, Prevention, and Personalized Treatment. *Curr. Diab. Rev.*, **6**, 42–51 (2010).
186. Gonzalez, E. L., Johansson, S., Wallander, M. A., and Rodriguez, L. A. Trends in the prevalence and incidence of diabetes in the UK: 1996–2005. *J Epidemiol Community Health*, **63**, 332–36 (2009).
187. Goodpaster, B. H. Subcutaneous abdominal fat and thigh muscle composition predict insulin sensitivity independently of visceral fat. *Diabetes.*, **46**, 1579–85 (1997).
188. Gossain, V. V. Insulin analogs and intensive insulin therapy in type 1 Diabetes. *Int. J. Diab. Dev. Coun.*, **23**, 26–36 (2003).
189. Gougeon, R., Marliss, E. B., Jones, P. J., Pencharz, P. B., and Morais, J. A. Effect of exogenous insulin on protein metabolism with differing nonprotein energy intakes in type 2 diabetes mellitus. *Int. J. Obes. Relat. Metab. Disord.*, **22**, 250–261 (1998).
190. Gougeon, R., Styhler, K., Morais, J. A., Jones, P. J., and Marliss, E. B. Effects of oral hypoglycemic agents and diet on protein metabolism in type 2 diabetes. *Diab. Care*, **23**, 1–8 (2000).
191. Gough, S.C., Walker, L. S., and Sansom, D. M. CTLA4 gene polymorphism and autoimmunity. *Immunol. Rev.*, **204**, 102–15 (2005).
192. Grant, S. F., Thorleifsson, G., Reynisdottir, I., Benediktsson, R., Manolescu, A., Sainz, J. et al.Variant of transcription factor 7 - like 2(TCF7L2) gene confers risk of type 2 diabetes. *Nat. Genet.*, **38**, 320–323 (2006).
193. Green, A., Gale, E. A. M., and Patterson, C. C. Incidence of childhood-onset insulin-dependent diabetes mellitus: the EURODIAB ACE Study. *Lancet*, **339**, 905–909 (1992).
194. Green, B. D., Flatt, P. R., and Bailey, C. J. Dipeptidyl peptidase IV (DPP IV) inhibitors: a newly emerging drug class for the treatment of type 2 diabetes. *Diabetes Vasc Dis Res.*, **3**, 159–165 (2006).

195. Gribble, F. M. and Reimann, F. Pharmacological modulation of K-ATP channels. *Biochem Soc Trans.*, **30**, 333–339 (2002).
196. Gross, J. L., de Azevedo, M. J., Silveiro, S. P., Canani, L. H., Caramori, M. L., and Zelmanovitz, T. Diabetic nephropathy: diagnosis, prevention, and treatment. *Diab. Care*, **28**, 164–176 (2005).
197. Grundy, S. M. Multifactorial causation of obesity: implications for prevention. *American Journal of Clinical Nutrition*, **67**(Suppl.), 563S–72S (1998).
198. Gu, D., Reynolds, K., Duan, X., Xin, X., Chen, J., and Wu, X., et al. InterASIA Collaborative Group. Prevalence of diabetes and impaired fasting glucose in the Chinese adult population: International Collaborative Study of Cardiovascular Disease in Asia (Inter ASIA). *Diabetologia*, **46**(9), 1190–1198 (2003).
199. Gu, Y., Zhang, Y., Shi, X., Li, X., Hong, J., Chen, J., Gu, W., Lu, X., Xu, G., and Ning, G. Effect of traditional Chinese medicine berberine on type 2 diabetes based on comprehensive metabonomics. *Talanta*, **81**(3), 766–772 (2010).
200. Guelfi, K. J., Ratnam, N., Smythe, G. A., Jones, T. W., and Fournier, P. A. Effect of intermittent high-intensity compared with continuous moderate exercise on glucose production and utilization in individuals with type 1 diabetes. *Am. J. Physiol. Endocrinol. Metab.*, **292**, E865–E870 (2007).
201. Guillemin, R. Hypothalamus, hormones, and physiological regulation. In *Claude Bernard and the Internal Environment: A Memorial Symposium.* E. Debbs-Robin (Ed.) New York, Dekker, pp. 137–56 (1978).
202. Guo, H., Ling, W., Wang, Q., Liu, C., Hu, Y., and Xia, M. Cyanidin 3-glucoside protects 3T3-L1 adipocytes against H2O2- or TNF-[α]-induced insulin resistance by inhibiting c-Jun NH2-terminal kinase activation. *Biochem. Pharmacol.*, **75**, 1393–1401 (2008).
203. Hales, C. N. The pathogenesis of NIDDM. *Diabetologia*, **37**, S162–8 (1994).
204. Hales, C. N. and Barker, D. J. The thrifty phenotype hypothesis. *Br. Med. Bull.*, **60**, 5–20 (2001).
205. Halford, W. K., Cuddihy, S., and Mortimer, R. H. Psychological stress and blood glucose regulation in type I diabetic patients. *Health Psychol.*, **9**, 516–528 (1990).
206. Haller, M. J., Atkinson, M. A., and Schatz, D. Type 1 diabetes mellitus: etiology, presentation, and management. *Pediatr. Clin. North Am.*, **52**, 1553–1578 (2005).
207. Halliwell, B. and Gutteridge, J. M. C. Oxygen radicals and nervous system. *Trends Neurosci.*, **8**, 22–26 (1996).
208. Hani, E. H., Stoffers, D. A., Chevre, J. C., Durand, E., Stanojevic, V., Dina, C., Habener, J. F., and Froguel, P. Defective mutations in the insulin promoter factor - 1 (IPF - 1) gene in late- onset T2D mellitus. *J. Clin. Invest.*, **104,** R41–48 (1999).
209. Hanis, C. L., Boerwinkle, E., Chakraborty, R., Ellsworth, D. L., Concannon, P., Stirling, B. et al. A genome-wide search for human non- insulin dependent (type 2) diabetes genes reveals a major susceptibility locus on chromosome 2. *Nat. Genet.*, **13**, 161–166 (1996).
210. Hansen, H. P., Tauber-Lassen, E., Jensen, B. R., and Parving, H. H. Effect of dietary protein restriction on prognosis in patients with diabetic nephr Salmeron opathy. *Kidney Int.*, **62**, 220–228 (2002).
211. Hasanain, B. and Mooradian, A. D. Antioxidant vitamins and their influence in diabetes mellitus. *Curr. Diab. Rep.*, **2**, 448–456 (2002).

212. Hauner, H. Managing type 2 diabetes mellitus in patients with obesity. *Treat. Endocrinol.*, **3**, 223–232 (2004).
213. Heilbronn, L. K., Noakes, M., and Clifton, P. M. Effect of energy restriction, weight loss, and diet composition on plasma lipids and glucose in patients with type 2 diabetes. *Diab Care.*, **22**, 889–895 (1999).
214. Heinemann, L., Hompesch, B., Linkeschova, R., Sedlak, M., Rave, K., and Heise, T. Time-action profile of the long-acting insulin analog Glargine (HOE901) in comparison with those of NPH insulin and placebo. Diab Care, **23**, 644–49 (2000).
215. Heinemann, L. and Richter, B. Clinical pharmacology of human insulin. *Diab. Care*, **16**(3) 90–100 (1993).
216. Herman, G. A., Stein, P. P., Thornberry, N. A., and Wagner, J. A. Dipeptidyl peptidase-4 inhibitors for the treatment of type 2 diabetes: focus on sitagliptin. *Clin Pharmacol Ther.*, **81**, 761–7 (2007).
217. Hermann, R., Bartsocas, C. S., Soltesz, G., Vazeou, A., Paschou, P., Bozas, E. et al. Genetic screening for individuals at high risk for type 1diabetes in the general population using HLA Class II alleles as disease markers: a comparison between three European populations with variable rates of disease incidence. *Diab. Metab. Res. Rev.*, **20,** 322–329 (2004).
218. Hermsmeier, D., Schittko, U., and Baldwin, I. T. Molecular interactions between the specialist herbivore Manduca sexta (Lepidoptera, Sphingidae) and its natural host Nicotiana attenuata. I. Large-scale changes in the accumulation of growhand defense-related plant mRNAs. *Plant Physiol.*, **125**, 683–700 (2001).
219. Hiatt, WR. Preventing atherothrombotic events in peripheral arterial disease: the use of antiplatelet therapy. *J. Intern. Med.*, **251**, 193–206 (2002).
220. Hidaka, H., Maekawa, S., Kashiwagi, A. et al. A change of NIDDM incidence in a population: a result of 15 years of the Aito study [in Japanese]. *J Japan Diabetes Soc.*, **39**, 217 (1996).
221. Hinchcliffe, M. and Illum, L. Intranasal insulin delivery and therapy. *Adv. Drug Deliv. Rev.*, **35**, 199–234 (1999).
222. Hirsch, I. Insulin analogues. *N. Engl. J. Med.*, **352**, 174–183 (2005).
223. Hitzman, C. J., Elmquist, W. F., and Wiedmann, T. S. Development of a respirable, sustained release microcarrier for 5-fluorouracil II: In vitro and in vivo optimization of lipid coated nanoparticles. *J. Pharm. Sci.*, **95**(5), 1127–1143 (2006).
224. Hjelm, K., Mufunda, E., Nambozi, G., and Kemp, J. Preparing nurses to face the pandemic of diabetes mellitus: a literature review. *J. Adva. Nurs*, **41**, 424–434 (2003).
225. Hoa, K. T., Shiaub, M. Y., Changc, Y. H., Chen, C. M., Yang, S. C., and Huang, C. N. Association of interleukin-4 promoter polymorphisms in Taiwanese patients with type 2 diabetes mellitus Metabol. *Clin. Experimental.*, **59**, 1717–1722 (2010).
226. Hod, M., Kitzmiller, J. L., Kjos, S. L., Oats, J. N., Pettitt, D. J., Sacks, D. A., and Zoupas, C. Summary and recommendations of the Fifth International Workshop-Conference on Gestational Diabetes Mellitus. *Diab Care.*, (2), S251–60 (2007).
227. Hoeldtke, R. D., Bryner, K. D., McNeill, D. R., Hobbs, G. R., Riggs, J. E., Warehime, S. S., Christie, I., Ganser, G., and Van Dyke, K. Nitrosative stress, uric acid, and peripheral nerve function in early type 1 diabetes. *Diabetes*, **51**, 2817–2825 (2002).

228. Hogge, J., Krasner, D., Nguyen, H., Harkless, L. B, and Armstrong, D. G. The potential benefits of advanced therapeutic modalities in the treatment of diabetic foot wounds. *J. Am. Podiatr. Med, Assoc.*, **90**, 57–65 (2000).
229. Holmkvist, J., Cervin, C., Lyssenko, V., Winckler, W., Anevski, D., Cilio, C. et al. Common variants in HNF-1 alpha and risk of T2D. *Diabetologia*, **49**, 2882–2891 (2006).
230. Holt, R. I., Coleman, M. A., and McCance, D. R. The implications of the new International Association of Diabetes and Pregnancy Study Groups (IADPSG) diagnostic criteriafor gestational diabetes. *Diabet Med.*, **28**, 382–5 (2011).
231. Hori, O., Yan, S. D., Ogawa, S., Kuwabara, K., Matsumoto, M., Stern, D., and Schmidt, A. M. The receptor for advanced glycation end-products has a central role in mediating the effects of advanced glycation end-products on the development of vascular disease in diabetes mellitus. *Nephrol. Dial. Transplant.*, **11**(5), 13–16 (1996).
232. Hotamisligil ,S., Arner, P., Caro, J. F., Atkinson, R. L., and Spiegelman, B. M. Increased adipose tissue expression of tumor necrosis factor-a in human obesity and insulin resistance. *J. Clin. Invest.*, **95**, 2409–2415 (1995).
234. Hotamisligil, G.; Spiegelman, B. Tumor necrosis factor α: a key component of the obesity-diabetes link. *Diabetes*, **43**, 1271–1278 (1994).
235. Hotamisligil, G. S. Inflammation and metabolic disorders. *Nature*, **444**, 860–867 (2006).
236. Hovind, P., Rossing, P., Tarnow, L., and Parving, H. H. Smoking and progression of diabetic nephropathy in type 1 diabetes. *Diab. Care*, **26**, 911–916 (2003).
237. Howey, D. C., Bowsher, R. R., Brunelle, R. L., and Woodworth, J. R. [Lys (B28), Pro (B29)]-human insulin. A rapidly absorbed analogue of human insulin. *Diabetes*, **43**, 396–402 (1994).
238. Hu, F. B. Globalization of Diabetes: The role of diet, lifestyle, and genes. *Diabetes Care*, **34**, 1249–1257 (2011).
239. Hu, F. B., Manson, J. E., Stampfer, M. J. et al. Diet, lifestyle, and the risk of type 2 diabetes mellitus in women. *N. Engl. J. Med.*, **345**, 790–797 (2001).
240. Hu, C.Y., Rodriguez-Pinto, D., Du, W., Ahuja, A., Henegariu, O., Wong, F. S., Shlomchik, M. J., and Wen, L. Treatment with CD20-specific antibody prevents and reverses autoimmune diabetes in mice. *J. Clin. Invest.*, **117**, 3857–3867 (2007).
241. Hu, F. B., Meigs, J. B., Li, T. Y., Rifai, N., and Manson, J. E. Inflammatory markers and risk of developing type 2 diabetes in women. *Diabetes*, **53**, 693–700 (2004).
242. Hu, F. B., Sigal, R. J., Rich-Edwards, J. W., Colditz, G. A., Solomon, C. G., Willett, W. C., Speizer, F. E., and Manson, J. E. Walking compared with vigorous physical activity and risk of type 2 diabetes in women: a prospective study. *JAMA*, **282**, 1433–1439 (1999).
243. Hu, F. B., Stampfer, M. J., Solomon, C., Liu, S., Colditz, G. A., Speizer, F. E., Willett, W. C., and Manson, J. E. Physical activity and risk for cardiovascular events in diabetic women. *Ann. Intern. Med.*, **134**, 96–105 (2001).
244. Hu, F. B., Li, T. Y., Colditz, G. A., Willett, W. C., and Manson, J. E. Television watching and other sedentary behaviors in relation to risk of obesity and type 2 diabetes mellitus in women. *JAMA*, **289**, 1785–1791 (2003).

245. Hu, F. B. and Malik, V. S. Sugar-sweetened beverages and risk of obesity and type 2 diabetes: epidemiologic evidence. *Physiol. Behav.*, **100**(1), 47–54 (2010).
246. Hunt, K. J. and Schuller, K. L. The Increasing Prevalence of Diabetes in Pregnancy Obstet. *Gynecol. Clin. North Am.*, **34**(2), 173–178 (2007).
247. Idris, I., Thomson, G. A., and Sharma, J. C. Diabetes mellitus and stroke. *Int. J. Clin. Pract.*, **60**, 48–56 (2006).
278. Iozzo, P. Viewpoints on the way to the consensus session. Where does insulin resistance start? The adipose tissue. *Diab Care.*, **32**(2), S168–S173.
249. Jain, D., Majumdar, D. K., and Panda, A. K. Insulin loaded eudragit L100 microspheres for oral delivery: preliminary *in vitro* studies. *J. Biomater. Appl.*, **21**, 195–211 (2006).
250. Jarvi, A. E., Karlstrom, B. K., Granfeldt, Y. E., Bjorck, I. M. E., Asp, N. G., and Vessby, B. O. H. Improved glycemic control and lipid profi le and normalized fibrinolytic activity on a low glycemic index diet in type 2 diabetes mellitus patients. *Diab Care*, **22**, 10–18 (1999).
251. Jun, H. S., Bae, H. Y., Lee, B. R., Koh, K. S., Kimc, Y. S., Leed, K. W., Kimd, H., and Yoona, J. W. Pathogenesis of non-insulin-dependent (type II) diabetes mellitus (NIDDM)-genetic predisposition and metabolic abnormalities. *Adv. Drug. Del. Rev.*, **35**, 157–177 (1999).
252. Jurgens, H., Haass, W., Castaneda, T. R., Schurmann, A., Koebnick, C., Dombrowski, F., Otto, B., Nawrocki, A. R., Scherer, P. E., Spranger, J., Ristow, M., Joost, H., Havel, P. J., and Tschop, M. H. Consuming fructose-sweetened beverages increases body adiposity in mice. *Obes. Res.*, **13**, 1146–1156 (2005).
253. Kahn, S. E., Andrikopoulos, S., and Verchere, C. B. Islet amyloid. A long-recognized but underappreciated pathological feature of type 2 diabetes. *Diabetes*, **48**, 241–53 (1999).
254. Kahn, S. E., D'Alessio, D. A., Schwartz, M. W., Fujimoto, W. Y, Ensinck, J. W., Taborsky, G. J. Jr., and Porte, D. Jr. Evidence of cosecretion of islet amyloid polypeptide and insulin by β-cells. *Diabetes.*, **39**, 634–638 (1990).
255. Kahn, S. E., Haffner, S. M., Heise, M. A., Herman, W. H., Holman, R. R., Jones, N. P., Kravitz, B. G., Lachin, J. M., O'Neill, M. C., Zinman, B., and Viberti, G. Glycemic durability of rosiglitazone, metformin, or glyburide monotherapy. *N. Engl. J. Med.*, **355**, 2427–2443 (2006).
256. Kahn, S. E., Hull, R. L., and Utzschneider, K. M. Mechanisms linking obesity to insulin resistance and type 2 diabetes. *Nature*, **444**, 840–846 (2006).
257. Kahn, S. E. The relative contributions of insulin resistance and beta-cell dysfunction to the pathophysiology of Type 2 diabetes. *Diabetologia*, **46**, 3–19 (2003).
258. Karvonen, M., Viik-Kajander, M., Moltchanova, E., Libman, I., LaPorte, R., and Tuomilehto, J. Incidence of childhood type 1 diabetes worldwide. Diabetes Mondiale (DiaMond) Project Group. *Diab. Care*, **23**, 1516–1526 (2000).
259. Kashiwagi, A., Harano, Y., Suzuki, M., Kojima, H., Harada, M., Nisho, Y., and Shigeta, Y. New α 2-adrenergic blocker (DG-5128) improves insulin secretion and in vivo glucose disposal in NIDDM patients. *Diabetes*, **35**, 1085–89 (1986).
260. Kato, H., Takada, T., Kawamura, T., Hotta, N., and Torii, S. The reduction and redistribution of plantar pressures using foot orthoses in diabetic patients. *Diab. Res. Clin. Pract.*, **31**, 115–118 (1996).

261. Kelley, D. E. and Simoneau, J. A. Impaired free fatty acid utilization by skeletal muscle in non- insulin-dependent diabetes mellitus. *J. Clin. Invest.*, **94**(6), 2349–56 (1994).
262. Kelly, D. J., Zhang, Y., Hepper, C., Gow, R. M., Jaworski, K., Kemp, B. E., Wilkinson-Berka, J. L., and Gilbert, R. E. Protein kinase C inhibition attenuates the progression of experimental diabetic nephropathy in the presence of continued hypertension. *Diabetes*, **52**, 512–518 (2003).
263. Kim, K. J., Lee, M. S., Jo, K., and Hwang, J. K. Piperidine alkaloids from Piper retrofractum Vahl. protect against high-fat diet-induced obesity by regulating lipid metabolism and activating AMP-activated protein kinase. *Biochem. Bioph. Res. Commun.*, **411**, 219–225 (2011).
264. Kim, K. S., Kim, S. K., Lee, Y. K., Park, S. W., and Cho, Y. W. Diagnostic value of glycated haemoglobin HbA(1c) for the early detection of diabetes in high-risk subjects. *Diabet Med.*, **25**, 997–1000 (2008).
265. Kim, S. M., Lee, J. S., Lee, J., Na, J. K., Han, J. H., Yoon, D. K., Baik, S. H., Choi, D. S., and Choi, K. M. Prevalence of diabetes and impaired fasting glucose in Korea: Korean National Health and Nutrition Survey 2001. *Diab Care.*, **29**(2), 226–231 (2006).
267. King, G. L. The Role of Inflammatory Cytokines in Diabetes and Its Complications. *J. Periodontol.*, (Suppl.), 1527–1534 (2008).
268. King, H., Aubert, R. E., and Herman, W. H. Global burden of diabetes, 1995–2025: prevalence, numerical estimates, and projections. *Diab. Care*, **21**, 1414–31 (1998).
269. King, H., Keuky, L., Seng, S., Khun T., Roglic, G., and Pinget, M. Diabetes and associated disorders in Cambodia: two epidemiological surveys. *Lancet*, **366**(9497), 1633–1639 (2005).
270. King, R. H. The role of glycation in the pathogenesis of diabetic polyneuropathy. *Mol. Pathol.*, **54**, 400–408 (2001).
271. Kissela, B. M., Khoury, J., Kleindorfer, D., Woo, D., Schneider, A., Alwell, K., Miller, R., Ewing, I., Moomaw, C. J., Szaflarski, J. P., Gebel, J., Shukla, R., Broderick, J. P. Epidemiology of ischemic stroke in patients with diabetes: the greater Cincinnati/Northern Kentucky Stroke Study. *Diab. Care*, **28**, 355–9 (2005).
272. Klonoff, D. C. Continuous Glucose Monitoring: Roadmap for 21st century diabetes therapy. *Diab. Care*, **28**(5), 1231–1239 (2005)
273. Klonoff, D. C. Personalized Medicine for Diabetes. *J. Diab. Sci. Technol.*, **2**(3), 335–341 (2008).
274. Knowles, E. A., Boulton, A. J. M. Do people with diabetes wear their prescribed footwear? *Diabet. Med.*, **13**, 1064–1068 (1996).
275. Ko, G. T., Chan, J. C., Woo, J., Lau, E., Yeung, V. T., Chow, C. C., andCockram, C. S. The reproducibility and usefulness of the oral glucose tolerance test in screening for diabetes and other cardiovascular risk factors. *Ann Clin Biochem.*, **35**, 62–67 (1998).
276. Kohn, A. D., Summers, S. A, Birnbaum, M. J., and Roth, R. A. Expression of a constitutively active Akt Ser/Thr kinase in 3T3-L1 adipocytes stimulates glucose uptake and glucose transporter 4 translocation. *J. Biol. Chem.*, **271**, 31372–31378 (1996).
277. Koivisto, V. A. The human insulin analogue insulin lispro. *Ann. Med.*, **30**, 260–66 (1998).

278. Kojima, I. and Umezawa, K. Conophylline: A novel differentiation inducer for pancreatic cells. *Int. J. Biochem. Cell Biol.*, **38**, 923–930 (2006).
279. Kosaka, K., Noda, M., and Kuzuya, T. Prevention of type 2 diabetes by lifestyle intervention: a Japanese trial in IGT males. *Diab. Res. Clin. Pract.*, **67**, 152–162 (2005).
280. Kotronen, A. and Yki-Järvinen, H. Fatty liver: a novel component of the metabolic syndrome. *Arterioscler. Thromb. Vasc. Biol.*, **28**, 27–38 (2008).
281. Krause, M. P., Hallage, T., Gama, M. P., Goss, F. L., Robertson, R., and da Silva, S. G. Association of adiposity, cardiorespiratory fitness, and exercise practice with the prevalence of type 2 diabetes in Brazilian elderly women. *Int. J .Med. Sci.*, **4,** 288–292 (2007).
282. Kriska, A. M., LaPorte, R. E., Pettitt, D. J., Charles, M. A., Nelson, R. G., Kuller, L. H., Bennett, P. H., and Knowler, W. C. The association of physical activity with obesity, fat distribution and glucose tolerance in Pima Indians. *Diabetologia*, **36**, 863–869 (1993).
283. Kroeger, K. M., Carville, K. S., and Abraham, L. J. The 308 tumor necrosis factor-alpha promoter polymorphism effects transcription. *Mol. Immunol.* **34**, 391–399 (1997).
284. Krook, A., Kawano, Y., Song, X. M., Efendic, S., Roth, R. A., Wallberg-Henriksson, H., and Zierath, J. R. Improved glucose tolerance restores insulin-stimulated Akt kinase activity and glucose transport in skeletal muscle from diabetic Goto-Kakizaki rats. *Diabetes*, **46**, 2110–2114 (1997).
285. Kuczmarski, R. J., Flegal, K. M., Campbell, S. M., and Johnson, C. L. Increasing prevalence of overweight among US adults. The National Health and Nutrition Examination Surveys 1960 to 1991. *JAMA*, **273**, 205–11 (1994).
286. Kumar, P. J. and Clark, M. Diabetes mellitus and other disorders of metabolism. *In: Textbook of Clinical Medicine*. Saunders, London, pp.1069–1121 (2005).
287. Kumar, S., Ashe, H. A., Parnell, L. N., Fernando, D. J., Tsigos, C., Young, R. J., Ward, J. D., and Boulton, A. J. The prevalence of foot ulceration and its correlates in type 2 diabetic patients: a population-based study. *Diabetic Med.*, **11**, 480–484 (1994).
288. Kunisaki, M., Bursell, S. E., Clermont, A. C., Ishii, H., Ballas, L. M., Jirousek, M. R., Umeda, F., Nawata, H., and King, G. L. Vitamin E prevents diabetes-induced abnormal retinal blood flow via the diacylglycerol protein kinase C pathway. *Am. J. Physiol.*, **269**, E239–E246 (1995).
289. Kutty, B. M. and Raju, T. R. New vistas in treating diabetes– Insight into a holistic approach. *Ind. J. Med. Res.*, **131**, 606–607 (2010).
290. Kuzuya, T. and Matsuda, A. Classification of diabetes on the basis of etiologies versus degree of insulin deficiency. *Diab. Care*, **20,** 219–220 (1997).
291. Lang, D. A., Matthews, D. R., Peto, J., and Turner, R. C. Cyclic oscillations of basal plasma glucose and insulin concentrations in human beings N. *Engl. J. Med.*, **301**, 1023–1027 (1979).
292. Langer, R. Drug delivery and targeting. *Nature*, **392**, 5–10 (1998).
293. Larsen, C.M., Faulenbach, M., Vaag, A., Volund, A., Ehses, J. A., Seifert, B., Mandrup-Poulsen, T., and Donath, M. Y. Interleukin-1-receptor antagonist in type 2 diabetes mellitus. *N. Engl. J. Med.*, **356**, 1517–1526 (2007).
294. Larsson, J., Agardh, C. D., Apelqvist, J., and Stenstrom, A. Long-term prognosis after healed amputation in patients with diabetes. *Clin. Orthop.*, **350**,149–158 (1998).

295. Lawrence, J. C. and Roach, P. J. New insights into the role and mechanism of glycogen synthase activation by insulin. *Diabetes*, **46,** 541–547 (1997).
296 Lawrence, J. M., Mayer-Davis, E. J., Reynolds, K., et al. Diabetes in Hispanic American youth: prevalence, incidence, demographics, and clinical characteristics: the SEARCH for Diabetes inYouth Study. *Diab care*,**32**(2), S123–S132 (2009).
297. Lebovitz, H. E. Alpha glucosidase inhibitors as agents in the treatment of diabetes. *Diab Rev.*, **6,** 132–145 (1998).
298. Lebovitz, H. E. Type 2 diabetes: an overview. *Clin Chem.*,**45**(8 Pt 2),1339–45 (1999).
299. Lebovitz, H. E. and Feinglos, M. N. Mechanism of action of the second-generation sulfonylurea glipizide. *Am. J .Med.*, **75**, 46–54 (1983).
300. Lee, Y. M., Haastert, B., Scherbaum, W., and Hauner, H. A phytosterol-enriched spread improves the lipid profile of subjects with type 2 diabetes mellitus- a randomized controlled trial under free-living conditions. *Eur. J. Nutr.*, **42**, 111–117 (2003).
301. Leiter, L. Insulin resistance. *Can. J. Cardiol.*, **15**(B), 20B–22B (1999).
032. Levin, M. E. An Overview of the Diabetic Foot: Pathogenesis, Management and Prevention of Lesions. *Int. J. Diab. Dev. Countries*, **14**, 39–47 (1994).
303. Levine, F. and Leibowitz, G. Towards gene therapy of diabetes mellitus. *Mol. Med*, **5**, 165–171 (1999).
304. Levitt, N. S. Diabetes in Africa: epidemiology, management and healthcare challenges. *Heart*, **94**, 1376–82 (2008).
305. Li, H. and Forsterman, U. Nitric oxide in the pathogenesis of vascular disease. *J. Pathol.*, **190**(3), 244–54 (2000).
306. Li, G., Zhang, P., Wang, J., Gregg, E. W., Yang, W., Gong, Q., Li, H., Li, H., Jiang, Y., An Y., Shuai, Y., Zhang, B., Zhang, J., Thompson, T. J., Gerzoff, R. B., Roglic, G., Hu, Y., and Bennett, P. H. The long-term effect of lifestyle interventions to prevent diabetes in the China Da Qing Diabetes Prevention Study: a 20-year follow-up study. *Lancet, 371*, 1783–1789 (2008).
307. Li, H., Fu, X., Ouyang, Y., Cai, C., Wang, J., and Sun, T. Adult bone marrow-derived mesenchymal stem cells contribute to wound healing of skin appendages. *Cell Tissue Res.*, **326**(3), 725–36 (2006).
308. Li, J. P., Wei, X., Yuan, Y., et al. Synthesis of magnetic nanoparticles composed by Prussian blue and glucose oxidase for preparing highly sensitive and selective glucose biosensor. *Sensors and Actuators B: Chemical*,**139**, 400–406 (2009).
309. Lie, B. A. and Thorsby, E. Several genes in the extended human MHC contribute to predisposition to autoimmune diseases. *Curr. Opin. Immunol.*, **17**(5), 526–31 (2005).
310. Lillioja, S., Mott, D. M., Spraul, M., Ferraro, R., Foley, J. E., Ravussin, E., Knowler, W. C., Bennett, P. H., and Bogardus, C. Insulin resistance and insulin secretory dysfunction as precursors of non-insulin-dependent diabetes mellitus: prospective studies of Pima Indians. *N. Engl. J. Med.*, **329,** 1988–1992 (1993)
311. Lin, C. D., Allori, A.C., Macklin, J. E., Sailon, A. M., Tanaka, R., Levine, J. P., Saadeh, P. B., and Warren, S. M. Topical lineage-negative progenitor-cell therapy for diabetic wounds. *Plast Reconstr Surg*, **122**(5), 1341–51 (2008).
312. Lindsay, R. S. Gestational diabetes: causes and consequences. *Br J Diab Vascular Dis*, **9**(1), 27–31 (2009)
313. Ling, C., Poulsen, P., Carlsson, E., Ridderstrale, M., Almgren, P., Wojtaszewski, J., Beck-Nielsen, H., Groop, L., and Vaag, A. Multiple environmental and genetic fac-

tors influence skeletal muscle PGC-1alpha and PGC-1beta gene expression in twins. *J. Clin. Invest.*, **114**(10), 1518–26 (2004).

314. Litzelman, D. K., Marriott, D. K., and Vinicor, F. The role of footwear in the prevention of foot lesions in patients with NIDDM: conventional wisdom or evidence-based practice? *Diab. Care*, **20**, 156–162 (1997).
315. Liu, D., Zhen, W., Yang, Z., Carter, J. D., Si, H., Reynold, K. A. Genistein acutely stimulates insulin secretion in pancreatic beta-cells through a cAMP-dependent protein Kinase pathway. *Diabetes*, **55**, 1043–1050 (2006).
316. Lloret, L. C., Pelletier, A. L., Czernichow, S., Vergnaud, A. C., Bonnefont-Rousselot, D., Levy, P., Philippe, R., and Eric, B. Acute Pancreatitis in a Cohort of 129 Patients Referred for Severe Hypertriglyceridemia. *Pancreas*, **37**, 13–8 (2008).
317. Lopez-Garcia, E., Schulze, M. B., Meigs, J. B., Manson, J. E., Rifai, N., Stampfer, M. J., Willett, W. C., Hu,F. B. Consumption of trans fatty acids is related to plasma biomarkers of inflammation and endothelial dysfunction. *J Nutr.*, **135**, 562–566 (2005).
318. Lorenzi, M. and Cagliero, E. Pathobiology of endothelial and other myocarvascular cells in diabetes mellitus. Call for data. *Diabetes*, **40**, 653–659 (1991).
319. Low, P. A., Nickander, K. K., and Tritschler, H. J.The roles of oxidative stress and antioxidant treatment in experimental diabetic neuropathy. *Diabetes*, **46**(2), S38–S42 (1997).
320. Lowe, C. E., Cooper, J. D., Brusko, T., et al. Large-scale genetic fine mapping and genotype-phenotype associations implicate polymorphism in the IL2RA region in type 1 diabetes. *Nat. Genet.*, **39**(9), 1074–82 (2007).
321. Lu, J., Li, Q., Xie, H., Chen, Z. J., Borovitskaya, A. E., Maclaren, N. K., Notkins, A. L., and Lan, M. S. Identifi cation of a second transmembrane protein tyrosine phosphatase, IA - 2beta, as an autoantigen in insulin – dependent diabetes mellitus: precursor of the 37-kDa tryptic fragment. *Proc. Natl. Acad.Sci.*, **93**, 2307–2311 (1996).
322. Lumeng, C. N., Deyoung, S. M., Bodzin, J. L., and Saltiel, A. R. Increased inflammatory properties of adipose tissue macrophages recruited during diet-induced obesity. *Diabetes*, **56**, 16–23 (2007).
323. Lyssenko, V., Lupi, R., Marchetti, P., Del Guerra, S., Ortho-Melander, M., Almgren, P., Sjogren, M., Ling, C., Eriksson, K. F., Lethagen, A. L., Mancarella, R., Berglund, G., Tuomi, T., Nilsson, P., Del Prato, S., Leif G., et al. Mechanisms by which common variants in the TCF7L2 gene increase risk of type 2 diabetes. *J. Clin. Invest.*, **117**, 2155–2163 (2007).
324. Maahs, D. M., Nadeau, K., Snell-Bergeon, J. K., Schauer, I., Bergman, B., et al.. Association of insulin sensitivity to lipids across the lifespan in people with Type 1 diabetes. *Diabet Med.*, **28**,148–5 (2011).
325. Maahs, D. M., West, N. A., Lawrence, J. M., and Mayer-Davis, E. J. Chapter 1: Epidemiology of Type 1 Diabetes. *Endocrinol. Metab. Clin. North Am.*, **39**(3), 481–497 (2010).
326. Maedler, K., Schumann, D. M., Sauter, N., Ellingsgaard, H., Bosco, D., Baertschiger, R., Iwakura, Y., Oberholzer, J., Wollheim, C. B., Gauthier, B. R., and Donath, M. Y. Low concentration of interleukin 1beta induces FLICE inhibitory protein mediated beta cell proliferation in human pancreatic islets. *Diabetes*, **55**, 2713–2722 (2006).
327. Maedler, K., Sergeev, P., Ris, F., Oberholzer, J., Joller-Jemelka, H. I., Spinas, G. A., Kaiser, N., Halban, P. A., and Donath, M. Y. Glucose induced beta cell production of

IL 1beta contributes to glucotoxicity in human pancreatic islets. *J. Clin. Invest.*, **110**, 851–860 (2002).

328. Maedler, K., Spinas, G. A., Lehmann, R., Sergeev, P., Weber, M., Fontana, A., Kaiser, N., and Donath, M. Y. Glucose induces beta - cell apoptosis via upregulation of the Fas receptor in human islets. *Diabetes*, **50**, 1683–1690 (2001).
329. Maier, L. M. and Wicker, L. S. Genetic susceptibility to type 1 diabetes. *Curr. Opin. Immunol*, **17**, 601–608 (2005).
330. Malandrino, N. and Smith, R. J. Personalized Medicine in Diabetes. *Clin Chem.*, **57**(2), 231–240 (2011).
331. Malik, V. S., Popkin, B. M., Bray, G. A., Despres, J. P., Willett, W. C., and Hu, F. B. Sugar-sweetened beverages and risk of metabolic syndrome and type 2 diabetes: a meta-analysis. *Diab. Care*, **33**, 2477–2483 (2010).
332. Mandrup-Poulsen, T. Interleukin-6 and Diabetes the Good, the Bad, or the Indifferent? *Diabetes*, **54**(2), S114–24 (2005).
333. Mandrup-Poulsen, T. The Role of Interleukin-1 in the Pathogenesis of Iddm. *Diabetologia*, **39**(9), 1005–1029 (1996).
334. Manson, J. E., Nathan, D. M., Krolewski, A. S., Stampfer, M. J., Willett, W. C., Hennekens, and C. H. A prospective study of exercise and incidence of diabetes among US male physicians. *JAMA*, **268**, 63–67 (1992).
335. Manson, J. E., Rimm, E. B., Stampfer, M. J., Colditz, G. A., Willett, W. C., Krolewski, A. S., Rosner, B., Hennekens, C. H., and Speizer, F. E. Physical activity and incidence of non-insulin-dependent diabetes mellitus in women. *Lancet*, **338**, 774–8 (1991).
336. Manyam, B. V. Diabetes mellitus, Ayurveda, and yoga. *J. Altern. Complement. Med.*, **10**, 223–225 (2004).
337. Margetic, S., Gazzola, C., Pegg, G. G., and Hill, R. A. Leptin: a review of its peripheral actions and interactions. *Int J Obes.*, **26**, 1407–1433 (2002).
338. Margolis, D. J., Allen-Taylor, L., Hoffstad, O., and Berlin, J. A. Diabetic neuropathic foot ulcers and amputation. *Wound Repair Regen*, **13**, 230–36 (2005).
339. Marhoffer, W., Stein, M., Maeser, E., and Federlin, K. Impairment of polymorphonuclear leukocyte function and metabolic control of diabetes. *Diab. Care*, **15**(2), 256–60 (1992).
340. Maritim, A. C., Sanders, R. A., and Watkins, J. B. Diabetes, Oxidative Stress, and Antioxidants: A Review. *Biochem. Molecular Toxicol.*, **17**(1), 24–38 (2003).
341. Marles, R. J. and Farnsworth, N. R. Antidiabetic plants and their active constituents. *Phy tomedecine*, **2**, 137–189 (1995).
342. Marliss, E. B. and Vranic, M. Intense exercise has unique effects on both insulin release and its roles in glucoregulation: implications for diabetes. *Diabetes*, **51**(1), S271–83 (2002).
343. Marron, M. P., Raffel, L. J., Garchon, H. J., et al. Insulin-dependent diabetes mellitus (IDDM) is associated with CTLA4 polymorphisms in multiple ethnic groups. *Hum. Mol. Genet.*, **6**(8), 1275–82 (1997).
344. Marschütz, M. K. and Bernkop-Schnürch, A. Oral peptide drug delivery: polymer-inhibitor conjugates protecting insulin from enzymatic degradation in vitro. *Biomaterials*, **21**(14), 1499–507 (2000).

345. Martin, B. C., Warram, J. H., Krolewski, A. S., Gergman, R. N., Soeldner, J. S., and Kahn, C. R. Role of glucose and insulin resistance in the development of type 2 diabetes mellitus: results of a 25-year follow-up study. *Lancet*, **340**, 925–929 (1992).
346. Martin, P. Wound healing- aiming for perfect skin regeneration. *Science*, **276**(5309), 75–81 (1997).
347. Maser, R. E., Mitchell, B. D., Vinik, A. I., and Freeman, R. The association between cardiovascular autonomic neuropathy and mortality in individuals with diabetes: a meta-analysis. *Diab. Care*, **26**, 1895–1901 (2003).
348. Mast, B. A. and Schultz, G. S. Interactions of cytokines: growth factors, and proteases in acute and chronic wounds. *Wound Repair Regen.*, **4**(4), 411–20 (1996).
349. Mather, H. M., Chaturvedi, N., and Fuller, J. H. Mortality and morbidity from diabetes in South Asians and Europeans: 11-year follow-up of the Southall Diabetes Survey, London, UK, *Diab. Med.*, **15**, 53–9 (1998).
350. Mathiowitz, E., Jacob, J. S, Jong, Y. S., Carino, G. P., Chickering, D. E., Chaturvedi, P., Santos, C. A., Vijayaraghavan, K., Montgomery, S., Bassett, M., and Morrell, C. Biologically erodable microspheres as potential oral drug delivery systems. *Nature*, **386**, 410–414 (1997).
351. Mathis, D. and Benoist, C. Back to central tolerance. *Immunity*, **20**, 509–516 (2004).
352. Mayer-Davis, E. J., Bell, R. A., Dabelea, D., et al. The many faces of diabetes in American youth: type 1and type 2 diabetes in five race and ethnic populations: the SEARCH for Diabetes in Youth Study. *Diab care*, **32**(2), S99–101 (2009).
353. Mbanya, J.C., Ngogang, J., Salah, J.N., Minkoulou, E, Balkau, B. Prevalence of NIDDM and impaired glucose tolerance in a rural and an urban population in Cameroon. Diabetologia 1997, 40, 824–829.
354. McCabe, C. J., Stevenson, R. C., and Dolan, A. M. Evaluation of a diabetic foot screening and prevention programme. *Diab. Med.*, **15**, 80–84 (1998).
355. McCarthy, M. I. and Hattersley, A. T. Learning from molecular genetics: novel insights arising from the definition of genes for monogenic and type 2 diabetes. *Diabetes*, **57**, 2889–98 (2008).
356. McCarty, D. J., Zimmet, P., Dalton, A., et al. *The rise and rise of diabetes in Australia: A review of statistics, trends, and costs.* Melbourne, International Diabetes Institute and Diabetes Australia (1996).
357. McDermott, M. M., Liu, K., Greenland, P., Guralnik, J. M., Criqui, M. H., Chan, C., Pearce, W. H., Schneider, J. R., Ferrucci, L.,, Celic, L.,, Taylor, L. M., Vonesh, E., Martin, G. J., Clark, E., et al. Functional decline in peripheral arterial disease: associations with the ankle brachial index and leg symptoms. *JAMA*, **292**,453–61 (2004).
358. McKnighta, A. J., Maxwella, A. P., Patterson, C. C., Bradyc, H. R., and Savage, D. A. Association of VEGF-1499CYT polymorphism with diabetic nephropathy in type 1 diabetes mellitus. *J. Diab and Its Complications*, **21**, 242–245 (2007).
359. McLarty, D. G., Athaide, I., Bottazzo, G. F., Swai, A. M., and Alberti, K. G. Islet cell antibodies are not specifi cally associated with insulin - dependent dia betes in Tanzanian Africans. *Diab. Res. Clin. Pract.*, **9**, 219–224 (1990).
360. McLennan, S. V., Heffernan, S., Wright, L., Rae, C., Fisher, E., Yue, D. K., and Turtle, J. R. Changes in hepatic glutathione metabolism in diabetes. *Diabetes*, **140**(3), 344–348 (1991).

361. McMahon, M. M. and Bistrian, B. R. Host defenses and susceptibility to infection in patients with diabetes mellitus. *Infect. Dis. Clin. North Am.*, **9**, 1–9 (1995).
362. MCveigh, G. E., Brennan, G. M., Johnston, G. D., MCdermott, B. J., MCgrath, L. T., Andrews, J. W., and Hayes, J. R. Impaired endothelium-dependent and independent vasodilation in patients with type II (non-insulin-dependent) diabetes mellitus. *Diabetologia*, **35**, 771–776 (1992).
363. McWhorter, L. S. Biological Complementary Therapies: A Focus on Botanical Products in Diabetes. Diab. *Spectrum*, **14**(4), 199–208 (2001).
364. Meloni, C., Morosetti, M., Suraci, C., Pennafina, M. G., Tozzo, C., Taccone-Gallucci, M., and Casciani, C. U. Severe dietary protein restriction in overt diabetic nephropathy: benefits or risks? *J. Ren. Nutr.*, **12**, 96–101 (2002).
365. Mendell, J. R.and Sahenk, Z. Painful sensory neuropathy. *N. Engl. J .Med.*, **248**, 1243–1255 (2003).
366. Metcalfe, K. A., Hitman, G. A., Rowe, R. E., et al. Concordance for type 1 diabetes in identical twins is affected by insulin genotype. *Diab. Care*, **24**(5), 838–42 (2001).
367. Metzger, B. E., Lowe, D. P., Dyer, A. R., Trimble, E. R., Chaovarindr, U., Coustan, D. R., et al. Hyperglycemia and adverse pregnancy outcomes. *N. Engl. J. Med.*, **358**, 1991–2002 (2008).
368. Meyer, C., Stumvoll, M., Nadkarni, V., Dostou, J., Mitrakou, A., and Gerich, J. Abnormal renal and hepatic glucose metabolism in type 2 diabetes mellitus. *J. Clin. Invest.*, **102**, 619–24 (1998).
369. Michalet, X., Pinaud, F. F., Bentolila, L. A., Tsav, J. M., Doose, S., Li, J. J., Sundaresan, G., Wu, A. M., Gambhir, S. S., and Weiss, S. Quantum dots for live cells, in vivo imaging, and diagnostics. *Science*, **307**, 538–544 (2005).
370. Mitra, A. Diabetes and Stress: A Review. *Ethno-Med.*, **2**(2), 131–135 (2008).
371. Modak, M., Dixit, P., Londhe, J., Ghaskadbi, S., and Devasagayam, T. P. A. Indian Herbs and Herbal Drugs Used for the Treatment of Diabetes. *J. Clin. Biochem. Nutr.*, **40**(3), 163–173 (2007).
372. Mohan, V., Sandeep, S., Deepa, R., Shah, B., and Varghese, C. Epidemiology of type 2 diabetes: Indian scenario. *Indian J Med Res* **125**, 217–230 (2007)
373. Moller, D. E. Potential role of TNF-a in the pathogenesis of insulin resistance and type 2 diabetes. *Trends Endocrinol. Metab.*, **11**, 212–217 (2000).
374. Mooradian, A. D., Bernbaum, M., and Albert, S. G. Narrative review: a rational approach to starting insulin therapy. *Ann. Intern. Med.*,**145**, 125–134 (2006).
375. Moore, D. J., Gregory, J. M., Kumah-Crystal, Y. A., and Simmons, J. H. Mitigating micro- and macro-vascular complications of diabetes beginning in adolescence. *Vascul. Health Risk Manage.*, **5**, 1015–1031 (2009).
376. Morran, M. P., McInerney, M. F., and Pietropaolo, M. Innate and adaptive autoimmunity in type 1 diabetes. *Pediatr. Diab.*, **9**, 152–161 (2008).
377. Moss, S. E., Klein, R., and Klein, B. E. K. The prevalence and incidence of lower extremity amputation in a diabetic population. *Arch. Intern. Med.*, **152**, 610–616.
378. Motala, A. A. Diabetes trends in Africa. *Diab. Metab. Res. Rev.*, **18**(3), S14–20 (2002).
379. Mottola, M. F. Prevention and Treatment of Gestational Diabetes Mellitus. *Current Diab Reports*, **8**, 299–304 (2008).

380. Moy, C. S., Songer, T. J., LaPorte, R. E., Dorman, J. S., Kriska, A. M., Orchard, T. J., Becker, D. J., and Darsh A. L. Insulin- dependent diabetes mellitus, physical activity, and death. *Am. J. Epidemiol.*, **137**, 74–81 (1993).
381. Mundargi, R. C., Rangaswamy, V., and Aminabhavi, T. M. pH-Sensitive oral insulin delivery systems using Eudragit microspheres. *Drug Develop. Indust. Pharmacy*, **37**(8), 977–985 (2011).
382. Murabito, J. M., D'Agostino, R. B., Silbershatz, H., and Wilson, W. F. Intermittent claudication: a risk profile from the Framingham Heart Study. *Circulation*, 9644–49 (1997).
383. Muraoka, O., Xie, W., Tanabe, G., Amer, M. F. A., Minematsu, T., and Yoshikawa, M. On the structure of the bioactive constituent from ayurvedic medicine Salacia reticulata: revision of the literature. *Tetrahedron Lett.*, **49**, 7315–7317 (2008).
384. Must, A., Jacques, P. F., Dallal, G. I., Pajema, C. J.,and Dietz, W. Long-term morbidity and mortality of overweight adolescents. A follow-up of the Harvard Growth Study of 1922 to 1935. *N. Engl. Med.*, **327**, 1350–1355 (1992).
385. Myers, J., Atwood, J. E., and Froelicher, V. Active Lifestyle and Diabetes. *Circulation.*, **107**, 2392–2394 (2003).
386. Myerson, M., Papa, J., Eaton, K., and Wilson, K. The total contact cast for management of neuropathic plantar ulceration of the foot. *J. Bone Joint Surg.*, **74**, 261–269 (1992).
387. Nathan, D. M., Cleary, P. A., Backlund, J. Y., Genuth, S. M., Lachin, J. M., Orchard, T. J., Raskin, P., and Zinman, B. Intensive diabetes treatment and cardiovascular disease in patients with type 1 diabetes. *N. Engl. J. Med.*, **353**, 2643–2653 (2005).
388. Nelson, R. G., Meyer, T. W., Myers, B. D., and Bennett, P. H. Clinical and pathological course of renal disease in non-insulindependent diabetes mellitus: the Pima Indian experience. *Semin Nephrol.*, **17**, 124–131 (1997).
389. Nerup, J., Platz, P., Andersen, O. O., Christy, M., Lyngsoe, J., Poulsen, J. E., Ryder, L. P., Thomsen, M., Nielsen, L. S., and Svejgaard, A. HL-A antigens and diabetes mellitus. *Lancet*, **2**, 864–866 (1974).
390. Neufeld ,G., Cohen, T., Gengrinovitch S., and Poltorak, Z.Vascular endothelial growth factor (VEGF) and its receptors. *FASEB J.*, **13**, 9–22 (1999).
391. Newman, J. D. and Turner, A. P. F. Home blood glucose biosensors: a commercial perspective. *Biosensors and Bioelectronics*, **20**, 2435–2453 (2005).
392. Ng, M. C., Park, K. S., Oh, B., Tam, C. H., Cho, Y. M., Shin, H. D., Lam, V. K., Ma, R. C., So, W. Y., Cho, Y. S., Kim, H. L., Lee, H. K., Chan, J. C., and Cho, N. H. Implication of genetic variants near TCF7L2, SLC30A8, HHEX, CDKAL1, CDKN2A/B, IGF2BP2, and FTO in type 2 diabetes and obesity in 6,719 Asians. *Diabetes*, **57**, 2226–2233 (2008).
393. Nielsen, E. M., Hansen, L., Carstensen, B., Echwald, S. M., Drivsholm, T., Glumer, C.,Thorsteinsson, B., Borch-Johnsen, K., Hansen, T., and Pedersen, O. The E23K variant of Kir 6.2 associates with impaired post-OGTT serum insulin response and increased risk of type 2 diabetes. *Diabetes*, **52**, 573–577 (2003).
394. Nilsson, P. M, Lind, L. Pollare, T., Berne, C., and Lithell, H. O. Increased level of hemoglobin A1c, but not impaired insulin sensitivity, found in hypertensive and normotensive smokers. *Metabol.*, **44**, 557–561 (1995).

395. Noble, J. A., Valdes, A. M., Bugawan, T. L., Apple, R. J., Thomson, G., and Erlich, H. A. The HLA class I`A locus affects susceptibility to type 1diabetes. Hum. *Immunol.*, **63**, 657–664 (2002).
396. Notkins, A. L. and Lernmark, A. Autoimmune type 1 diabetes: resolved and unresolved issues. *J. Clin, Invest.*, **108**, 1247–1252 (2001).
397. Oates, P. J. Polyol pathway and diabetic peripheral neuropathy. *Int. Rev. Neurobiol.* **50**,325–392 (2002).
398. Oberley, L. W. Free radicals and diabetes. Free Radic. *Biol. Med.*, **5**,113–124 (1988).
399. Odegaard, A. O., Koh, W. P., Arakawa, K., Yu, M. C., and Pereira, M. A. Soft drink and juice consumption and risk of physician-diagnosed incident type 2 diabetes: the Singapore Chinese Health Study. *Am. J. Epidemiol.*, **171**,701–8 (2010).
400. Oikawa, Y., Shimada, A., Kasuga, A., Morimoto, J., and Osaki, T. Systemic administration of IL- 8 promotes diabetes development in young nonobese diabetic mice. *J. Immunol.*, **171**, 5865–5875 (2003).
401. Okada, T., Kawano, Y., Sakakibara, T., Hazeki, O., and Ui, M. Essential role of phosphatidylinositol 3-kinase in insulin-induced glucose transport and antilipolysis in rat adipocytes. Studies with a selective inhibitor wortmannin. *J. Biol. Chem.*, **269**, 3568–3573 (1994).
402. Olsen, N. J. and Heitmann, B. L. Intake of calorically sweetened beverages and obesity. *Obes. Rev.*, **10**, 68–75 (2008).
403. Olsson, A. K., Dimberg, A., Kreuger, J., and Claesson-Welsh, L. VEGF receptor signalling-in control of vascular function. *Mol .Cell Biol.*, **7**, 351–371 (2006).
404. Omar, M., Seedat, M., Motala, A., Dyer, R., and Becker P. The prevalence of diabetes mellitus and impaired glucose tolerance in a group of urban South African blacks. *SAMJ*, **83** 641–643 (1993).
405. Onengut-Gumuscu, S., Ewens, K. G., Spielman, R. S., and Concannon, P. A. Functional polymorphism (1858C/T) in the PTPN22 gene is linked and associated with type I diabetes in multiplex families. *Genes Immun.*, **5**(8), 678–80 (2004).
406. O'Rahilly, S., Turner, R. C., and Matthews, D. R. Impaired pulsatile secretion of insulin in relatives of patients with non-insulin-dependent diabetes. *N. Engl. J. Med.*,**318**, 1225–1230 (1988).
407. Owens, D. R. New horizons- alternative routes for insulin therapy. *Nature Rev. Drug Discov.*,**1**, 529–540 (2002).
408. Owens, D. R., Zinman B., and Bolli G. B. Insulins today and beyond. *Lancet*, **358**, 739–46 (2001).
409. Pan, D. A., Lillioja, S., Kriketos, A. D., Milner, M. R., Baur, L. A., Bogardus C., Jenkins, A. B., and Storlien, L. H. Skeletal muscle triglyceride levels are inversely related to insulin action. *Diabetes*, **46**(6), 983–8 (1997).
410. Pan, X. R., Yang, W. Y., Li, G. W., and Liu, J. Prevalence of diabetes and its risk factors in China, 1994. *Diab Care*, **20**, 1664–9 (1997).
411. Panagiotopoulos, C., Qin, H., Tan, R., and Verchere, C. B. Identification of a beta-cell-specific HLA class I restricted epitope in type 1 diabetes. *Diabetes*, **52**, 2647-2651.
412. Paris, C. A., Imperatore, G., Klingensmith, G., Petitti, D., Rodriguez, B., Anderson, A. M., Schwartz, I. D., Standiford, D. A., and Pihoker, C. Predictors of insulin regimens

and impact onoutcomes in youth with type 1 diabetes: the SEARCH for Diabetes in Youth study. *J. Pediatr.*, **155**, 183–189 (2009).
413. Parker, D. R., Weiss, S. T., Troisi, R., Cassano, P. A., Vokonas, P. S., and Landsberg L. Relationship of dietary saturated fatty acids and body habitus to serum insulin concentrations: the Normative Aging study. *Am. J. Clin. Nutr.*, **58**, 129–36 (1993).
414. Parks, W. C. Matrix metalloproteinases in repair. *Wound Repair Regen*, **7**(6), 423–32 (1999).
415. Patterson, C. C., Dahlquist, G., Gyurus, E., Green, A., and Soltesz, G. EURODIAB Study Group. Incidence trends for childhood type 1 diabetes in Europe during 1989–2003 and predicted new cases 2005–20: A multicentre prospective registration study. *Lancet*, **373**, 2027–2033 (2009).
416. Paul, W. E. Interleukin 4: signaling mechanisms and control of T cell differentiation. *Ciba und Symp.*, **204**, 208–16 (1997).
417. Payton, M. A., Hawkes, C. J., and Christie, M. R. Relationship of the 37,000- and 40,000 - M(r) tryptic fragments of islet antigens in insulin-dependent diabetes to the protein tyrosine phosphatase - like molecule IA - 2 (ICA512). *J. Clin. Invest.*, **96**, 1506–1511 (1995).
418. Pearson, E. R. Pharmacogenetics in diabetes. *Curr. Diab. Rep.*, **9**, 172–81 (2009).
419. Pearson, E. R., Starkey, B. J., Powell, R. J., Gribble, F. M., Clark, P. M., and Hattersley, A. T. Genetic causes of hyperglycaemia and response to treatment in diabetes. *Lancet*, **362**, 1275–1281 (2003).
420. Pescovitz, M. D., Greenbaum, C. J., Krause-Steinrauf. H., Becker. D. J., and Gitelman, S. E. Rituximab, B-lymphocyte depletion, and preservation of beta-cell function. *N Engl J Med.*, **361**, 2143–2152 (2009).
421. Petersen, K. and Shulman, G. Etiology of insulin resistance. *Am. J. Med.*, **119**,10S–16S (2006).
422. Pfeifer, M. A., Weinberg, C. R., Cook, D. L., Reenan, A., Halter, J. B., Ensinck, J. W., and Porte, D. Jr. Autonomic neural dysfunction in recently diagnosed diabetic subjects. *Diab. Care*, **7**, 447–453 (1984).
423. Pickup, J. C., Freeman, S. C., and Sutton, A. J. Glycaemic control in type 1 diabetes during real time continuous glucose monitoring compared with self monitoring of blood glucose: metaanalysis of randomised controlled trials using individual patient data. *BMJ*, **343**, d3805 (2011).
424. Pijls, L. T., de Vries, H., van Eijk, J. T., and Donker, A. J. Protein restriction, glomerular fi ltration rate and albuminuria in patients with type 2 diabetes mellitus: a randomized trial. *Eur. J. Clin. Nutr.*, **56**, 1200–1207 (2002).
425. Pinent, M., Castell, A., Baiges, I., Montagut, G., and Arola, L. Bioactivity of flavonoids on insulin-secreting cells. *Compr. Rev. Food. Sci. Food Safety*, **7**, 299–308 (2008).
426. Pinkse G. G., Tysma, O. H., Bergen, C. A., Kester, M. G., Ossendorp, F., van Veelen, P. A., Keymeulen, B., Pipeleers, D., Drijfhout, J. W., and Roep, B. O. Autoreactive CD8 T cells associated with beta cell destruction in type 1 diabetes. *Proc. Natl. Acad. Sci.*, **102**, 18425–18430 (2005).
427. Potts, R. O., Tamada, J. A., and Tierney, M. J. Glucose monitoring by reverse iontophoresis. *Diab. Metab. Res. Rev.*, **18**, S49–S53 (2002).

428. Pradhan, A. D., Manson, J. E., Rifai, N., Buring, J. E., and Ridker, P. M. C-reactive protein, interleukin 6, and risk of developing type 2 diabetes mellitus. *JAMA*, **286**, 327–334 (2001).
429. Pratley, R. E. and Gilbert, M. Targeting incretins in type 2 diabetes: role of GLP-1receptor agonists and DPP-4 inhibitors. *Rev Diabet Stud.*, **5**, 73–94 (2008).
430. Pratley, R. E. and Salsali, A. Inhibition of DPP-4: A new therapeutic approach for the treatment of type 2 diabetes. *Curr. Med. Res. Opin.*, **23**, 919–931 (2007).
431. Prentice, A. M. and Jebb, S. A. Fast foods, energy density and obesity: a possible mechanistic link. *Obes Rev.*, **4**, 187–194 (2003).
432. Pugliese, A. Pathogenesis of type 1 diabetes: genetics. *Int. Diab. Monitor.*, **22**(3), 101–111 (2010).
433. Pugliese, A., Zeller, M., Fernandez, A. J., et al. The insulin gene is transcribed in the human thymus and transcription levels correlated with allelic variation at the INS VNTR-IDDM2 susceptibility locus for type 1 diabetes. *Nat. Genet.*, **15**(3), 293–7 (1997).
434. Qiu, J. D., Zhou, W. M., Guo, J., Wang, R., Liang, R. P., et al. Amperometric sensor based on ferrocene modified multiwalled carbon nanotube nanocomposites as electron mediator for the determination of glucose. *Anal. Biochem.*, **385**, 264–269 (2009).
435. Rabinovitch, A. and Suarez-Pinzon, W. L. Role of cytokines in the pathogenesis of autoimmune diabetes mellitus. *Rev Endocr Metab Disord.*, **4**, 291–299 (2003).
436. Rahim, M.A., Hussain, A., Azad Khan, A. K., Sayeed M. A, Keramat Ali, S. M., Vaaler S. Rising prevalence of type 2 diabetes in rural Bangladesh: a population based study. *Diab. Res. Clin. Pract.*, **77**(2), 300–305 (2007).
437. Rahiman, S. and Tantry, B. A. Nanomedicine Current Trends in Diabetes Management. *J. Nanomed. Nanotechol.*, **3**(5), 2–7 (2012).
438. Rains, J. L and Jain, S. K. Oxidative stress, insulin signaling, and diabetes. *Free Radic Biol Med.*, **50**(5), 567–75 (2011)
439. Ramsey, S. D., Newton, K., Blough, D., McCulloch, D. K., Sandhu, N., Reiber, G. E., and Wagner, E. H. Incidence, outcomes, and cost of foot ulcers in patients with diabetes. *Diab. Care*, **22**, 382–87 (1999).
440. Rasmussen, S. K., Urhammer, S. A., Jensen, J. N., Hansen, T., Borch-Johnsen, K., and Pedersen, O. The 238 and 308 G?A polymorphisms of the tumor necrosis factor a gene promoter are not associated with features of the insulin resistance syndrome or altered birth weight in Danish Caucasians. *J. Clin. Endocrinol. Metab.*, **85**, 731–1734 (2000).
441. Rasool, N., Yasin, T., Heng, J. Y. Y., and Akhter, Z. Synthesis and characterization of novel pH, ionic strength and temperature-sensitive hydrogel for insulin delivery. *Polymer*, **51**, 1687–1693 (2010).
442. Ravussin, E. and Swinburn, B. A. *Pathophysiology of obesity. Lancet*, **340**, 404–8 (1992).
443. Reach, G. and Wilson, G. S. Can continuous glucose monitoring be used for the treatment of diabetes. *Anal. Chem.*, **64**(6), 381A–386A (1992).
444. Redondo, M. J., Fain, P. R., and Eisenbarth G. S. Genetics of type 1A diabetes. *Recent Prog. Horm. Res.*, **56**, 69–89 (2001).

445. Reiber, G. E. Epidemiology of foot ulcers and amputations in the diabetic foot. *In: The Diabetic Foot*, J. H. Bowker and M. Pfeifer (Eds.), Mosby, St. Louis., pp. 13–32 (2001).
446. Reiber, G. E., Vileikyte, L., Boyko, E. J., del Aguila, M., Smith, D. G., Lavery, L. A., and Boulton, A. J. Causal pathways for incident lower extremity ulcers in patients with diabetes from two settings. *Diab. Care*, **22**, 157–162 (1999).
447. Ridker, P. M., Cushman, M., Stampfer, M. J., Tracy, R. P., and Hennekens, C. H. Plasma concentration of C-reactive protein and risk of developing peripheral vascular disease. *Circulation*, **97**, 425–8 (1998).
448. Rieck, M., Arechiga, A., Onengut-Gumuscu, S., Greenbaum, C., Concannon, P., and Buckner, J. H. Genetic variation in PTPN22 corresponds to altered function of T and B lymphocytes. *J. Immunol.*, **179**(7), 4704–10 (2007).
449. Rizkalla, S. W., Taghrid, L., Laromiguiere, M., Huet, D., Boillot, J., Rigoir, A. et al. Improved plasma glucose control, whole-body glucose utilization, and lipid profile on a low- glycemic index diet in type 2 diabetic men: a randomized controlled trial. *Diab. Care*, **27**, 1866–1872 (2004).
450. Robertson, R. P., Olson, I. K., and Zhang, H. J. Differentiating glucose toxicity from glucose desensitization: a new message from the insulin gene. *Diabetes*, **43**, 1085–1089 (1994).
451. Roden, M., Price, T. B., Perseghin, G., Petersen, K. F, Rothman, D. L, Cline, G. W., Shulman, and G. I. Mechanism of free fatty acid-induced insulin resistance in humans. *J Clin Invest*, **97**(12), 2859–65 (1996).
452. Roep, B. O., Kallan, A. A., Hazenbos, W. L., Bruining, G. J., Bailyes, E. M., Arden, S. D., Hutton, J. C., and de Vries, R. R. T-cell reactivity to 38 kD insulin-secretory-granule protein in patients with recent-onset type 1 diabetes. *Lancet*, **337**, 1439–1441 (1991).
453. Rosenheck, R. Fast food consumption and increased caloric intake: a systematic review of a trajectory towards weight gain and obesity risk. *Obes. Rev.*, **9,** 535–547 (2008).
454. Rossetti, L., Giaccari, A., and DeFronzo, R. A. Glucose toxicity. *Diab. Care*, **13**, 610–630 (1990).
455. Rossing, K., Jacobsen, P., Pietraszek, L., and Parving, H. H. Renoprotective effects of adding angiotensin II receptor blocker to maximal recommended doses of ACE inhibitor in diabetic nephropathy: a randomized double-blind crossover trial. *Diab. Care*, **26**, 2268–2274 (2003).
456. Rotenstein, L. S., Kozak, B. M., Shivers, J. P., Yarchoan, M., Close, J., and Close, K. L. The Ideal Diabetes Therapy: What Will It Look Like? How Close Are We? *Clin. Diab.*, **30**(2), 44–3 (2012).
457. Rovin, B. H., Lu, L., and Zhang, X. A novel interleukin-8 polymorphism is associated with severe systemic lupus erythematosus nephritis. *Kidney Int.*, **62**, 261–265 (2002).
458. Rovira, A. Treating diabetes:a holistic approach. *Av. Diabetol.*, **18**, 161–167.
459. Ruggenenti, P. and Remuzzi, G. Nephropathy of type-2 diabetes mellitus. *J. Am. Soc. Nephrol.*, **9**, 2157–2169 (1998).
460. Rull, J. A. and Aguilar-Salinas, C. A. Epidemiology of type 2 diabetes in Mexico. *Arch. Med. Res.*, **36**, 188–96 (2005).

461. Sacco, R. L., Benjamin, E. J., Broderick, J. P., Dyken, M.,Easton, J. D., Feinberg, W. M.,Goldstein, L. B.,Gorelick, P. B.,Howard, G., Kittner, S. J., Manolio, T. A., Whisnant, J. P., and Wolf, P. A. American Heart Association Prevention Conference. IV. Prevention and Rehabilitation of Stroke. Risk factors. *Stroke*, **28**, 1507–17 (1997).
462. Sacks, D. B., Bruns, D. E. , Goldstein, D. E. , Maclaren, N. K., McDonald, J. M., and Parrott, M. Guidelines and recommendations for laboratory analysis in the diagnosis and management of diabetes mellitus. *Clin.Chem.*, **48**, 436–472 (2002).
463. Sadikot, S. M., Nigam, A., Das, S., Bajaj, S., Zargar, A. H., and Prasannakumar, K. M et al. The burden of diabetes and impaired glucose tolerance in India using the WHO 1999 criteria: prevalence of diabetes in India study (PODIS), *Diab Res. Clin. Pract.*, **66**(3), 301–307, (2004).
464. Sahu, N.,Mahato, S. B.,Sarkar, S. K., and Poddar, G. Triterpenoidsaponins from Gymnemasylvestre. *Phytochem.*, 41, 1181–1185 (1996).
465. Salmeron, J., Ascherio, A., Rimm, E. B., Colditz, G. A., Spiegelman, D., and Jenkins, D. J et al. Dietary fiber, glycemic load, and risk of NIDDM in men. *Diab. Care*, 20,545– 50 (1997).
466. Sander, D., Sander, K., and Poppert, H. Stroke in type 2 diabetes.*Br. J. Diab. Vas Dis.*, 8, 222–229 (2008).
467. Sanke, T., Hanabusa, T., Nakano, Y., Oki C., Okai, K., Nishimura, S.,Kondo, M., and Nanjo, K. Plasma islet myloid polypeptide (amylin) levels and their responses to oral glucose in type 2 (non - insulin - dependent) diabetic patients. *Diabetologia.*, 34, 129–132 (1991).
468. Santhosh, P., Manesh, K. M., Uthayakumar, S., Gopalan, A. I., Lee, K. P. Hollow spherical nanostructured polydiphenylamine for direct electrochemistry and glucose biosensor. Biosens. *Bioelectron.*, 24, 2008– 2014 (2009).
469. Sathish. R., Madhavan, R., Vasanthi, H. R., and Amuthan, A. *In-vitro* alpha-glucosidase inhibitory activity of abragachendhooram, a Siddha drug. *Int. J. Pharmacol. Clinl. Sci.*, **1**(3), 79–81 (2012).
470. Saudek, C. D., Herman, W. H., Sacks, D. B., Bergenstal, R. M., Edelman, D., and Davidson, M. B. A new look at screening and diagnosing diabetes mellitus. *J. Clin. Endocrinol.Metab.*, 93, 2447–2453 (2008).
471. Saxena A. and Vikram, N. K. Role of selected Indian plants in management of type 2 diabetes: A review. *J. Altern. Complement. Med.*, 10, 369–378 (2004).
472. Saxena, A. K., Srivastava, P., Kale R. K., and Baquer, N. Z. Impaired antioxidant status in diabetic rat liver. Effect of vanadate. *Biochem. Pharmacol.*, **45**(3), 539–542 (1993).
473. Saxena, R., Voight, B. F., Lyssenko, V., Burtt. N. P., de Bakker, P. I., Chen, H., Roix, J. J., Kathiresan, S., Hirschhorn, J. N., Daly, M. J., et al. Genome-wide association analysis identifies loci for type 2 diabetes and triglyceride levels. *Science.*, 316, 1331–1336 (2007).
474. Scanlon, P. H. Diabetic Retinopathy. In *Textbook of Diabetes*, 4th edition., R. Holt, C. Cockram, A. Flyvbjerg, and B. Goldstein, (Eds.), Wiley-Blackwell., pp.581–583 (2010).
475. Scheen A. Is there a role for alpha-glucosidase inhibitors in the prevention of type 2 diabetes mellitus? Drugs, **63**(10), 933–51 (2003).

476. Schleicher, E. D. and Weigert C. Role of the hexosamine biosynthetic pathway in diabetic nephropathy. *Kidney Int.*, **58**(Suppl 77), S13–S18 (2000).
477. Schranz, D. B. and Lernmark, A. Immunology in diabetes: An update. *Diab.Metab. Rev.*, 14, 3–29 (1998).
478. Schrauwen, P. and Hesselink, M. K. Oxidative capacity, lipotoxicity, and mitochondrial damage in type 2 diabetes. *Diabetes.*, 53(6), 1412–7 (2004).
479. Schrijvers, B. F., Flyvbjerg, A., and De Vriese A. S. The role of vascular endothelial growth factor (VEGF) in renal pathophysiology. *Kidney Int.*, **65**(6), 2003–2017 (2004).
480. Schulze, M. B., Hoffmann K., Manson J. E.,Willett, W. C., Meigs, J. B., Weikert, C., Heidemann C., Colditz, G. A., and Hu, F. B. Dietary pattern, inflammation, and incidence of type 2 diabetes in women. *Am. J. Clin. Nutr.*, 82, 675–684 (2005).
481. Schulze, M. B., Manson, J. E., Ludwig, D. S., Colditz, G. A., Stampfer, M. J., Willett, W. C., and Hu, F. B. Sugar-sweetened beverages, weight gain and incidence of type 2 diabetes in young and middle-aged women. *JAMA.*,292, 927–34 (2004).
482. Schulze, M. B., Schulz, M.,Heidemann, C., Schienkiewitz, A., Hoffmann, K., and Boeing, H. Carbohydrate intake and incidence of type 2 diabetes in the European prospective investigation into cancer and nutrition (EPIC)-Potsdam study. *Br. J. Nutr.*, 99, 1107–16 (2008).
483. Schulze, M. B., Schulz, M., Heidemann, C., Schienkiewitz, A., Hoffmann, K., and Boeing, H. Fiber and magnesium intake and incidence of type 2 diabetes: a prospective study and metaanalysis. *Arch. Intern.Med.*, 167, 956–65 (2007).
484. Schuster, D. P. Obesity and the development of type 2 diabetes:the effects of fatty tissue inflammation: Diabetes, Metabolic Syndrome and Obesity. *Targets and Therapy.*, 3, 253–262 (2010).
485. Schwanstecher, C. and Schwanstecher, M. Nucleotide sensitivity of pancreatic ATP-sensitive potassium channels and type 2 diabetes. *Diabetes.*,**51**(Suppl), 3S358–S362 (2002).
486. Schwartz, S. and Modi, P. Pharmacodynamics of oral insulin in healthy volunteers. *Diabetologia.*, **43**(Suppl. 1), A202 (2000).
487. Selvin, E., Marinopoulos, S., Berkenblit, G., Rami, T., Brancati, F. L., Powe, N. R., and Golden, S. H. Meta-analysis: glycosylated hemoglobin and cardiovascular disease in diabetes mellitus. *Ann. Intern. Med.*, 141, 421–31 (2004).
488. Semple, R. K., Chatterjee, V. K., and O' Rahilly S. PPAR gamma and human metabolic disease. *J. Clin. Invest.*, 116, 581–589 (2006).
489. Sesti, G. Pathophysiology of insulin resistance. *Best Pract. Res. Clin. Endocrinol. Metab.*, 20,665–679 (2006).
490. Seyfert-Margolis V., Gisler T. D., Asare A. L., Wang R. S., Dosch H. M., Brooks-Worrell B., Eisenbarth, G. S., Palmer, J. P., Greenbaum, C. J., Gitelman, S. E., Nepom, G. T., Bluestone, J. A., and Herold, K. C. Analysis of T-cell assays to measure autoimmune responses in subjects with type 1 diabetes: results of a blinded controlled study. *Diabetes.*, 55, 2588–94 (2006).
491. Shah, P., Vella A., Basu A., Basu R., Schwenk, W. F., and Rizza, R. A. Lack of suppression of glucagon contributes to postprandial hyperglycemia in subjects with type 2 diabetes mellitus. *J. Clin. Endocrinol. Metab.*, 85, 4053–4059 (2000).

492. Shankar, R. and Singhal, R. K. Clinical studies of the effect of abraka(mica) chendooramin the treatment of diabetes mellitus (neerazhivu). *J. Res. Ayu. Siddha.*, 16, 108–17 (1995).
493. Sharma, H. and Chandola, H. M. Ayurvedic Concept of Obesity, Metabolic Syndrome and Diabetes Mellitus. Part 1- Etiology, Classification, and Pathogenesis. *J. Altern Complement. Med.*, **17**(6), 549–552 (2011).Sharma, H., Chandola, H. M., Singh, G., and Basisht, G. Utilization of Ayurveda in health care: An approach for prevention, health promotion, and treatment of disease. Part 2-Ayurveda in Primary Health Care. *J. Altern. Complement. Med.*, **13**(10), 1011–1019 (2007).
494. Sharma, H. M. Contemporary Ayurveda. In *Fundamentals of Complementary and Alternative Medicine*, 4th ed., M. S. Micozzi, (ed.), St. Louis, Saunders Elsevier., pp.495–508 (2011).
495. Shaw, J. E., Sicree, R. A., and Zimmet, P. Z. Global estimates of the prevalence of diabetes for 2010 and 2030. *Diab. Res. Clin. Pract.*, 87, 4–14 (2010).
496. Sheehy, M. J., Scharf, S. J., Rowe, J. R., Neme de Gimenez, M. H., Meske, L. M., Erlich, H. A., and Nepom, B. S. A diabetes-susceptible HLA haplotype is best defined by a combination of HLA-DR and –DQ alleles. *J. Clin. Invest.*,83, 830–835 (1989).
497. Shichiri, M., Kawamori, R., Yamasaki, Y., Hakui, N., and Abe, H. Wearable artificial endocrine pancrease with needle-type glucose sensor. *Lancet*, 2, 1129–1131 (1982).
498. Shimabukuro, M., Zhou, Y. T., Levi, M., and Unger, R. H. Fatty acid induced b cell apoptosis: A link between obesity and diabetes. *Proc. Natl. Acad. Sci.*, 95, 2498–502 (1998).
499. Shoelson, S. E., Lee, J., and Goldfine, A. B. Inflammation and insulin resistance. *J. Clin. Invest.*, 116, 1793–1801 (2006).
500. Shu, L., Sauter, N. S., Schulthess, F. T., Matveyenko, A. V., Oberholzer, J., and Maedler, K. TCF7L2 regulates -cell survival and function in human pancreatic islets. *Diabetes.*, 7, 645–653 (2008).
501. Sierra, G. N The global pandemic of diabetes. *Afri. J. Diab. Med.*, 4, 4–8 (2009).
502. Sigal, R. J., Kenny, G. P., Wasserman, D. H., Castaneda-Sceppa, C., and White, R. D. Physical activity/exercise and type 2 diabetes: a consensus statement from the American Diabetes Association. *Diab. Care.*, 29, 1433–1438 (2006).
503. Sillesen, H. H. Peripheral Vascular Disease. In *Textbook of Diabetes*, 4th edition., R. Holt, C. Cockram, A. Flyvbjerg, B. Goldstein, (Eds.), Wiley-Blackwell: West Sussex., pp.710–711 (2010).
504. Silvio, E. and Darren K. McGuire New Drugs for the Treatment of Diabetes: Part II. Incretin-Based Therapy and Beyond. *Circulation.*, 117,574–584 (2008).
505. Simmons, D. The epidemiology of diabetes and its complications in New Zealand. *Diabet Med.*, 13,371–5 (1996).
506. Singh, J., Cumming, E. L., Manoharan, G., Kalasz, H., and Adeghate, E. Medicinal Chemistry of the Anti-Diabetic Effects of Momordica Charantia: Active Constituents and Modes of Actions. *Open Medicinal Chem J.*, **5**(Supple 2-M2), 70–77 (2011).
507. Skyler, J. S. Update on worldwide efforts to prevent type 1 diabetes. *Ann. N. Y. Acad. Sci.*,1150, 190–196 (2008).
508. Sladek, R., Rocheleau, G., Rung, J., Dina, C., Shen, L., Serre, D., Boutin, P., Vincent, D., Belisle, A., Hadjadj, S., and et al. A genome-wide association study identifies novel risk loci for type 2 diabetes. *Nature.*, 445, 881–885 (2007).

509. Slavens, E. R. and Slavens, M. L. Therapeutic Footwear for Neuropathic Ulcers. *Foot Ankle Int.*, **16**(10),663–6 (1995).
510. Slavin, J. L., Martini, M. C., Jacobs, D. R Jr., and Marquart, L. Plausible mechanisms for the protectiveness of whole grains. *Am. J. Clin. Nutr.*, 70, 459S–63S (1999).
511. Smyth, D., Cooper, J. D., Collins, J. E., and et al. Replication of an association between the lymphoid tyrosine phosphatase locus (LYP/PTPN22) with type 1 diabetes, and evidence for its role as a general autoimmunity locus. Diabetes 2004, 53(11), 3020–3.
512. Soulier, S. The use of running shoes in the prevention of plantardiabetic ulcers. *Am J Pod.*,76,395–9 (1986).
513. Southam, L., Soranzo, N., Montgomery, S. B., Frayling, T. M., McCarthy, M. I., Barroso, I., and Zeggini, E. Is the thrifty genotype hypothesis supported by evidence based on confirmed type 2 diabetes- and obesitysusceptibility variants? *Diabetologia.*, 52, 1846–1851 (2009).
514. Spellman, C. W. Pathophysiology of Type 2 Diabetes: Targeting Islet Cell Dysfunction. *J. Am. Osteopath. Assoc.*, **110**(3 suppl 2), S2–S7 (2010).
515. Sprangler, J., Kroke, A., Mohlig, M., Bergmann, M. M., Ristow, M., Boeing, H., and Pfeiffer, A. F. H. Adiponectin and protection against type 2 diabetes. *Lancet.*, 361,226–228 (2003).
516. Spruce, M. C., Potter, J., and Coppini, D. V. The pathogenesis and management of painful diabetic neuropathy. *Diab. Med.*,20, 88–98 (2003).
517. Staal, S. P. Molecular cloning of the akt oncogene and its human homologues AKT1 and AKT2: amplification of AKT1 in a primary human gastric adenocarcinoma. *Proc. Natl. Acad. Sci.* ,84, 5034–5037 (1987).
518. Staels, B. and Fruchart, J. Therapeutic roles of peroxisome proliferator -activated receptor genes. *Diabetes.*, 54, 2460–2470 (2005).
519. Stafford, J. M. and Elasy, T. Treatment update: Thiazolidenediones in combination with metformin for the treatment of type 2 diabetes. *Vasc.Health Risk Manag.*, 3,503–510 (2007).
520. Staiger, H., Machicao, F., Fritsche, A., and Haring H. U. Pathomechanisms of type 2 diabetes genes. *Endocr. Rev.*, **30**(6), 557–585 (2009).
521. Staiger, H., Machicao, F., Fritsche, A., and Haring, H. U. Pathomechanisms of type 2 diabetes genes. *Endocr. Rev.*, **30**(6), 557–585 (2009).
522. Stanhope, K. L. and Havel, P. J. Fructose consumption: potential mechanisms for its effects to increase visceral adiposity and induce dyslipidemia and insulin resistance. *Curr.Opinion Lipidol.*, **19**(1), 16–24 (2008).
523. Stanhope, K. L. and Havel, P. J. Fructose consumption: recent results and their potential implications. *Ann. NY Acad. Sci.*, **1190**(1), 15–24 (2010).
524. Stefan, N., Fritsche, A., Haring, H., and Stumvol, L. M . Effect of experimental elevation of free fatty acids on insulin secretion and insulin sensitivity in healthy carriers of the Pro12Ala polymorphism of the peroxisome proliferator - activated receptor-gamma 2 gene. *Diabetes.*,50, 1143–1148 (2001).
525. Steil, G. M., Rebrin, K., Darwin, C., Hariri, F., and Saad, M. F. Feasibility of automating insulin delivery for the treatment of type 1 diabetes. *Diabetes.*, 55, 3344–3350 (2006).

526. Steinthorsdottir, V., Thorleifsson, G., Reynisdottir, I., Benediktsson, R., Jonsdottir, T., Walters, G. B., and et al. A variant in CDKAL1 influences insulin response and risk of type 2 diabetes. *Nat. Genet.*, 39, 770–775 (2007).
527. Steyn, N. P., Mann, J, Bennett, P. H., Temple, N., Zimmet, P., Tuomilehto, J., Lindstrom, J., and Louheranta, A . Diet, nutrition and the prevention of type 2 diabetes. *Pub.Health Nutr.*, **7**(1A), 147–165 (2004).
528. Stitt, A. W., Gardiner, T. A., and Archer, D. B. Histological and ultrastructural investigation of retinal microaneurysm development in diabetic patients. *Br. J. Ophthalmol.*, 79, 362– 367 (1995).
529. Stocker, R. Antioxidant defenses in the vascular wall. P.27.47. In *Oxidative stress and vascular disease*, J. F. Keaney, Jr., (Ed.), Dordrecht, Kluwer Academic Publishers, pp. 373 (1999).
530. Stumvoll, M., Goldstein, B. J., and Haeften, T. W. Type 2 diabetes: principles of pathogenesis and therapy. *Lancet.*, 365, 1333–1346 (2005).
531. Stumvoll, M., Goldstein, B. J., and van Haeften, T. W. Pathogenesis of type 2 diabetes. *Endocr. Res.*, 32, 19–37 (2007).
532. Stunkard, A. J., Sorensen, T. I., Hanis, C., Teasdale, T. W., Chakraborty, R., Schull, W. J., and Schulsinger, F. L. An adoption study of human obesity.*N. Engl. J. Med.*, 314,193–198 (1986).
533. Summers, S. A. Ceramides in insulin resistance and lipotoxicity. *Prog.Lipid. Res.*, **45**(1), 42–72 (2006).
534. Sun, S. Z., Anderson, G. H., Flickinger, B. D., Patricia, S., Williamson-Hughes, and Empie, M. W. Fructose and non-fructose sugar intakes in the US population and their associations with indicators of metabolic syndrome. *Food Chem. Toxicol.*, 49, 2875–2882 (2011).
535. Sundkvist, G., Dahlin, L. B., Nilsson, H., Eriksson, K. F., Lindgarde, F., Rosen. I, Lattimer, S. A., Sima, A. A., Sullivan, K., and Greene, D. A. Sorbitol and myo-inositol levels and morphology of sural nerve in relation to peripheral nerve function and clinical neuropathy in men with diabetic, impaired, and normal glucose tolerance. *Diab. Med.*, 17, 259–268 (2000).
536. Sundkvist, G., Lind, P., Bergstrom, B., Lilja, B., and Rabinowe, S. L. Autonomic nerve antibodies and autonomic nerve function in type 1 and type 2 diabetic patients. *J. Intern. Med.* 229,505–510 (1991).
537. Surwit, R. S., van Tilburg, M. A., Zucker, N., McCaskill, C. C., Parekh, P., Feinglos, M. N., Edwards, C. L., Williams, P., and Lane, J. D. Stress management improves long-term glycemic control in type 2 diabetes. *Diab.Care.*, **25**(1), 30–4 (2002).
538. Surwit, R. S. and Williams P. G. Animal Models Provide Insight Into Psychosomatic Factors in Diabetes. Animal Models Provide Insight Into Psychosomatic Factors in Diabetes. *Psychosomatic Med.*, 58,582–589 (1996).
539. Tajima, N. The epidemiology of Diabetes in Japan. In: *Diabetes in the new millennium*, J. R. Turtle, T. Kaneko, and S. Osato (Eds.), Pot Still Press, Sydney, pp. 23–30 (1999).
540. Tanasescu, M., Cho, E., Manson, J. E., and Hu, F. B. Dietary fat and cholesterol and the risk of cardiovascular disease among women with type 2 diabetes. *Am. J. Clin. Nutr.*, **79**, 999–1005 (2004).

541. Tang, Q., Henriksen, K. J., Bi, M., Finger, E. B., Szot, G., Ye, J., Masteller, E. L., McDevitt, H., Bonyhadi, M., and Bluestone, J. A. In vitro-expanded antigen-specific regulatory T cells suppress autoimmune diabetes. *J. Exp. Med.*, **199**, 1455–1465 (2004).
542. Tanne, D., Koren-Morag, N., Goldbourt, U. Fasting plasma glucose and risk of incident ischemic stroke or transient ischemic attacks: a prospective cohort study. Stroke 2004, 35, 2351–5.
543. Tariq, S. H., Karcic, E., Thomas, D. R., Thomson, K., Philpot, C., Chapel, D. L., et al. The use of a no concentrated sweets diet in the management of type 2 diabetes in nursing homes. *J. Am. Diet. Assoc.*, **101**, 1463–1466 (2001).
544. Tashiro, K., Koyanagi, I., Saitoh, A., Shimizu, A., Shike, T., Ishiguro, C., Koizumi, M., Funabiki, K., Horikoshi, S., Shirato, I., and Tomino, Y. Urinary levels of monocyte chemoattractant protein-1 (MCP-1) and interleukin-8 (IL-8), and renal injuries in patients with type 2 diabetic nephropathy. *J. Clin. Lab Anal.*, **16**, 1–4 (2002).
545. Taylor, C. G. Zinc, the pancreas, and diabetes: insights from rodent studies and future directions. *Biometals*, **18**, 305–312 (2005).
546. Teft, W. A., Kirchhof, M. G., and Madrenas J. A molecular perspective of CTLA-4 function. *Annu. Rev. Immunol.*, **24**, 65–97 (2006).
547. Thiyagarajan, R. Introduction, Apparatus, Drugs, Nine gem stones. In Siddha Materia Medica (Mineral & Animal section), A. R. Anandan and M. Thulasimani (Eds.), 1st ed. Chennai, Dept of Indian Medicine and Homeopathy, pp.515–25 (2008).
548. Thomas P. K. Classification, differential diagnosis, and staging of diabetic peripheral neuropathy. *Diabetes*, **46**(2), S54–S57 (1997).
549. Thomson, A. G. Pandemic diabetes: a threat we cannot ignore. *Pract. Diab. Int.*, **23**, 324 (2007).
550. Thunander, M., Petersson, C., Jonzon, K., Fornander, J., Ossiansson, B., Torn, C., Edvardsson, S., and Landin-Olsson, M. Incidence of type 1 and type 2 diabetes in adults and children in Kronoberg, Sweden. *Diab. Res. Clin. Pract.*, **82**, 247–255 (2008).
551. Tian, L. Y., Bai, X., Chen, X. H., Fang, J. B., Liu, S. H., Chen, J. C. Anti-diabetic effect of methylswertianin and bellidifolin from Swertia punicea Hemsl. and its potential mechanism. *Phytomed.*, **17**, 533–539 (2010).
552. Tinker, L. F, Heins, J. M, and Holler, H. J. Commentary and translation: 1994 nutrition recommendations for diabetes. *J. Am. Diet. Assoc.*, **94**, 507–511 (1994).
553. Tirosh, A., Potashnik, R., Bashan, N., and Rudich, A. Oxidative stress disrupts insulin-induced cellular redistribution of insulin receptor substrate-1 and phosphatidylinositol 3-kinase in 3T3-L1 adipocytes. A putative cellular mechanism for impaired protein kinase B activation and GLUT4 translocation. *J. Biol. Chem.*, **274**, 10595–10602 (1999).
554. Toeller, M. and Mann, J. I. Nutrition in the etiolgy and management of type 2 diabetes . In Type 2 Diabetes Principles and Practice, 2nd edition, B. J. Goldstein and D. Muller-Wieland (Eds.), New York/London, *Informa Healthcare*., 59–71 (2008).
555. Toeller, M. *Lifestyle Issues: Diet. In Textbook of Diabetes, 4th edition*, R. Holt, C. Cockram, A. Flyvbjerg, B. Goldstein (Eds.), Wiley-Blackwell, West Sussex, p. 353 (2010).

556. Toeller, M., Buyken, A., Heitkamp, G., Bramswig, S., Mann, J., Milne, R., Gries, F. A., and Keen, H. Protein intake and urinary albumin excretion rates in the EURO-DIAB IDDM Complications Study. *Diabetologia*, **40**, 1219–1226 (1997).
557. Torn, C., Mueller, P. W., Schlosser, M., Bonifacio, E., and Bingley, P. J. Diabetes Antibody Standardization Program: evaluation of assays for autoantibodies to glutamic acid decarboxylase and islet antigen-2. *Diabetologia*, **51**, 846–852 (2008).
558. Travis, L. *Stress, hyperglycemia, and ketosis. In Diabetes Mellitus in Children and Adolescents*, L. Travis, B. H. Brouhard, and B. D. Schreiner (Eds.), Philadelphia, Saunders, 137–146 (1987).
559. Tsai, E. C., Hirsch, I. B., Brunzell, J. D., and Chait, A. Reduced plasma peroxyl radical trapping capacity and increased susceptibility of LDL to oxidation in poorly controlled IDDM. *Diabetes* **43**(8), 1010–1014 (1994).
560. Tuomi, T., Groop, L. C., Zimmet, P. Z., Rowley, M. J., Knowles, W., and Mackay, I. R. Latent autoimmune diabetes mellitus in adults with a non-insulin dependent onset of disease. *Diabetes* **42**, 359–362 (1993).
561. Ubeda, M., Rukstalis, J. M., and Habener, J. F. Inhibition of cyclin-dependent kinase 5 activity protects pancreatic beta cells from glucotoxicity. *J. Biol. Chem.*, **281**, 28858–28864 (2006).
562. Uccioli, L., Faglia, E., Montocine, G., Favales, F., Durola, L., Aldeghi, A., Quarantiello, A., Calia, P., and Menzinger, G. Manufactured shoes in the prevention of diabetic foot ulcers. *Diab. Care*, **18**, 1376–1378 (1995).
563. Unger, R. H, Grundy, S. Hyperglycaemia as an inducer as well as a consequence of impaired islet cell function and insulin resistance: implication for the management of diabetes. *Diabetologia*, **28**, 119–121 (1985).
564. Vaag, A., Henriksen, J. E., Madsbad, S., Holm, N., and Beck-Nielsen, H. Insulin secretion, insulin action, and hepatic glucose production in identical twins discordant for non-insulin dependent diabetes mellitus. J Clin Invest., 95,690–8 (1995).
565. Valdes, A. M., Erlich, H. A., and Noble, J. A. Human leukocyte antigen class I B and C loci contribute to type 1 diabetes (T1D) susceptibility and age at T1D onset. Hum Immunol,66, 301–313 (2005).
566. Vang, T., Congia, M., Macis, M. D., et al. Autoimmune-associated lymphoid tyrosine phosphatase is a gain-of-function variant. Nat. Genet., 37(12), 1317–19 (2005).
567. Varshosaz, J. Insulin Delivery Systems for Controlling Diabetes..Recent Patents on Endocrine, Metabol Immun Drug Discovery, 1, 25–40 (2007).
568. Vashist, S. K. Non-invasive glucose monitoring technology in diabetes management: A review. Analytica Chimica Acta.,750, 16–27 (2012).
569. Vazeou, A. Continuous blood glucose monitoring in diabetes treatment. Diab. Res. Clin. Pract., 93, S125–S130 (2011).
570. Vella, A., Cooper, J. D., Lowe, C. E., Walker, N., and Nutland, S. Localization of a type 1 diabetes locus in the IL2RA/CD25 region by use of tag single-nucleotide polymorphisms. Am. J. Hum. Genet., 76, 773–779 (2005)
571. Vilsboll, T., Krarup, T., Deacon, C. F., Madsbad, S., and Holst, J. J. Reduced post-prandial concentrations of intact biologically active glucagon-like peptide 1 in type 2 diabetic patients. Diabetes, 50, 609–13 (2001).
572. Vinik, A. I., Maser, R. E., Mitchell, B. D., and Freeman R. Diabetic autonomic neuropathy (Technical Review). Diab. Care, 26, 1553–1579 (2003).

573 .Vinik, A. I. Diagnosis and management of diabetic neuropathy. Clin. Geriatr. Med., 15, 293–320 (1999).
574. Vinik, A. I. and Erbas, T. Recognizing and treating diabetic autonomic neuropathy. Cleve. Clin. J. Med., 68, 928–944 (2001).
575. Waden, J., Forsblom, C., Thorn, L. M., Saraheimo, M., Rosengard- Barlund, M., and Heikkila, O. FinnDiane Study Group. Physical activity and diabetes complications in patients with type 1 diabetes: the Finnish Diabetic Nephropathy (FinnDiane) Study. *Diab Care*, **31,** 230–232 (2008).
576. Waldhausl, W., Bratusch-Marrain, P., Gasic, S., Korn, A., and Nowotny, P. Insulin production rate, hepatic insulin retention, and splanchnic carbohydrate metabolism after oral glucose ingestion in hyperinsulinemic type II (non-insulin dependent) diabetes mellitus. *Diabetologia*, **23**, 6–15 (1982).
577. Walston, J., Seibert, M., Yen, C. J., Cheskin, L. J., and Andersen, R. E . Tumor necrosis factor-a 238 and 308 polymorphisms do not associate with traits related to obesity and insulin resistance. *Diabetes*, **48**, 2096–2098 (1999).
578. Wang J. Glucose Biosensors: 40 Years of Advances and Challenges. *Electroanalysis*, **13**(12), 983–988 (2001).
579. Wang, J. Electrochemical Glucose Biosensors. *Chem. Rev*., **108**, 814–825 (2008).
580. Wang, Y., Campbell, T., Perry, B., Beaurepaire, C., and Qin, L. Hypoglycemic and insulin-sensitizing effects of berberine in high-fat diet- and streptozotocin-induced diabetic rats. *Metab. Clin. Exp*., **60** (2), 298–305 (2010).
581. Wang, Y., Mi, J., Shan, X. Y., Wang, Q. J., and Ge, K. Y. Is China facing an obesity epidemic and the consequences? The trends in obesity and chronic disease in China. *Int J Obes*., **31**,177–188 (2007).
582. Warram, J. H., Martin, B. C., Krolewski, A. S., Soeldner, J. S., and Kahn, C. R. Slow glucose removal rate and hyperinsulinemia precede the development of type II diabetes in the offspring of diabetic patients. *Ann. Intern. Med*., **113**, 909–915 (1990).
583. Watanabe, R. M., Allayee, H., Xiang, A. H., Trigo, E., Hartiala, J., Lawrence, J. M., and Buchanan, T. A. Transcription factor 7-like 2 (TCF7L2) is associated with gestational diabetes mellitus and interacts with adiposity to alter insulin secretion in Mexican Americans. *Diabetes*, **56**, 1481–1485 (2007).
584. Watkins P. J. *Retinopathy. BMJ*, **326**, 924–926 (2003).
585. Weber, A. E. Dipeptidyl peptidase IV inhibitors for the treatment of diabetes. *J Med Chem*, **47**, 4135–4141 (2004).
586. Wei, M., Gibbons, L. W., Kampert, J. B., Nichaman, M. Z., and Blair, S. N. Low cardiorespiratory fitness and physical inactivity as predictors of mortality in men with type 2 diabetes. *Ann. Intern. Med*., **132**, 605–611 (2000).
587. Weinberg, M. S., Kaperonis, N., and Bakris, G. L. How high should an ACE inhibitor or angiotensin receptor blocker be dosed in patients with diabetic nephropathy? *Curr Hypertens Rep*., **5**, 418–425 (2003).
588. Weinzimer, S. A., Steil, G. M., Swan, K. L., Dziura, J., Kurtz, N., and Tamborlane, W. V. Fully automated closed - loop insulin delivery versus semiautomated hybrid control in pediatric patients with type 1 diabetes using an artificial pancreas. *Diab. Care*, **31,** 934–939 (2008).

589. Weiss, R., Yegorchikov, Y., Shusterman ,A., and Raz, I. *Diab. Technol. Ther.*, pp 968–74 (2007).
590. Weitz, J. I., Byrne, J., Clagett, P, et al. Diagnosis and treatment of chronic arterial insufficiency of the lower extremities: a critical review. *Circulation.*, **94**, 3026–49 (1996).
591. Wenzlau, J. M., Juhl, K., Yu, L., Moua, O., Sarkar, S. A., Gottlieb, P., Rewers, M., Eisenbarth, G. S., Jensen, J., Davidson, H. W., and Hutton, J. C. The cation efflux transporter ZnT8 (Slc30A8) is a major autoantigen in human type 1 diabetes. *Proc. Natl. Acad. Sci.*, **104**, 17040–17045 (2007).
592. Weyer, C., Bogardus, C., Mott, D. M., and Pratley, R. E. The natural history of insulin secretory dysfunction and insulin resistance in the pathogenesis of type 2 diabetes mellitus. *J. Clin. Invest.*, **104**(6), 787–794 (1999).
593. White, K. E. and Bilous, R. W. Type 2 diabetic patients with nephropathy show structural- unctional relationships that are similar to type 1 disease. *J Am Soc Nephrol.*, **11**, 1667–1673 (2000).
594. Wicker, L. S., Clark, J., Fraser, H. I., Garner, V. E., and Gonzalez-Munoz, A. Type 1 diabetes genes and pathways shared by humans and NOD mice. *J. Autoimmun.*, **25** (Suppl), 29–33 (2005).
595. Wild, S., Roglic G., Green A., Sicree R., and King H. Global prevalence of diabetes: estimates for the year 2000 and projections for 2030. *Diab Care*, **27**, 1047–1053 (2004).
596. Wilkinson, C. P., Ferris, F. L 3rd.; Klein, R. E., Lee, P. P., Agardh, C. D., Davis, M., Dills, D., Kampik, A., Pararajasegaram, R., and Verdaguer, J. T. Global Diabetic Retinopathy Project Group. Proposed international clinical diabetic retinopathy and diabetic macular edema disease severity scales. *Ophthalmol.*, **110**, 1677–1682 (2003).
597. Willcox, A., Richardson, S. J., Bone, A. J., Foulis, A. K., and Morgan, N. G. Analysis of islet inflammation in human type 1 diabetes. *Clin. Exp. Immunol.*, **155**, 173–181 (2009).
598. Willi, C., Bodenmann, P., Ghali, W. A., Faris, P. D., and Cornuz, J. Active smoking and the risk of type 2 diabetes: a systematic review and meta-analysis. *JAMA*, **298**, 2654–2664 (2007).
599. Willi, C., Bodenmann, P., Ghali, W. A., Faris, P. D., and Cornuz, J. Active smoking and the risk of type 2 diabetes: a systematic review and meta-analysis. *JAMA*, **298**, 2654–2664 (2007).
600. Williams, S. B., Cusco, J. A., Roddy, M. A., Johnstone, M. T., and Creager, M. A. Impaired nitric oxide-mediated vasodilation in patients with non-insulin dependent diabetes mellitus. *J. Am. Coll. Cardiol.*, **27**,567–74 (1996).
601. Witt, C. M., Ludtke, R., Mengler, N., and Willich, S. N. How healthy are chronically ill patients after eight years of homeopathic treatment? - results from a long term observational study. *BMC Public Health*, **17**(8), 413 (2008).
602. Woodcock, J. The prospects for personalized medicine in drug development and drug therapy. *Clin. Pharmacol. Ther.*, **81**,164–9 (2007).
603. Woodfield S. L., Lundergan C. F., Reiner J. S., Greenhouse S. W., Thompson M. A., Rohrbeck S. C., Deychak Y., Simoons M. L., Califf R. M., Topol E. J., and Ross A. M. Angiographic findings and outcome in diabetic patients treated with thrombolytic

therapy for acute myocardial infarction: the GUSTO-I experience *J. Am. Coll. Cardiol.*, **28**, 1661–1669 (1996).

604. Woodgett J. R. Recent advances in the protein kinase B signalling pathway. *Curr. Opinion Cell Biol.*, **17**, 150–157 (2005).
605. Wu, Y., Li, H., Loos, R. J., Yu, Z., Ye, X., Chen, L., Pan, A., Hu, F. B, and Lin, X. Common variants in CDKAL1, CDKN2A/B, IGF2BP2,SLC30A8, and HHEX/IDE genes are associated with type 2 diabetes and impaired fasting glucose in a Chinese Han population. *Diabetes*, **57**, 2834–2842 (2008).
606. Wu, Y., Wang, J., Scott, P. G., and Tredget, E. E. Bone marrow-derived stem cells in wound healing: a review. *Wound Repair Regen.*, **15**(1), S18–26 (2007).
607. Yadav, N., Morris, G., Harding, S. E., Ang, S., and Adams, G. G. Various Non-Injectable Delivery Systems for the Treatment of Diabetes Mellitus. *Endocrine, Metabolic & Immune Disorders - Drug Targets*, **9**, 1–13 (2009).
608. Yang, Q, Graham, T. E, Mody, N, Preitner, F, Peroni, O. D, Zabolotny, J. M, Kotani, K, Quadro, L, and Kahn, B. B. Serum retinol binding protein 4 contributes to insulin resistance in obesity and type 2 diabetes. *Nature*, **436**, 356–362 (2005).
609. Yang, W., Lin, L., Qi, J., Yu, Z., Pei, H., He, G., Yang, Z., Wang, P., Li, G., and Pan, X. The preventive effect of acarbose and metformin on the progression to diabetes mellitus in the IGT population: a 3-year multicenter prospective study. Chin. *J. Endocrinol. Metab.*, **17**, 131–136 (2001).
610. Yang, W., Lu, J., Weng, J., et al. China National Diabetes and Metabolic Disorders Study Group. Prevalence of diabetes among men and women in China. *N. Engl. J. Med.*, **362**, 1090–1101 (2010).
611. Yang, X. D. and McDevitt, H. O. Role of TNF-alpha in the development of autoimmunity and the pathogenesis of insulin-dependent diabetes mellitus in NOD mice. *Circ. Shock*, **43**, 198–201 (1994).
612. Yasir, M., Shrivastava, R., Jain, P., and Das, D. Hypoglycemic and Antihyperglycemic Effects of Different Extracts and Combinations of Withania coagulans Dunal and Acacia arabica Lamk in Normal and Alloxan Induced Diabetic Rats. *Pharmacog. Commun.*, **2**(2), 61–66 (2012).
613. Yasuda, K., Miyake, K., Horikawa, Y., et al.Variants in KCNQ1 are associated with susceptibility to type 2 diabetes mellitus. *Nat. Genet.*, **40**, 1092–1097 (2008).
614. Yin, J., Xing, H., and Ye, J. Efficacy of berberine in patients with type 2 diabetic mellitus. *Metab.*, **57**(5), 712–717 (2008).
615. Yki-Jarvinen, H. Role of insulin resistance in the pathogenesis of NIDDM. Diabetologia, **38**, 1378–1388 (1995).
616. Yoon, J. W., Austin, M., Onodera, T., and Notkins, A. L. Isolation of a virus from the pancreas of a child with diabetic ketoacidosis. *N. Engl. J. Med.*, **300**, 1173–1179 (1979).
617. Yoon, K. H., Lee, J. H., Kim, J. W., Cho, J. H., Choi, Y. H., Ko, S. H., Zimmet, P., and Son, H. Y. Epidemic obesity and type 2 diabetes in Asia. *Lancet*, ***368***, 1681–1688 (2006).
618. Zdychova, J. and Komers, R. Emerging role of Akt Kinase/Protein Kinase B Signaling in pathophysiology of diabetes and its Complications. *Physiol. Res.*, **54**, 1–16 (2005).

619. Zeggini, E., Weedon, M. N., Lindgren, C. M., Frayling, T. M., Elliott, K. S., Lango, H., Timpson, N. J., Perry, J. R.,, Rayner, N. W., Freathy, R. M., et al. Replication of genome-wide association signals in UK samples reveals risk loci for type 2 diabetes. **Science**, **316**, 1336–1341 (2007).
620. Zhang, P., Zhang, X., Brown, J., Vistisen, D., Sicree, R., Shaw J., and Nichols G. Global healthcare expenditure on diabetes for 2010 and 2030. Diabetes Res Clin Pract., **87**, 293–301 (2010).
621. Zimmet, P., Alberti, K. G., and Shaw, J. Global and societal implications of the diabetes epidemic. Nature, **13**, 782–7 (2001).

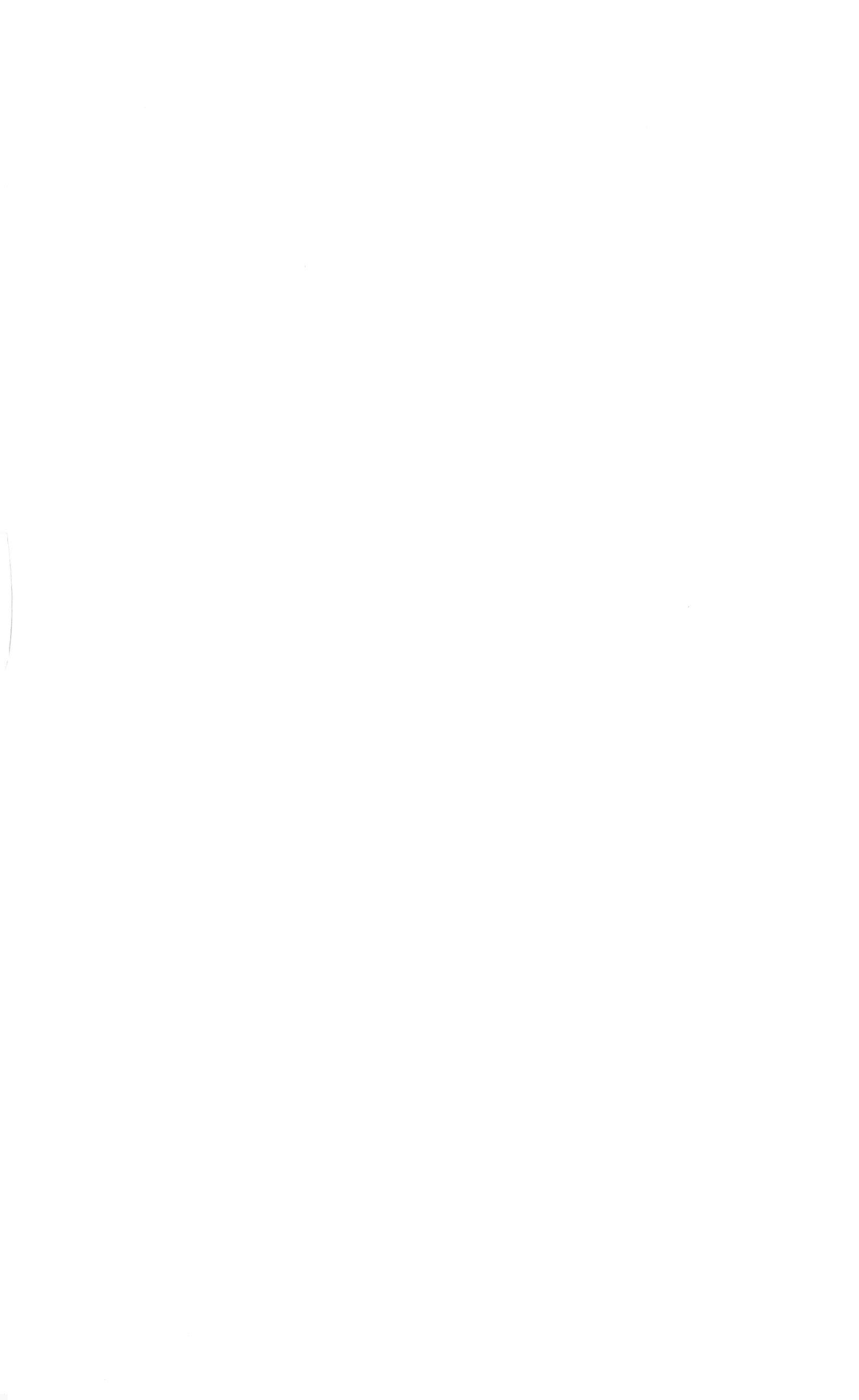

CHAPTER 2

WITHANIA COAGULANS DUNAL: AN OVERVIEW ON ITS UP TO DATE ANTIDIABETIC INVESTIGATIONS

S. HEMALATHA, SATYENDRA K. PRASAD, MANISH KUMAR, and S. D. DUBEY

CONTENTS

ABSTRACT

The fruits of *Withania coagulans* (*W. coagulans*) Dunal (Solanaceae), commonly known as *panner*, is widely used by the local population for the treatment of diabetes in Northern parts of India especially in Varanasi. In Ayurvedic system of medicine, the plant *W. coagulans* comes under *Rsyagandha*. The fruits are taken in the form of infusion (10 fruits in one glass of water with overnight soaking) in empty stomach. It posseses wide range of medicinal importance such as hepatoprotective, anti-inflammatory, antidiabetic, hypolipidemic, antioxidant, antifungal, antibacterial, cardio tonic, and wound healing activities. Recently, *W. coagulans* has gained immense popularity in the treatment of diabetes therefore, this chapter provides up to date information about the various investigations conducted confirming it to be a potential antidiabetic tool. It shown that aqueous extract of fruits of *W. coagulans* (1 g/kg: p.o.) have significantly lowered the blood sugar, serum cholesterol, serum LPO, and hepatic LPO levels. Investigation on effect of *W. coagulans* on glucose uptake by rat hemi-diaphragm justified its potential in peripheral utilization of glucose. Its hypoglycemic activity at the same dose was also confirmed through glucose tolerance test, normoglycemic studies, and chronic treatment. A new withanolide that is coagulanolide (4) along with four known withanolides (1–3) and (5) have been isolated from fruits, which have shown to possess significant antihyperglycemic and antidyslipidemic activity comparable to metformin. The recent investigation has depicted its role in diabetic wound healing which was evident through a significant increase in the rate of wound contraction and levels of collagen, protein, deoxyribonucleic acid (DNA), superoxide dismutase (SOD), catalase (CAT), and decrease in level of hexosamine. A clinical study using aqueous extract of *W. coagulans* (*Sitakasaya*) showed significant results in type II diabetic patients. Thus, this chapter will act as a source of valuable information and as awareness for diabetic patients about the clinical significance of *W. coagulans* in treatment of diabetes.

2.1 INTRODUCTION

In India, Ayurveda is the most ancient health care system of medicines involving Atharveda (around 1200 BC), *Charak samhita* and *Sushrut Samhita* (100–500 BC) (Dash and Sharma, 2001) describing details of more than 700 herbs. This system of medicines have provided researches of various fields like pharmacognosy, pharmacology, chemistry, and therapeutics of various pharmaceutical corporation to renew their strategies in favor of natural products drug discovery which resulted in incorporation of many of such drugs in international pharmacopoeia on the basis of their ethnopharmacological and traditional reports (Waxler, 1988). With the estimated 10–100 million species or organisms and higher plants form a group of some 2,50,000 species, only 6% of the plants and 15% of their chemicals have been investigated for biological activities. The current estimate shows that about 80% of people in developing countries still rely on traditional medicine from plant or animal source. Among all the drugs sold in worldwide market 30% of drugs belong to the plant source (Abourashed, et al., 2004).

Because of their high biological activity, high safety margin, and lesser cost than the synthetic drugs, there is a great demand for herbal medicine in developed as well as in developing countries (Gadro et al., 2001). The importance of medicinal plants from antiquity to date has led herbal therapy, over the years, to become one of the pillars of areas like pharmacy, medicine, natural product chemistry, and others. All these scientific disciplines now recognize the importance of plants as sources of medicines and have initiated active research program either to isolate new lead compounds or to produce standardized extracts (Prasad et al., 2010b).

Diabetes mellitus is defined as a group of disorders characterized by hyperglycemia, altered metabolism of lipids, carbohydrates, and proteins (Warjeet, 2004; Pareek et al., 2009). It is considered to be third "killer" of mankind's health along with cancer, cardiovascular, and cerebrovascular diseases (Chauhan et al., 2010). It may also be caused either due to insufficient insulin secretion, insulin action, or both. The common symptoms of diabetes mellitus are increased thirst, increased urinary output, ketonaemia, and ketouria. The prevalence of diabetes mellitus is expected to reach up to 4.4% by 2030 with maximum contribution from India, China, and

USA. Among all the types of diabetes, type 2 diabetes (non-insulin-dependent diabetes mellitus) is the most common which covers around 90–95% of all cases where body is unable to produce enough insulin or properly use it (Balaraman et al., 2010; Li et al., 2004). The World Health Organization has estimated that, diabetic population is likely to increase up to 300 million or more by the year 2025 (Sy et al., 2005; Meenakshi et al., 2008). Recently, diabetes mellitus has resulted in rapid rise in unhealthy life style, urbanization, and aging leading to significant increase in morbidity and mortality attributed to microvascular (retinopathy, neuropathy, and nephropathy) and macrovascular (heart attack, stroke, and peripheral vascular disease) complications (Bagria et al., 2009).

Therapies available for diabetes include insulin and various oral antidiabetic agents such as sulfonylureas, biguanides, and glinides where many of them have a number of serious adverse effects. Therefore, it focused on antidiabetic agents from plant source aiming for more effective and safer antidiabetic agents (Saxena and Vikram, 2004). The traditional medicines from readily available medicinal plants offer great potential for the discovery of new antidiabetic drugs (Jung et al., 2006). The attributing factor for antihyperglycemic activity of plants lies mainly due to their ability to restore the function of pancreatic tissues by causing an increase in insulin output or inhibit the intestinal absorption of glucose or facilitation of metabolites in insulin dependent processes. The main class of phytochemicals responsible for antidiabetic activity includes phenols, glycosides, alkaloids, terpenoids, flavonoids, saponins, tannins, and cartenoids (Malviya et al., 2010).

Withania coagulans Dunal is one of such plant which has recently gained remarkable importance majorly in relation to botanical, commercial, ethnopharmacological, phytochemical, pharmacological, and toxicological studies that appears in the literature. *W. coagulans* belongs to family Solanaceae and is distributed in the East of the Mediterranean region and extends up to South Asia. It shows the presence of esterases, lignan, alkaloids, free amino acids, fatty oils, essential oils, and withanolides (Kiritikar and Basu, 1999). The different parts of this plant have been reported to possess a variety of biological activities. It possesses potent antidiabetic, hypolipidemic, antioxidant (Hemalatha et al., 2004), wound healing (Hemalatha et al., 2008), antimicrobial (Gaind and Budhiraja, 1967), and cardio tonic activities (Budhiraja et al., 1983). The fruit, berries are used for commercial purposes like milk coagulation (Kiritikar and Basu, 1999). As the plant has recently gained vast therapeutic and commercial value therefore, this chapter highlights into one of its most popular therapeutic identity that is a potential antidiabetic agent. This chapter gives us up to date information on different investigations carried out on the fruits of plant as a potential tool for the treatment of diabetes.

2.2 PLANT PROFILE

2.2.1 GEOGRAPHICAL DISTRIBUTION

It is grown mainly in the Eastern parts of Mediterranean regions like Sutlej valley, Sindh, Afghanistan, and extends up to South Asia. In India it is grown in the Northern plains of Punjab and also in the hilly regions of Simla, Kumaun, and Garhwal (Kiritikar and Basu, 1999).

2.2.2 TAXONOMICAL DESCRIPTION

Kingdom	Plantae, Plants
Subkingdom	Tracheobionta, Vascular plants
Super division	Spermatophyta, Seeds plants
Division	Angiosperms
Class	Dicotyledons
Order	Tubiflorae
Family	Solanaceae
Genus	*Withania*
Species	*Withania coagulans* Dunal

2.2.3 SYNONYMS (KIRITIKAR AND BASU, 1999)

Hindi	*Dudha panir, Bimputakah, Akri, Punir*
Punjabi	*Panir, Kharmjaria, Khumazare*

Tamil	*Amukkra*
Telugu	*Pennerugadd*a
Urdu	*Kakamaj*

2.2.4 BOTANICAL DESCRIPTION (CHADHA, 1976; KIRITIKAR AND BASU, 1999)

Withania coagulans is a rigid, gray under shrub, 60–120 cm high, and the plant flowers during November–April and the berries ripen during January–May. The natural regeneration is from the seed. The flowers are dioceous, in auxiliary clusters, pedicil 0.6 mm long, deflexed, and slender. Calyx is 6 mm long, campanulate, and clothed with fine stellate greay tomentum; teeth triangular, and 2.5 mm long. Corolla are 8 mm long stellately mealy outside and divided about 1/3 the way down; lobes ovate-oblong and sub acute. In male flowers stamens are in about level with the top of the corolla tube with filament 2 mm long, glabrous, and anthers 3–4 mm long while in female flowers, stamens scarcely reaches 1/2 way up the corolla tube; filaments are about 0.85 mm long; anther smaller than in the male flowers and are sterile. Ovary is ovoid, gabalaras, style gal-abrous, stigma mushroom-shaped, and 2-lamellate. Berries are 6–8 mm globose, smooth, closely girt by the enlarged membranous calyx, which is scurfy-pubescent outside. Seeds are 2.5–3.0 mm in diameter, somewhat ear shaped, and glabrous (Figure 1).

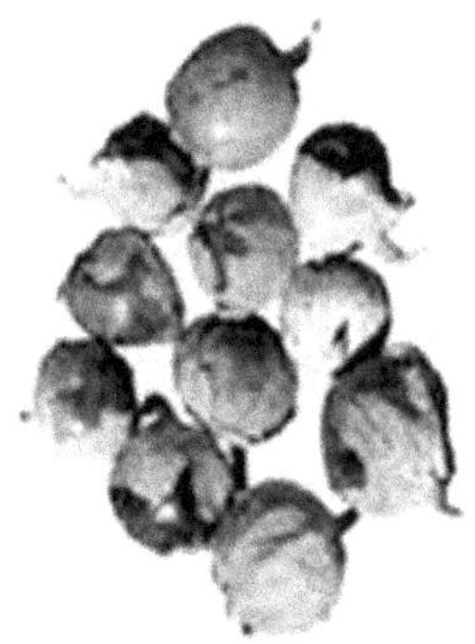

FIGURE 1 Fruits of *W. coagulans* Dunal (Prasad et al., 2010b).

2.2.5 MACROSCOPICAL AND MICROSCOPICAL DESCRIPTION OF FRUITS

The fruits are superior, indehiscent, and many seeded berry type. It is pedicellate, round to globous in shape, 4–6 mm in diameter, yellow to brown in colour, and closed in leathery persistent calyx mostly with pedicel. The fruits have an indistinct odour with a slightly bitter taste (Figure 1). The transverse section of the pedicel shows a single layered epidermis covered with a large number of branched and unbranched trichomes, followed by cortex constituting 6–10 layers of collenchymatous cells. The pericycle shows the presence of pericyclic fibers with intervening parenchymatous cells, whereas the central region represents a continuous narrow band of phloem encircling the xylem beneath which is a ring of intraxylary phloem. The centre most region is consist of hollow pith surrounded by parenchymatous cells with a few thick walled lignified fibers towards the intraxylary phloem. The calyx shows a single layer of thin walled cells in upper and lower epidermis with a few branched and more unicellular covering trichomes similar to the pedicel which are present only in the upper epidermis, followed by the presence of few candelabra-type trichomes. The mesophyll is represented by spongy parenchyma traversed by a number of small veins covered with a bundle sheath of thin walled parenchymatous cells (Figure 2).

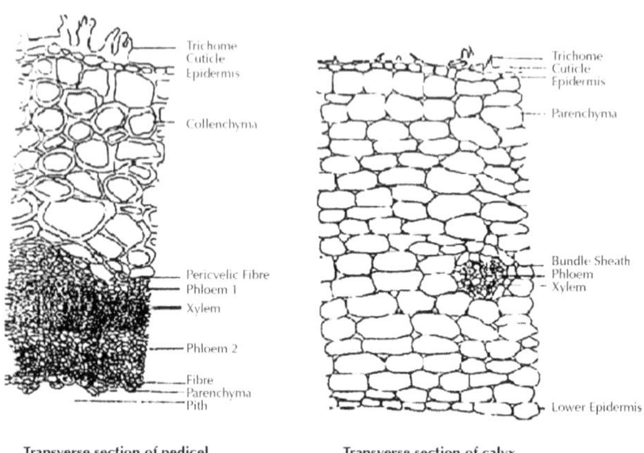

FIGURE 2 Microscopical characters of pedicel and calyx of fruit of *W. coagulans* (Prasad et al., 2010b).

The transverse section of fruit shows the presence of exocarp which represents a single layer while mesocarp shows a wide zone of parenchymatous cells with strong cellulosic thickening. The endocarp is similar to that of exocarp but at some places the cells are flattened and collapsed. The seeds in transverse section show a single layer of epidermis followed by a layer of highly flattened thin walled sub-epidermal cells. Beneath the sub-epidermis there is a layer of highly lignified palisade-like cells with narrow lumen. The inner epidermis of the seed coat comprise of 1–2 layer of thin-walled parenchymatous cells which at places are collapsed showing hyaline like structure. The endosperm is represented by cells showing strong cellulosic thickening filled with aluerone grains without any globoide. The cotyledon shows thin-walled radially elongated cells enclosing a wide zone of round to oval to polyhedral parenchymatous cells (Figure 3).

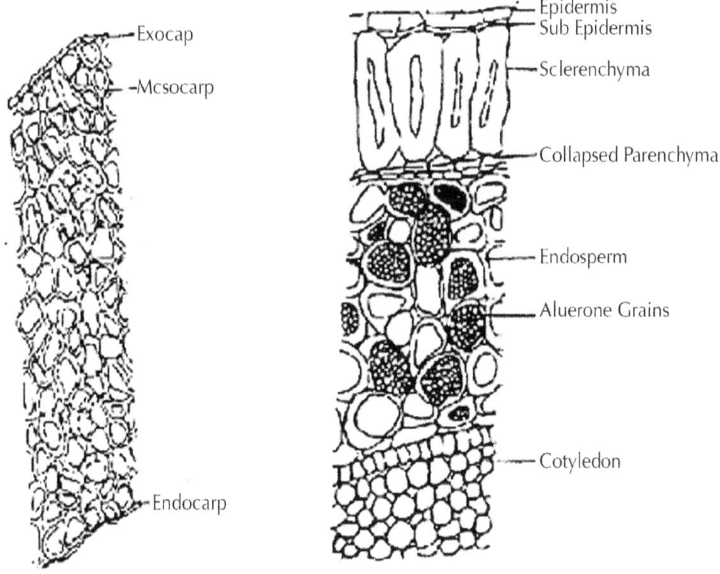

FIGURE 3 Microscopical characters of pericarp and seed of fruit of *W. coagulans* (Prasad et al., 2010b).

The powder characteristic of the fruits of *W. coagulans* is demonstrated in Figure 4 (A), which shows a large number of parenchymatous cells of cotyledons (a), fragments of pericarp showing parenchymatous cells (b–c), thick walled endosperm cells showing aluerone grains (d–e), epidermal cells of calyx with unicellular covering trichomes (f) and few xylem vessels with spiral thickening (p) (Figure 4(B)).

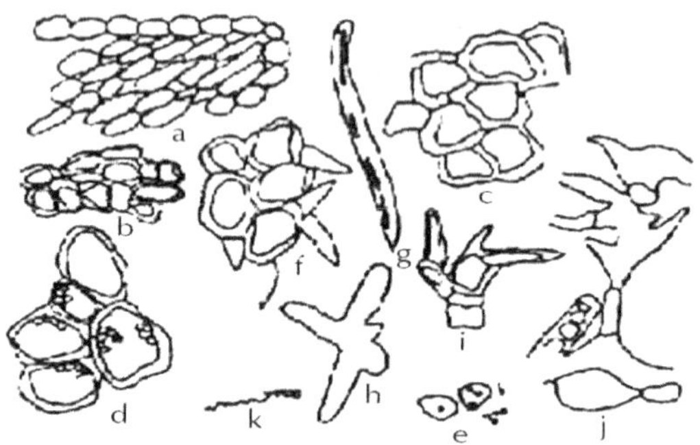

Powder characteristics of fruits
A

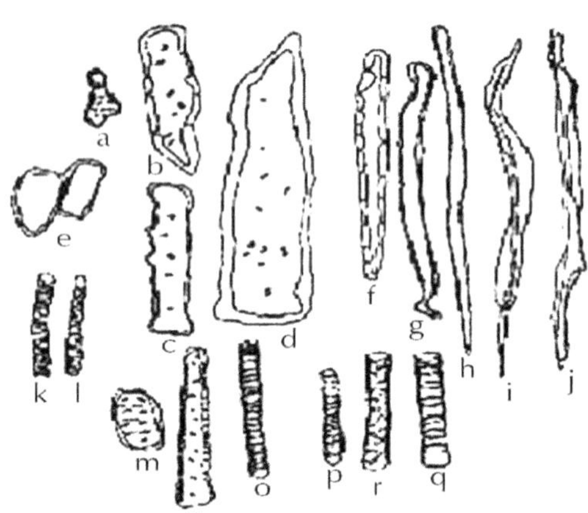

Isolated elements of fruits
B

FIGURE 4 Powder characteristics (A) and isolated elements (B) of fruits of *W. Coagulans*.

In Figure 4(A) a: Portion of cotyledon, b–c: Pericarp in surface view, d–e: Endosperm cells with aluerone grains, f: Upper epidermis of calyx, g: Fibre, h–j: Trichome, k: Xylem vessel. In Figure 4(B) a–d: Tracheids, e: Parenchyma, f–j: Fibre, k–r: Tracheidal vessels (Prasad et al., 2010b).

2.2.6 PHYTOCHEMISTRY

Phytochemical investigation of *W. coagulans* showed the presence of mainly steroids that is withanoloid. It also showed the presence of alkaloids, phenolic compounds, saponins, and carbohydrates. The major constituents isolated from the fruits of the plant includes Withaferin A, 3β-hydroxy-2,3-dihydrowithanolide F, β-Sitosterol-3-β-D-glucoside, 14β,15β-epoxywithanolide I, Enzymes-esterase, Amino acids, Coagulin B–R, Withacoagulin, Coagulanonide 4, 17β-hydroxywithanolide K, Withanolide F, and (17S,20S,22R)-14α,15α,17β,20β-tetrahydroxy-1-oxowitha-2,5,24-trienolide (Hemalatha et al., 2008; Maurya et al., 2010). Different phytoconstituents isolated from the different parts of the plants are represented in Table 1.

TABLE 1 Phytoconstituents isolated from *W. coagulans*

Phytoconstituents	Structure	Isolated from part of plant/ extract	References
5α, 20α (R) Dihydroxy-6α,7α-epoxy-1-oxo witha-2, 24-dienolide	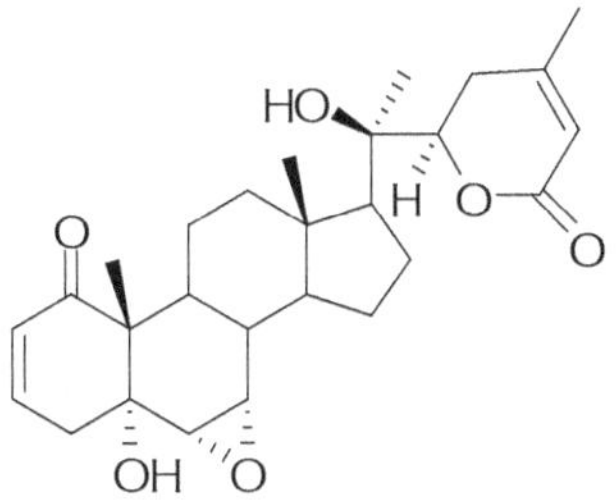 HO, H, O, O, O, OH, O	Fruit	(Anonymous, 1996)

TABLE 1 *(Continued)*

5α, 17α Dihydroxy-1-oxo-6α, 7α-epoxy-22 R-witha-2, 24-dienolide	OH, O, O, OH, O	Fruit	(Anonymous, 1996)
Withaferin	OH, O, O, O, HO, O	Fruit	(Neogi, et al., 1988)
Chlorogenic acid	HO, COOH, O, HO, O, HO, OH, OH	Leaves	(Karthikar and Basu, 1993)
Linoleic acid	$H_3C-(CH_2)-(CH=CH)_2-CH_2-(CH_3)_6-C(=O)OH$	Seed	(Anonymous, 1996)
β-Sitosterol	H_3C, H_3C, H_3C, H_3C, CH_3, H_3C, H, H, HO	Seed	(Anonymous, 1996)

TABLE 1 *(Continued)*

D-Galactose	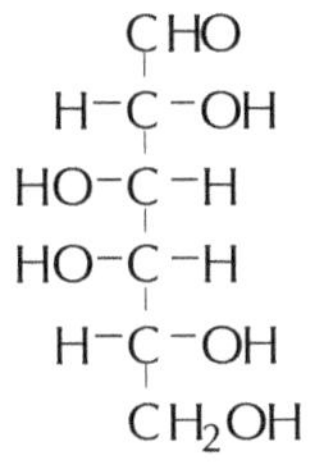 CHO H–C–OH HO–C–H HO–C–H H–C–OH CH_2OH	Seed	(Anonymous, 1996)
D-Arabinose	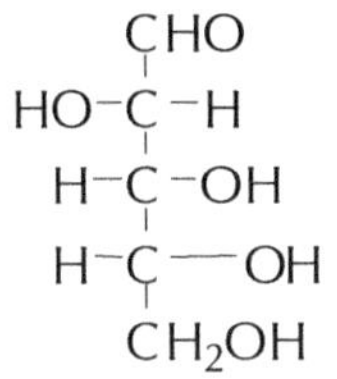 CHO HO–C–H H–C–OH H–C–OH CH_2OH	Seed	(Anonymous, 1996)
5α, 27-Dihydroxy-6α,7α-epoxy-1-oxo witha-2, 24-dienolide	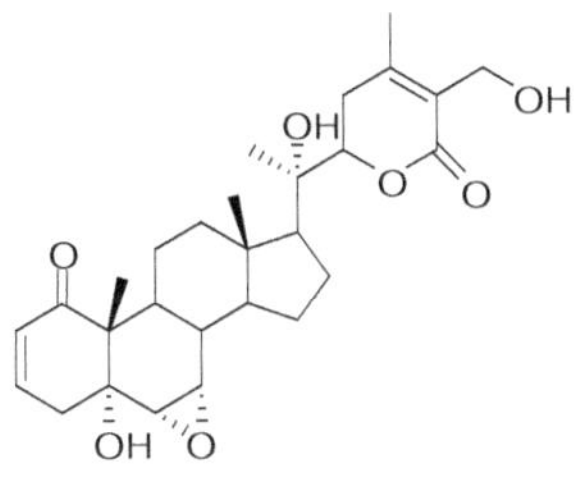	Fruit	(Anonymous, 1996)
Withaferin A	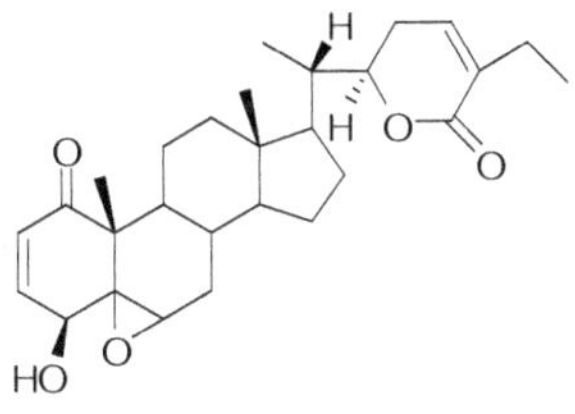	Root	(Subramanian, et al., 1969)
3β-Hydroxy-2,3-dihydrowithanolide F	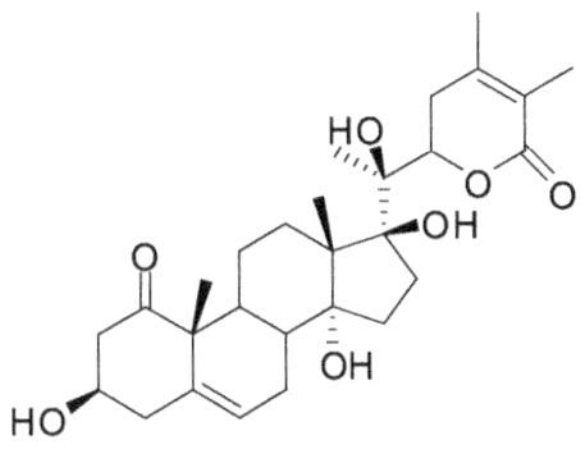	Fruit	(Budhiraja et al., 1983)

TABLE 1 *(Continued)*

5,20 α (R)-Dihydroxy-6 α ,7 α -epoxy-1-oxo-(5 α)-witha-2,24-dienolide	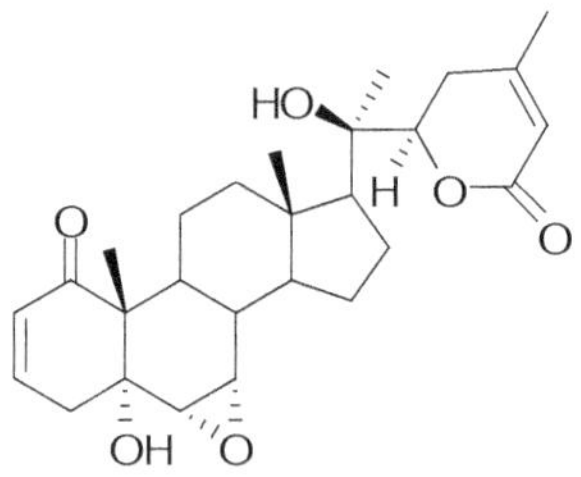	Dry leaves	(Subramanian et al., 1971)
Ergosta-5,25-dien-3 β, 24-ε diol	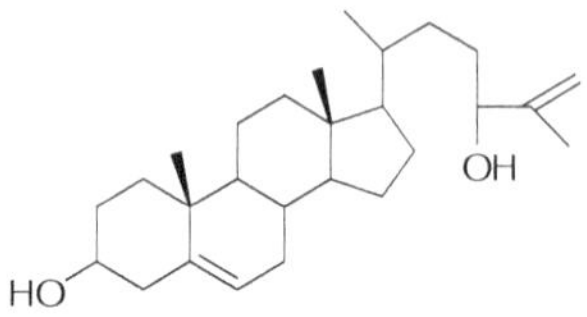	Fruit	(Vincent et al., 1983)
β-Sitosterol-3- β-D- glucoside	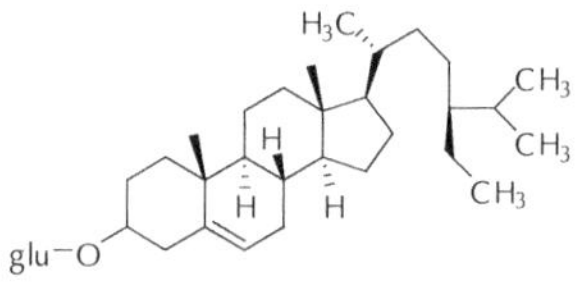	Fruit	(Vincent et al., 1983)
3α, 14α, 17 β, 20 α-Tetrahydroxy-1-oxo-20 S, 22R-with-5, 24-dienolide	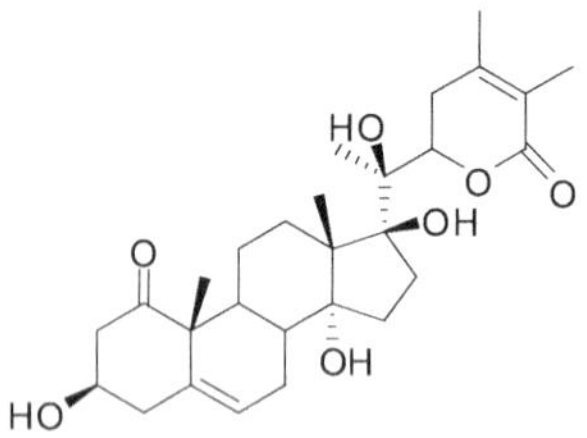	Fruit	(Vincent et al., 1983)
Fatty acid	CH_3-$(CH_2)_n$-CH_2-CH_2-COOH	Seed	(Sattar et al., 1988)
Withacoagin	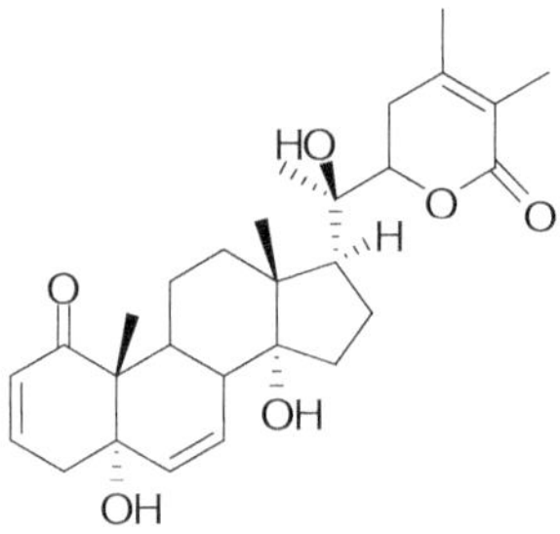	Root	(Neogi, et al., 1988)

TABLE 1 *(Continued)*

(20 R, 22R) 6α, 7α-Epoxy-5α,20-dihydroxy-1-oxo-witha-2, 24-dienolide		Root	(Neogi, et al., 1988)
(20 S, 22R) 6α, 7α-Epoxy-5α-hydroxy-1-oxo- witha-2, 24-di-enolide		Root	(Neogi, et al.., 1988)
17β, 27 Dihydroxy-14, 20-epoxy-1-oxo-22R-witha-3, 5, 24-trienolide	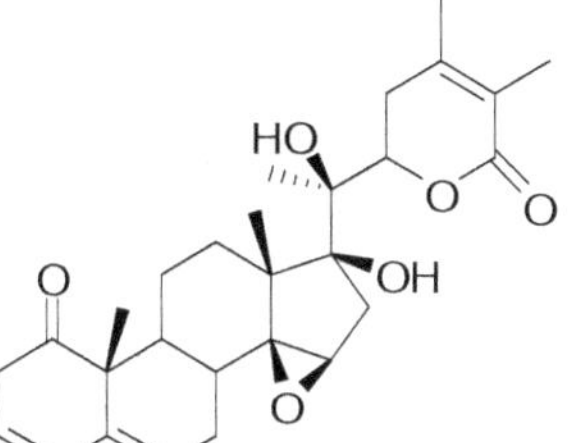	Whole plant	(Atta-ur-Rahman et al., 1993)
14β, 15β-Epoxywithanolide I		Whole plant	(Chaudhary et al.., 1995)

TABLE 1 *(Continued)*

17β, 20β- Dihydroxy-1-oxo-witha-2,5,24-trienolide	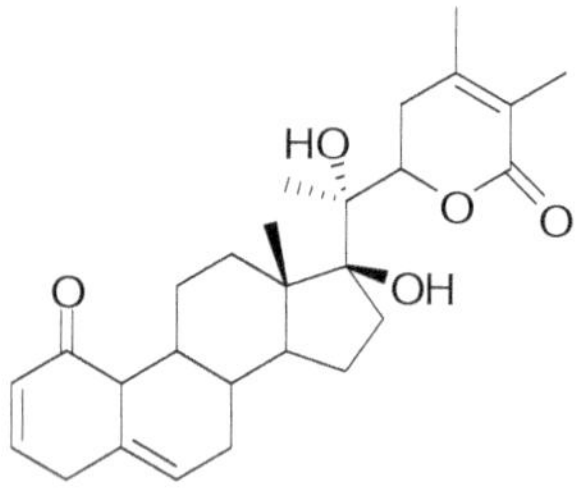	Whole plant	(Chaudhary et al., 1995)
Enzymes-esterase, Amino acids	-	Fruit	(Anonymous, 1996)
Coagulin B	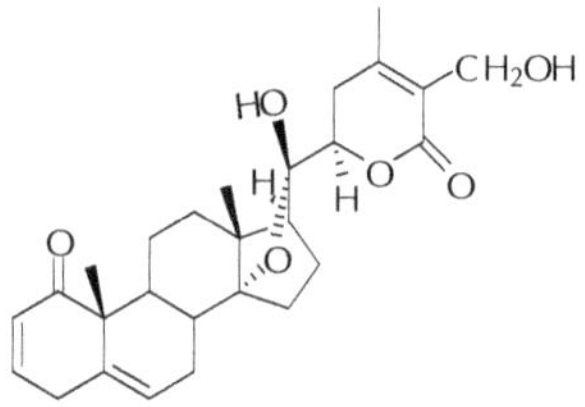	Aerial parts of plant	(Atta-ur-Rahman et al., 1998a)
Coagulin C	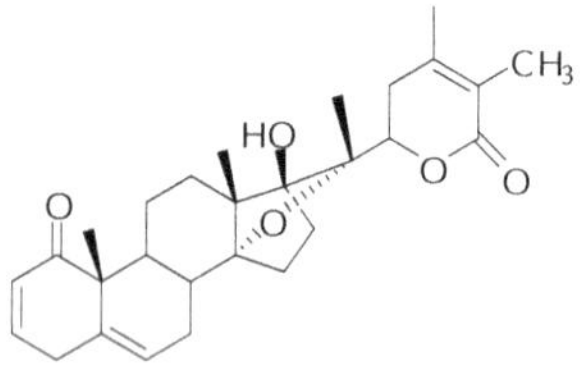	Aerial parts of plant	(Atta-ur-Rahman et al., 1998a)
Coagulin D	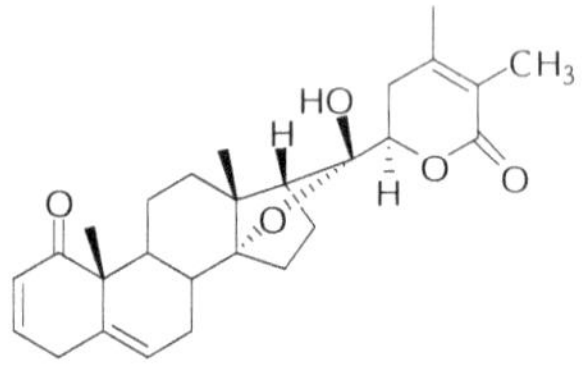	Aerial parts of plant	(Atta-ur-Rahman et al., 1998a)
Coagulin E	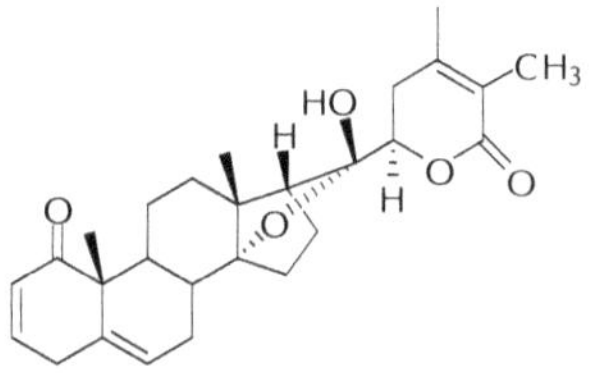	Aerial parts of plant	(Atta-ur-Rahman et al., 1998a)

TABLE 1 *(Continued)*

Coagulin F 27-hydroxy-14,20-epoxy-1-oxo-(22R)-witha-3,5,24-trienolide	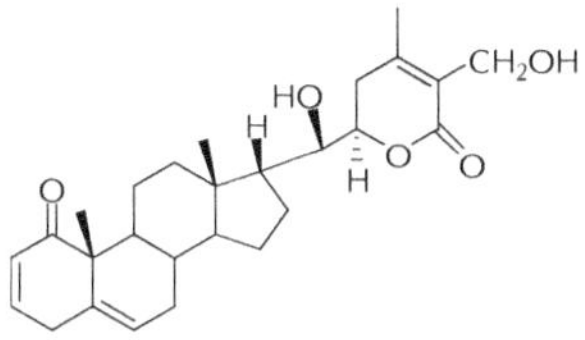	Whole plant	(Atta-ur-Rahman et al., 1998b)
Coagulin G 17β,27-dihydroxy-14,20-epoxy-1-oxo-(22R)-witha-2,5,24-trienolide	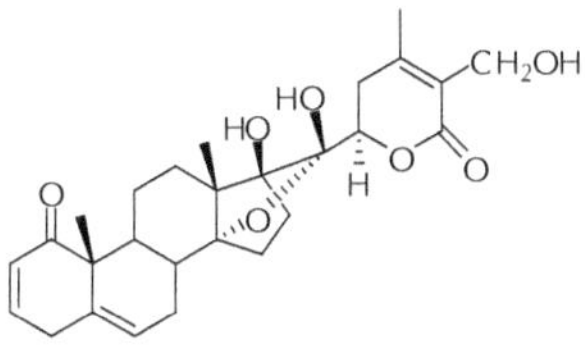	Whole plant	(Atta-ur-Rahman et al., 1998b)
Coagulin H 5 α ,6β,14 α ,15 α ,17,20-hexahydroxy-1-oxowitha-2,24-dienolide	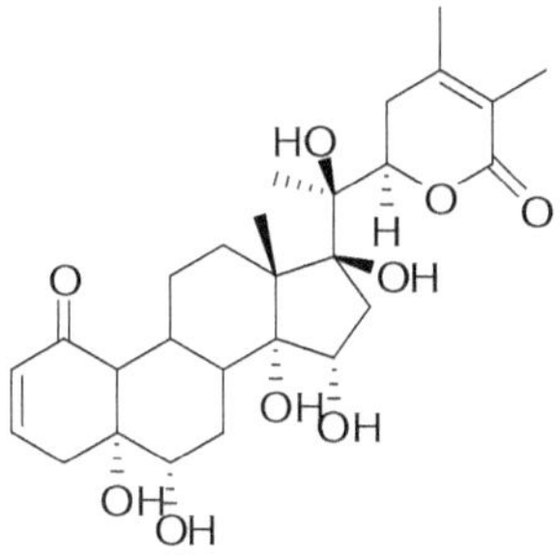	Whole plant	(Atta-ur-Rahman et al., 1998c)
Coagulin I 5 α ,6 β ,17-trihydroxy-14,20-epoxy-1-oxowitha-2,24-dienolide	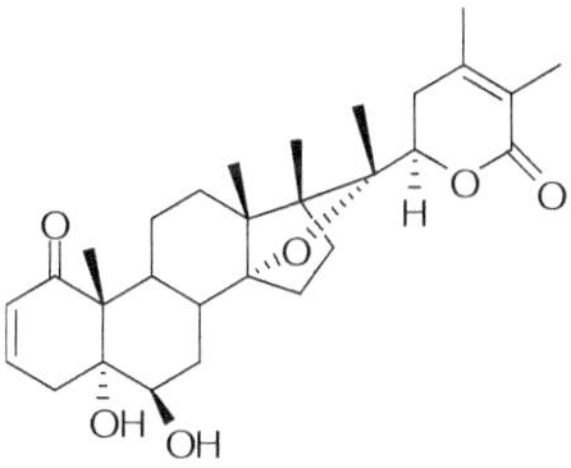	Whole plant	(Atta-ur-Rahman et al., 1998c)
Coagulin J 3 β ,27-dihydroxy-14,20-epoxy-1-oxowitha-5,24-dienolide	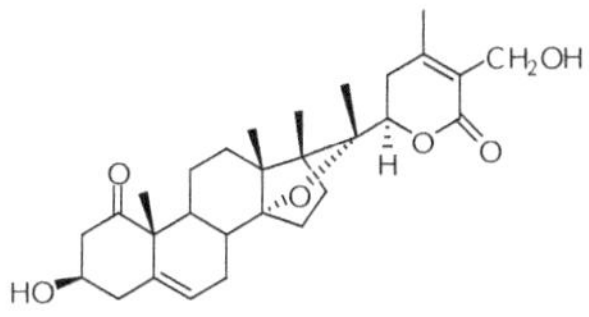	Whole plant	(Atta-ur-Rahman et al., 1998c)

TABLE 1 *(Continued)*

Coagulin K 14,20-epoxy-3 β -(O- β -D-glucopyranosyl)-1-oxowitha-5,24-dienolide	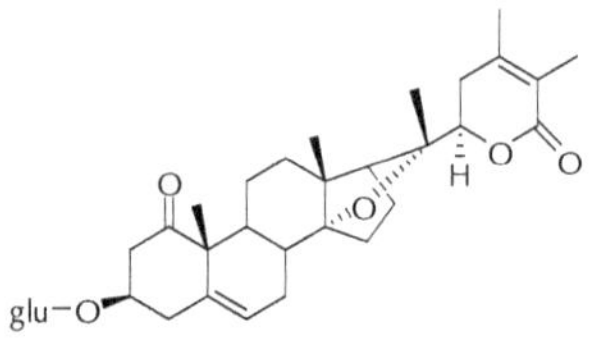	Whole plant	(Atta-ur-Rahman et al., 1998c)
Coagulin L 14,17,20-trihydroxy-3 β -(O- β -D-glucopyranosyl)-1-oxowitha-5,24-dienolide	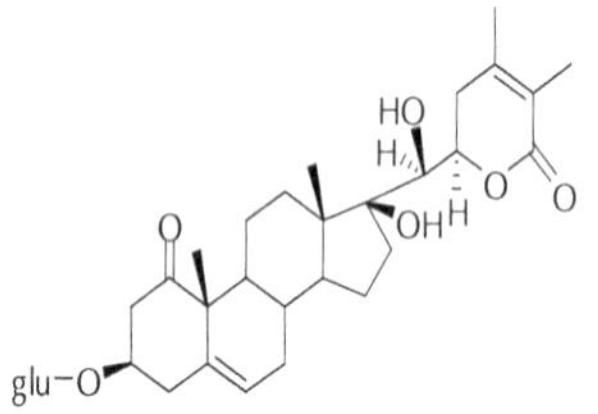	Whole plant	(Atta-ur-Rahman et al., 1998c)
Coagulin M 5 α ,6 β ,27-trihydroxy-14,20-epoxy-1-oxo-witha-24-enolide	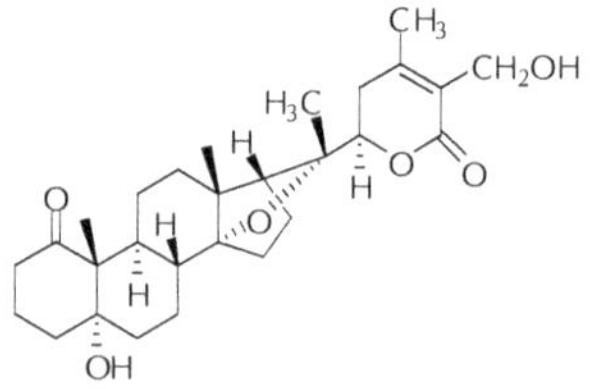	Whole plant	(Atta-ur-Rahman et al., 1998d)
Coagulin N 15 α ,17-dihydroxy-14,20-epoxy-3 β -(O- β -D-glucopyranosyl)-1-oxowitha-5,24-dienolide	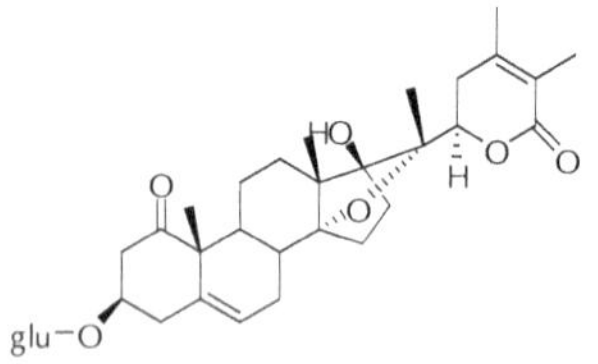	Whole plant	(Atta-ur-Rahman et al., 1998d)
Coagulin O 14,20-dihydroxy-3 β -(O- β -D-glucopyranosyl)-1-oxowitha-5,24-dienolide	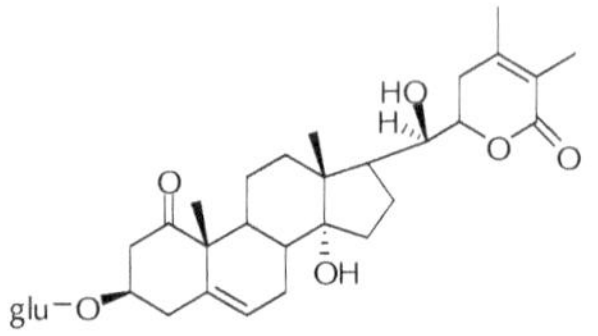	Whole plant	(Atta-ur-Rahman et al., 1998d)
Coagulin P 20,27-dihydroxy-3 β -(O-b-D-glucopyranosyl)-1-oxo-(20S,22R)-witha-5,14,24-trienolide,	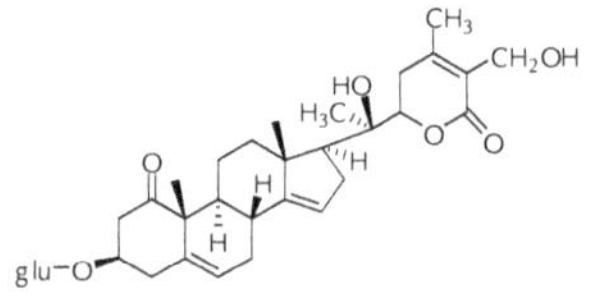	Whole plant	(Atta-ur-Rahman et al., 1999)

TABLE 1 *(Continued)*

Coagulin Q 1 α, 20-Dihydroxy-3 β -(O- β -D-Glucopyranosyl)-(20S,22R)-witha-5,24-dienolide	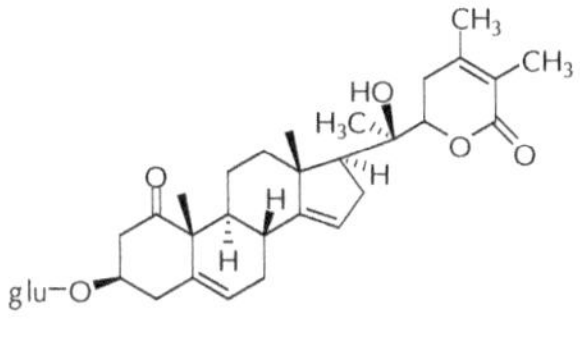	Whole plant	(Atta-ur-Rahman et al., 1999)
Coagulin R 3 β,17 β -Dihydroxy-14,20-epoxy-1-oxo-(22R)-witha-5,24-dienolide	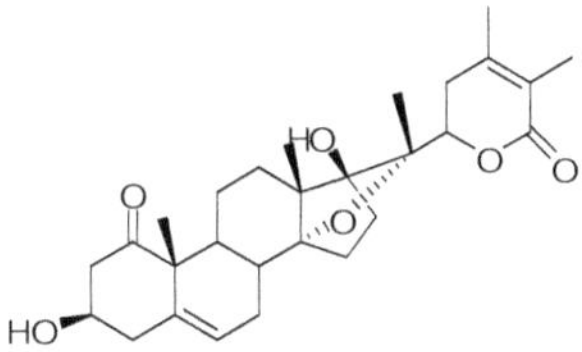	Whole plant	(Atta-ur-Rahman et al., 1999)
20β, Hydroxy-1-oxo-(22R)-witha-2,5,24-trienolide	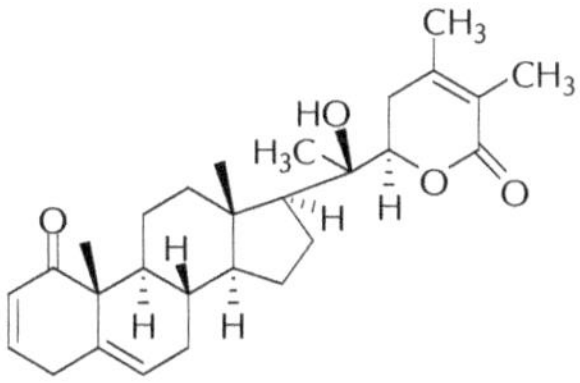	Fruit	(Atta-ur-Rahman et al., 2003)
Withacoagulin	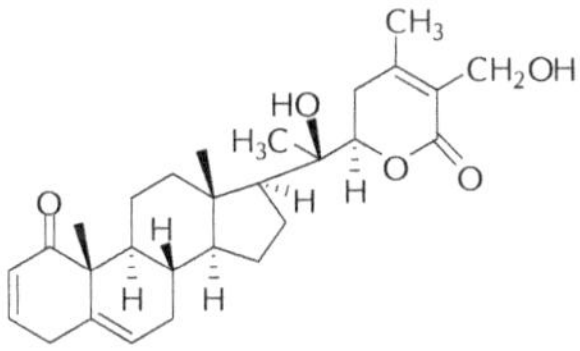	Fruit	(Atta-ur-Rahman et al., 2003)
Coagulin S (20S*,22R*)-5 α ,6 β ,14 α ,15 α ,17 β ,20,27-Heptahydroxy-1-oxowith-24-enolide	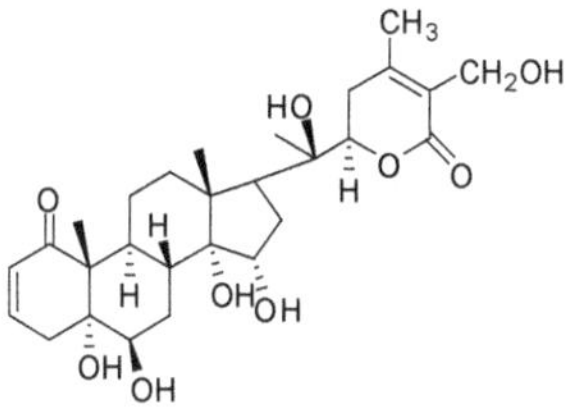	Fruit	(Nur-E-Alam et al., 2003)
17b-Hydroxywithanolide K	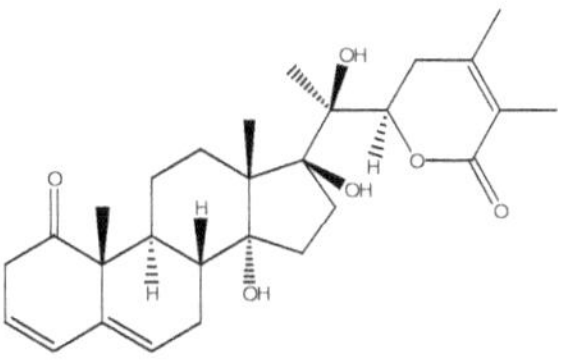	Fruits	(Maurya et al., 2008)

TABLE 1 *(Continued)*

Withanolide F	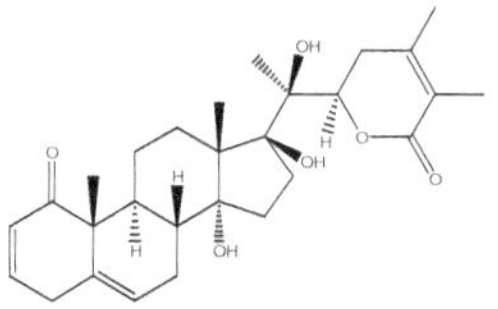	Fruits	(Maurya et al., 2008)
Coagulanonide 4 ((17S,20S,20S,22R)-14α,15α,17β,20β-Tetrahydroxy-1-oxowitha-2,5,24-trienolide))	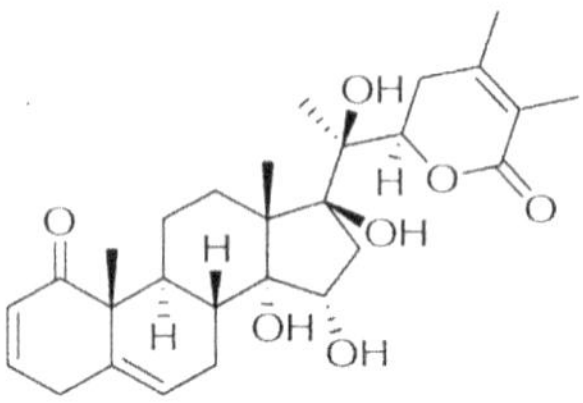	Fruits	(Maurya et al., 2008)

2.2.7 ETHNOMEDICINAL IMPORTANCE

Ethnoomedically the fruits of the plant possess sedative, emetic, and diuretic action and are used in dyspepsia, flatulent, asthma, biliousness, and as a blood purifier. It is also used in the treatment of ulcers, rheumatism, and dropsy, which is well known in the traditional system of medicines. The twigs are chewed for cleaning teeth and the smoke of the plant is inhaled for relief in toothache. In Pakistan, leaves are used as vegetable, and fodder for camels and sheep. The fruits are applied to wound, while leaves are used as febrifuge. The seeds are useful in ophthalamia, and lessen the inflammation of piles (Hemalatha et al., 2008).

2.2.8 ECONOMICAL IMPORTANCE

Since the fruits and leaves of *W. coagulans* have properties to coagulate milk therefore, it is commonly known as '*paneer*', 'cheese maker' or 'vegetable rennet' in Northern parts of India. The above properties of the fruit may be attributed to the presence of an enzyme in pulp and husk of berries, which has milk coagulating activity. A decoction is made from one ounce fruit of *W. coagulans* and one quart of boiling water, one table spoonful of which coagulate a gallon of warm milk in about an hour (Dymock et al., 1972). In Punjab, the berries of *W. coagulans* are used as the source of coagulating enzyme for clotting the milk and therefore, are called as '*paneer*'. Buffalo or sheep milk is warmed to about 1000°F and crushed berries of plant, tied in a cloth, are dipped in it. The milk takes 30–40 min to curdle (Kiritikar and Basu, 1999).

2.2.9 PHARMACOLOGICAL IMPORTANCE

The different parts of the plants have been evaluated for numerous pharmacological activities. Treatment with aqueous extract of fruits of *W. coagulans* at 1 g/kg p.o. for 7 days has shown to possess hypoglycemic activity in normal and streptozotocin (STZ)-induced diabetic rats. The results depicted a significant reduction in the elevated blood glucose, cholesterol, and lipid peroxidation (LPO) levels in diabetic rats (Hemalatha et al., 2004). A potential free radical scavenging activity of aqueous extract of *W. coagulans* was evaluated in an *in vitro* system using 1,1-diphenyl-2-picrylhydrazyl (DPPH) (Hemalatha et al., 2004). Aqueous extract of fruits of *W. coagulans* at 1 g/kg; p.o. was administered to high fat diet (HFD) induced hyperlipidemic and triton induced hypercholesterolemic rats which significantly reduced elevated serum cholesterol, triglycerides, lipoprotein, and LPO levels (Hemalatha et al., 2006). Hydroalcoholic fraction of *W. coagulans* showed significant wound healing activity in normal as well as diabetic rats showing an accelerated collagen, mucopolysaccharides, DNA, and protein synthesis (Hemalatha et al., 2008; Prasad et al., 2010a).

Essential oil obtained from petroleum ether extract of the fruits showed potential activity against *Micrococcus pyrogenes* var. aureus and *Vibrio cholerae*. Different extracts of the fruits of *W. coagulans* showed a potential antibacterial activity against *Staphylococcus aureus, Escherichia coli,* and *Vibrio cholera* and was also reported to have anthelminic activity (Gaind and Budhiraja, 1967). Ethanolic extract of leaves and stem of *W. coagulans* have also been reported to have antibacterial activity (Khan et al., 1993). A significant antifungal activity of a steroidal lactone 17β-hydroxywithanolide K [(20S, 22R) 14α, 17β, 20β-trihydroxy-1-oxowitha-2,5, 24-trienolide] isolated from the ethanolic extract of whole plant of *W. coagulans* was reported by Choudhary et al. (1995).

A withanolide isolated from fruits of *W. coagulans* has shown to posses cardiovascular effects at a dose of 5 mg/kg showing a moderate fall of blood pressure in dogs (34 ± 2.1 mm Hg), while in case of rabbits it produced myocardial depressant effects but in perfused frog heart it produced mild positive inotropic and chronotropic effects (Budhiraja et al., 1983). Root extract of *W. coagulans* had shown significant effect on the withdrawal syndrome which was evident through morphine induced withdrawal jump in mice (Karami et al., 2006). The 3β-hydroxy-2, 3-dihydrowithanolide F, isolated from the fruits of *W. coagulans* has shown protective effect against CCl_4 induced hepatotoxicity (Budhiraja et al., 1984).

Budhiraja et al. (1984) has reported anti-inflammatory activity of a withanolide from *W. coagulans* showing marked effects in sub-acute inflammation in experimental rats. A significant anti-inflammatory activity was observed with hydroalcoholic extract of the berries of *W. coagulans* in carrageenan induced rat paw edema model (Rajurkar et al., 2001). Withaferin A, even at a low dose of 10 mg/kg has been reported for their immunoactivating as well as immunosuppressive activities (Bahr and Hansel, 1982). The immunoactivation property may be attributed to an inducing proliferation of peritoneal macrophages in mice and not in splenocytes (Shohat and Joshua, 1971). A study has revealed immunosuppressive action of withaferin A on human B and T lymphocytes as well as on mice thymocytes. At very low concentrations, it has also shown to inhibit erythrocyte (E) rosettes and erythrocyte-antibody-complement (EAC) rosette formation by normal human T and B lymphocytes (Shohat et al., 1978). 5,20a(R)-dihydroxy-6a,7a-epoxy-1-oxo-(5a)-witha-2,24-dienolide isolated from the plant has shown to possess immunosuppressant activity in spleen cell culture by inhibiting proliferation of murine spleen cell cultures (Bahr and Hansel, 1982). Coagulin H exhibited an inhibitory effect on lymphocyte proliferation and expression of interleukin-2 (IL-2) cytokine which also completely suppressed phytohaemagglutinin-activated T-cells at ≥2.5 μg/mL. Docking studies have revealed that coagulin H binds more effectively than prednisolone to receptor binding site of IL-2 (Mesaik et al., 2006).

The alcoholic extract, total alkaloids and aqueous extract of *W. coagulans* fruits at a dose of 1 g/kg, 200–400 mg/kg, and 5 mg/100 g demonstrated a significant central nervous system (CNS) depressant activity in albino rats which was characterized by sedation, reduced exploratory, spontaneous activity, and hypothermia. The extract also potentiated the pentobarbitone sleeping time in rats when administered at the same dose, 30 min before a hypnotic (Budhiraja et al., 1977). The compound 3β -hydroxy-2,3-dihydro-withanolide F was tested for its CNS depressant activity, where it did not show any analgesic, hypothermic or local anesthetic activity (Budhiraja and Sudhir, 1987).

The aqueous extract of *W. coagulans* was evaluated for anti cytotoxic activity in lymphocytes of healthy broiler chickens. The extract at concentration of 600 mg/ml depicted a significant protection against dimethyl sulfoxide (DMSO) induced cytotoxicity, reduction in cell viability, and decreased mitochondrial succinate dehydrogenase level. The *W. coagulans* also inhibited the production of tumor necrosis factor alpha (TNFα) thus, preventing its cytotoxic effect on pancreatic cells adding an evidence to its antidiabetic potential (Chattopadhyay et al., 2007). The 3β-hydroxy-2,3-dihydro-withanolide F isolated from the plant was reported to posses significant anti tumor activity (Chattopadhyay et al., 2007). Withaferin A has demonstrated tumour-inhibitory activity in an *in-vitro* model against cells derived from human carcinoma of the nasopharynx (Kupchan et al., 1965). It inhibited ribonucleic acid (RNA) synthesis of Sarcoma-180 ascites tumour cells by inhibiting transcription and translation processes of these cells (Chowdhury and Neogy, 1975). It also has been reported to inhibit human umbilical vein endothelial cell (HUVEC) sprouting in three-dimensional collagen-I matrix through a process associated with the inhibition of cyclin D1 expression (Mohan et al., 2004).

2.3 DIABETES RELATED INVESTIGATIONS

2.3.1 HYPOGLYCEMIC ACTIVITY

The aqueous extract of fruits of *W. coagulans* was tested at three different dose levels that is 100, 500, and 1000 mg/kg p.o. in STZ induced diabetic and normal rats. The results depicted a significant ($P < 0.001$) reduction in fasting blood glucose levels of diabetic rats on treatment with aqueous extract of *W. coagulans* at the dose of 1 g/kg; p.o. after 7 days (Table 2), whereas the lower dose dint had any significant blood glucose lowering effect. The extract also demonstrated a significant decline in serum cholesterol and serum as well as hepatic LPO in STZ injected diabetic rats (Table 3). Normal rats, when treated with aqueous extract of *W. coagulans* (1 g/kg; p.o.) for 7 days showed a significant fall in blood glucose level as compared to untreated rats (Table 4). In addition, the aqueous extract of *W. coagulans* (2 mg/ml) showed free radical scavenging activity in an *in vitro* system using DPPH (Hemalatha et al., 2004). It is also reported that the extract at a concentration of 25 mg/mL showed a significant ($P < 0.001$) increase in glucose uptake in isolated rat hemi diaphragm (Hemalatha et al., 2005). Thus, the overall effect of extract may be similar to insulin and may also be attributed to an increase in the uptake of glucose by peripheral tissue and thereby presumably decreased the blood glucose levels. The observed LPO lowering activity and free radical scavenging activity in aqueous extract of *W. coagulans* may provide protection to some degree against oxidative damage to beta cells of pancreas, and can also help in reducing the known complication of diabetes mellitus (Hemalatha et al., 2004). The above findings were justified by histopathological studies which depicted regeneration of β-cells in rats treated with extract, glibenclamide which were found to be intact and also preserved islets thus, confirming the protective effect of extract (Figure 5).

TABLE 2 Effect of aqueous extract of *W. coagulans* in STZ induced diabetic rats

Groups	**Blood glucose level (mg%)**	
	1st day	**7th day**
Normal	45.37 ± 2.7	46.51 ± 2.4
Diabetic	269.60 ± 3.2	259.09 ± 4.2 (ns)
WC 100 mg/kg p.o.	257.91 ± 2.2	247.90 ± 2.4 (ns)
WC 500 mg/kg p.o.	257.50 ± 3.4	249.51 ± 2.2 (ns)
WC 1 g/kg p.o.	259.90 ± 10.4	43.64 ± 7.3*

Values are mean ±S.E.M. (n = 6). Where ns: not significant and ∗ P< 0.001 compared with diabetic control.

TABLE 3 Effect of aqueous extract of *W. coagulans* (1 g/kg; p.o.) on cholesterol and LPO

Groups	Serum cholesterol (mg/dl)	Serum LPO (nmol/ml)	Liver LPO (nmol/g of wet tissues)
Normal rats	87.67 ± 3.03	22.57 ± 1.17	344.79 ± 5.00
Diabetic rats	200.71 ± 3.40	43.94 ± 2.22	479.98 ± 5.50
WC 1 g/kg p.o.	89.67 ± 3.82*	23.87 ± 0.44∗	328.34 ± 8.20∗

Values are mean ±S.E.M. (n = 6). Where ∗ P< 0.001 compared with diabetic rats.

TABLE 4 Effect of aqueous extract of *W. coagulans* in normal rats

Groups	Blood glucose level (mg%)	
	1st day	7th day
Normal (vehicle)	52.04 ± 2.9	48.08 ± 4.6
WC 1 g/kg p.o.	58.16 ± 2.6	26.80 ± 1.7*

Values are mean ± S.E.M. (n = 6). Where ∗ P< 0.001 compared with normal r

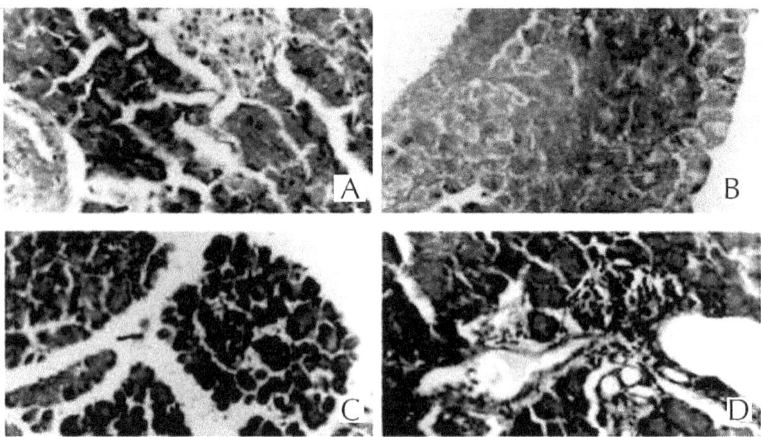

FIGURE 5 Photographs of pancreas of *W. coagulans* treated rats. Where (A): Normal rat pancreas, (B): STZ induced diabetic rat pancreas, (C): Glibenclamide treated rat pancreas, and (D): *W. coagulans* treated rat pancreas.

2.3.2 ANTIDIABETIC POTENTIAL

The antidiabetic potential of aqueous extract of *W. coagulans* along with the role of minerals in its glycemic potential was determined in this study. Laser induced breakdown spectroscopic analysis was used for glycemic element detection. The effect on blood glucose levels of normal, sub, mild, and severely diabetic rats were assessed for fasting blood glucose, glucose tolerance test, and post prandial glucose studies. The results depicted a significant reduction in fasting blood glucose level maximum by 33.2% at 4 hr in normal rats at a dose level of 1 g/kg p.o. Glucose tolerance test studies of normal, sub, and mild diabetic rats showed the maximum reduction of 15.7, 28.9, and 37.8% at 3 hr in same dose. Chronic treatment for 30 days in case of severely diabetic rats showed reduction of 52.9% and 54.1% in fasting blood glucose and post prandial glucose levels. The observed hypoglycemic and antidiabetic potential of fruits of *W. coagulans* may be attributed to presence of significant amount of Mg and Ca in the extract which plays a vital role in diabetes management, as Ca^{2+} ion activates insulin gene expression *via* calcium responsive element binding (CREB) protein responsible for exocytosis of stored insulin (Jaiswal, et al., 2009).

In another investigation combined use of aqueous and chloroform extracts of *W coagulans* fruits, were evaluated for its effects on blood glucose, lipid profile, and body weight in type 2 diabetic rats. The extracts were prepared by simple maceration and hot refluxing using Soxhlet apparatus, and were administered orally singly and as combination, once daily, at a dose of 1 g/kg p.o. for 14 days to normoglycemic and hyperglycemic rats. The results depicted a highly significant ($p < 0.01$) decrease in the blood glucose (52%), triglycerides (TG), total cholesterol (TC), low density lipoprotein (LDL) and very low density lipoprotein (VLDL) level and highly significant ($p < 0.01$) increase in high density lipoprotein (HDL) level on treatment with aqueous extract which showed slightly superior (6%) antihyperglycemic effect compared to metformin. The combination of both extracts showed highly significant ($p < 0.01$) effect in all the above mentioned parameters and was found to have better antihyperglycemic effect than Metformin, and aqueous extracts by 9% and 3%, respectively (Hoda et al., 2010).

2.3.3 HYPOLIPIDEMIC ACTIVITY

The aqueous extract of fruits of *W. coagulans* (1 g/kg; p.o.) was administered to HFD induced hyperlipidemic rats for 7 weeks. The results illustrated a significant decrease in body weight, serum cholesterol, triglycerides, and lipoproteins, whereas no significant decrease in the atherogenic index, hepatic cholesterol, and hepatic LPO was observed (Table 5). The extract at same dose level also showed a 15% reduction in serum cholesterol level in triton induced hyperlipidemic rats compared with untreated animals. Histopathological studies of hepatic tissues revealed that aqueous extract of *W. coagulans* and the reference drug *Navaka guggulu* considerably prevented degenerative changes along with micro vesicular fatty changes in tissues (Figure 6). The above antihyperlipidemic activity of extract may be due to the presence of phytoconstituents that is β-sitosterol and linoleic acid, earlier reported in the seeds of *W. coagulans* (Hemalatha et al., 2006).

TABLE 5 Effect of *W. coagulans* on lipid profile on HFD induced hyperlipidemic rats

S. No.	Serum cholesterol (mg/dl)	HDL (mg/dl)	Triglyceride (mg/dl)	LDL (mg/dl)	VLDL (mg/dl)	AI %	Liver cholesterol (mg/g of tissue)	Liver LPO (n moles/g of tissue)
HFD	398.77 ± 60.88	164.54 ± 42.03	80.51 ± 8.37	318.12 ± 21.17	18.10 ± 1.67	2.48 ± 0.314	26.04 ± 1.9752	1565.14 ± 296.72
W. Coagulans	193.19 ± 5.8^{a}	79.19 ± 10.5^{a}	61.25 ± 6.8^{a}	101.75 ±5.5^{a}	12.25 ± 1.5^{a}	2.44 ±0.5^{ns}	27.46 ± 2.50^{ns}	1284.21 ± 25.0^{ns}
Navaka guggulu	183.12 ± 49.14^{a}	88.28 ± 30.49^{a}	41.26 ± 7.32^{a}	86.59 ± 20.69^{a}	8.25 ± 1.46^{a}	2.12 ± 0.2209^{ns}	25.17 ± 2.29^{ns}	962.74$^{<}$ ± 189.77^{b}

Values are mean ± S.E.M. (n = 6). Where a: P< 0.001 compared with HFD, b: P< 0.01 compared with HFD and ns: Non significant.

TABLE 6 Effect of compound 5 on the plasma lipid profile in C57BL/KsJ-db/db mice

Lipid profiles of db/db mice	Control (1% gum acacia)	Compound 5 (50 mg/kg)	Fenofibrate (50 mg/kg)
TG (mg/dl)	140.8 ± 6.07	120.0 ± 4.48 (–14.7%)	118.0 ± 4.02 (–16.2%)*
CHOL (mg/dl)	160.4 ± 5.17	119.1 ± 2.01 (–25.7%) **	110.9 ± 3.71 (–30.8%)**
HDL-C (mg/dl)	56.6 ± 2.52	70.6 ± 3.50 (+24.7%)**	63.6 ± 4.01 (+12.4%)
LDL-C (mg/dl)	146.3 ± 4.28	115.2 ± 2.13 (–21.2%)**	110.5 ± 4.11 (–24.5%)**
VLDL-C (mg/dl)	28.2 ± 0.56	23.8 ± 0.34 (–15.6%)*	22.1 ± 0.19 (–21.6%)**

Values are expressed as mean ± SEM, N = 5, $p < 0.05$ and $p < 0.01$ compared to control. - denotes decrease in parameter compared to vehicle-treated control group. + denotes increase in parameter compared to vehicle-treated control group.

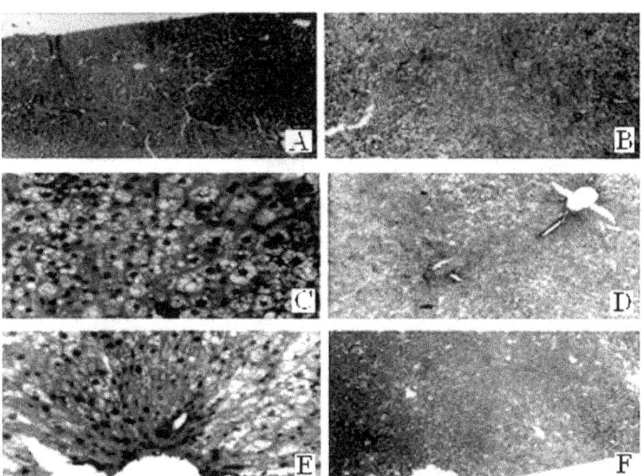

FIGURE 6 Photomicrographs of liver on treatment with *W. coagulans.* Where (A): Normal rat liver architecture, (B): Hyperlipidemic rat liver, (C): High power view of hyperlipidemic rat liver, (D): *W. coagulans* treated hyperlipidemic rat liver. (E): High power view of *W. coagulans* treated hyperlipidemic rat liver, and (F): *Navaka Guggulu* treated hyperlipidemic rat liver (Hemalatha et al., 2006).

2.3.4 DIABETIC WOUND HEALING ACTIVITY

As *W. coagulans* has been reported to possess hypoglycemic, free radical scavenging, and wound healing activity therefore, the study was performed to assess its diabetic wound healing potential. The hydroalcoholic fraction of methanolic extract of *W. coagulans* which was standardized by withaferin-A using high performance thin layer chromatography (HPTLC) was applied/administered in the form of 10% w/w ointment topically and orally at a dose of 500 mg/kg p.o. to STZ-induced diabetic rats. The obtained results were compared with the diabetic control and reference drug used for the study was *Aloe barbadensis* Miller (*Aloe vera* L.) (Liliaceae). This study included determination of rate of wound contraction and estimation of various biochemical parameters such as collagen, hexosamine, total protein, total DNA, SOD, and CAT levels in the granulation tissues. The quantity of withaferin-A present in the methanolic extract was reported to be 3.67 mg/g of the extract. A significant increase in rate of wound contraction was observed in both cases that is topically and orally treated rats (higher in case of orally treated rats), which may be as a result of enhanced activity of fibroblasts mediated through specialized myofibroblasts, found in the granulated tissues (Figure 7).

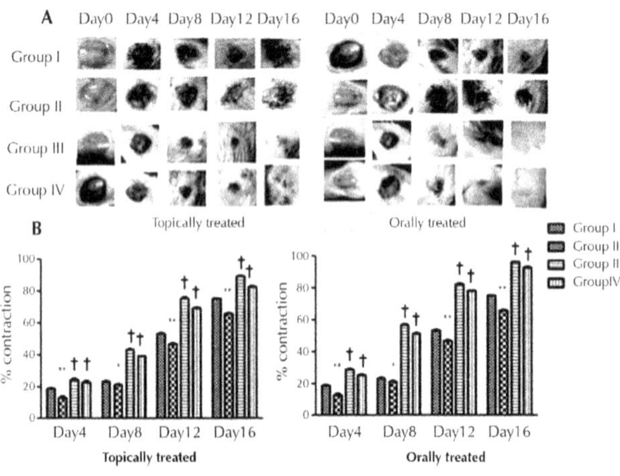

FIGURE 7 Images of wounds on topical and oral treatment of hydroalcoholic fraction of *W. coagulans* (A) and its effect on wound contraction (B). Where Group I: Normal control, Group II: Diabetic control, Group III: Diabetic treated with *Aloe vera*, and Group IV: Diabetic treated with hydroalcoholic fraction of *W. coagulans* (Prasad et al., 2010a).

The rate of contraction is directly proportional to the amount of collagen deposited, where the results depicted a significant increase in the collagen content and reduction in hexosamine level of both topically and orally treated rats reaching their maximum level on 8th day (Figure 8). The collagen gets embedded on highly hydrated gel-like ground substances that is glycosaminoglycans and proteoglycans (major components of hexosamine), and provides strength and integrity to tissue matrix during the various phases of healing that is epithelialization, remodelling resulting in decreased erythema, and scar marks around wound and maintains homeostasis (Figure 8). Significant increase in protein and DNA content in the granulation tissues justified higher cellular proliferation showing better healing of diabetic wounds. As compared to untreated groups, there was a significant increase in SOD and CAT level which plays a major role in detoxifying free radicals and other cytotoxic chemical species, which resulted in potentiation of healing processes. These free radicals at low concentration inhibit proliferation and migration of various cell types, like Keratinocytes, and at high concentrations induces severe tissue damage and can even lead to neoplastic transformation which is more commonly observed in disease states such as diabetes and age associated biochemical phenomenon.

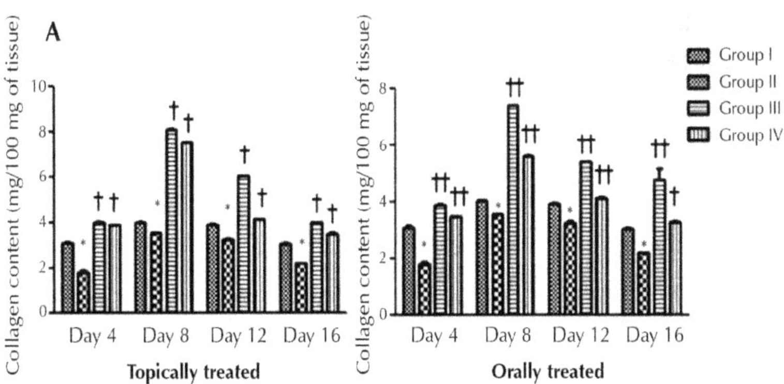

Values are given as mean ± SEM (n=6). * indicates $p<0.001$, compared to normal control; indicates $p<0.001$, compared to diabetic control incase of topically treated whereas † and †† indicate p<p0.01 and $p<0.001$ respectively, compared to diabetic control in case of orally treated.

FIGURE 8 *(Continued)*

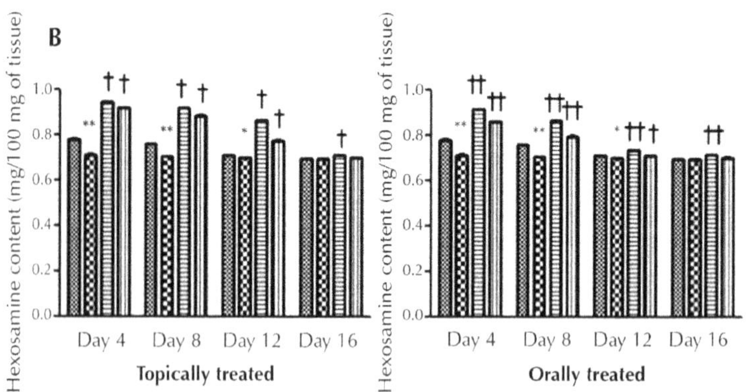

Values are given as mean ±SEM (n=6). * and ** indicatep<0.01 and p<0.001 respectively, compared to normal controll † indicates p<0.001, compared to diabetic control in case of topically treated whereas † and† † indicate p<0.01 and p<0.001 respectively, compared to diabetic control in case of orally treated.

FIGURE 8 Effect of topical and oral treatment of hydroalcoholic fraction of *W. coagulans* on collagen (A) and hexosamine (B) content (Prasad et al., 2010a).

The observed diabetic wound healing effect of the hydroalcoholic fraction of the extract may be attributed to the presence of phenols and tannins which potentiate the wound healing by quenching or chelation of free radicals, promoting contraction of wound, increasing the formation of capillary vessels and fibroblasts, and it also induces Keratinocytes proliferation. The activity may also be due to its hypoglycemic and lowering of LPO level thus, protecting oxidative damage to β cells of pancreas resulting in reduced blood glucose level (Prasad et al., 2010a).

2.3.5 ANTIHYPERGLYCEMIC POTENTIAL OF ISOLATED COMPOUNDS

A new withanolide, (17S,20S,22R)-14α,15α,17β,20β-tetrahydroxy-1-oxowitha-2,5,24-trienolide named coagulanolide 4 (compound 4) along with four known withanolides that is coagulin C (compound 1), 17β-hydroxywithanolide K (compound 2), Withanolide F (compound 3), and Coagulin L (compound 5) were isolated from fruits of *W. coagulans* (Table 1). The structures of these isolated compounds were elucidated by different spectroscopic techniques. All the isolated compounds 1–5 significantly reduced the postprandial rise in hyperglycemia in post-sucrose loaded normoglycemic rats and in STZ-induced diabetic rats. The db/db mice administered with compound 5 at a dose of 50 mg/kg p.o. for 10 days, showed a significant decline in postprandial blood glucose level by 22.7% ($p < 0.01$), compared to vehicle treated control group . Treatment with compound 5 for 10 days significantly ($p < 0.05$) improved glucose tolerance compared to untreated group showing maximum inhibition in rise of postprandial blood glucose level at time interval of 90 min and 120 min. Also compound 5 at a dose of 50 mg/kg p.o. showed significant improvement in plasma lipid profiles (reduction in plasma TG, TC, LDL-C, VLDL-C, and rise in HDL-C level) of dyslipidemic db/db mice after 10 days of consecutive treatment (Table 6). Median effective dose of the compound 5 was determined which was found to be around 25 mg/kg p.o. in STZ-induced diabetic rats, which is considered to be better than metformin. Therefore, compound 5 can be developed as potential antidiabetic agent for treatment of diabetes (Maurya et al., 2008).

2.3.6 IN VITRO α-GLUCOSIDASE AND ALDOSE REDUCTASE INHIBITORY ACTIVITY

A chronic study was conducted for about 30 days on treatment with ethanol extract of *W. coagulans* and various biochemical parameters like blood glucose, glycylated hemoglobin, insulin, liver glycogen, and urinary albumin levels were measured in normal and STZ induced diabetic rats. The results depicted a significant ($P < 0.05$) reduction in fasting blood glucose level after 30 days of treatment with ethanol extract of *W. coagulans* (100 mg/kg p.o.). The study revealed a 59.6% inhibition in α-glucosidase inhibition at 30 μg/mL. In case of aldose reductase inhibitory activity a 98.6% inhibition was reported at a concentration of 30 μg/mL. The results also demonstrated a significant increase in glycated hemoglobin, liver glycogen, and insulin level in diabetic treated rats (Lamba et al., 2011).

2.3.7 CLINICAL STUDY

A clinical study was performed to assess the antidiabetic potential of *W. coagulans* in the Department of Dravyaguna, Faculty of Ayurveda, Institute of Medical Sciences, Banaras Hindu University (Varanasi). 100 patients were selected for this clinical study. The patients were administered *Sitakasaya* prepared from fruits of *W. coagulans* by soaking sufficient quantity (15 g) in six time volume of water followed by filtration. The above preparation was administered orally to the patients with type II diabetes mellitus daily before breakfast. All the parameters observed, showed a highly significant (P< 0.001) effect justifying its antidiabetic potential (Table 7). However, this study was a preliminary and a pilot study along with a deep thorough research is needed to evaluate the efficacy that may benefit people with diabetes (Mishra and Dubey, 2008).

TABLE 7 Clinical study on *W. coagulans*

Treatment (Sitakasaya prepared by overnight soaking the fruits of *W. coagulans* in six times volume of water)	**Effect observed in 80 patients (mean ± SD)**	
	Initial	**Final (After three months)**
Fasting blood glucose level (mg/dl)	140.30 ± 13.25	107.60 ± 8.45*
Post prandial blood glucose level (mg/dl)	230.10 ± 11.67	153.10 ± 6.60*
Serum cholesterol (mg/dl)	208.00 ± 20.83	161.30 ± 4.51*
Glycylated Hb (Hb AIC%)	8.50 ± 1.00	6.55 ± 1.19*

Values are mean ± S.D. (n = 80). Where *: P < 0.001 versus. Initial reading.

2.4 CONCLUSION

Thus, this chapter brings an insight into the various antidiabetic investigations performed on fruits of *W. coagulans*. All the investigations support the traditional use of *W. coagulans* as a potential antidiabetic agent by the traditional medical practitioners. In addition to its antidiabetic potential, the plant has also been proven to solve the secondary complications associated with diabetes. The isolated compounds 1–5 from fruits have shown significant hypoglycemic and antihyperglycemic activity among which compound 5 (most potent) could act as a lead molecule in developing a new antidiabetic drug and can become a major area of interest for scientist in determining the exact mechanism of action for antidiabetic potential of *W. coagulans*.

KEYWORDS

- **Anti-inflammatory activity**
- **Diabetes mellitus**
- **Dimethyl sulfoxide**
- **Withaferin A**
- ***Withania coagulans***

REFERENCES

1. Abourashed, E. A., Koetter, U., and Brattstrom, A. *Phytomedicine.* **11**, 633–638 (2004).
2. Anonymous. *The Wealth of India*, Publication and Information Directorate, CSIR, New Delhi (1996).
3. Atta-ur-Rahman, Abbas, S., Dur-e-Shahwar, Jamal, S. A., and Choudhary, M. I. *J. Nat. Prod.*, **56**, 1000–1006 (1993).
4. Atta-ur-Rahman, Choudhary, M. I., Qureshi, S., Gul, W., and Yousaf, M. *J. Nat. Prod.*, **61**, 812–814 (1998b).
5. Atta-Ur-Rahman, Choudhary, M. I., Yousaf, M., Gul, W., and Qureshi, S. *Chem. Pharm. Bull.*, **46**, 1853–1856 (1998d).
6. Atta-ur-Rahman, Dur-e-Shahwar, D., Naz, A., and Choudhary, M. I. *Phytochemistry.*, **63**, 387–390 (2003).
7. Atta-ur-Rahman, Shabbir, M., Dur-e-Shahwar, D., Choudhary, M. I., Voelter, W., and Hohnholz, D. *Heterocycles.*, **47**, 1005–1012 (1998a).
8. Atta-ur-Rahman, Shabbir, M., Yousaf, M., Qureshi, S., Dur-e-Shahwar, D., Naz, A., and Choudhary, M. I. *Phytochemistry.*, **52**, 1361–1364 (1999).

9. Atta-Ur-Rahman, Yousaf, M., Gul, W., Qureshi, S., Choudhary, M. I., Voelter, W., Hoff, A., Jens, F., and Naz, A. *Heterocycles.*, **48**, 1801–1811 (1998c).
10. Bagri, P., Alia, M., Aeri, V., Bhowmik, M., and Sultana, S. *Food Chem. Toxicol.*, **47**, 50–54 (2009).
11. Bahr, V. and Hansel, R. *Planta Med.*, **44**, 32–33 (1982).
12. Balaraman, A. K., Singh, J., Dash, S., and Maity, T. K. *Saudi Pharm. J.*, **18**, 173–178 (2010).
13. Budhiraja, R. D., Sudhir, S., Garg, K. N., and Arora, B. C. *Planta Med.*, **50**, 134–136 (1984).
14. Budhiraja, R. D., Sudhir, S., and Garg, K. N. *Indian J. Phys. Pharmacol.*, **27**, 129–134 (1983).
15. Budhiraja, R. D., Sudhir, S., and Garg, K. N. *Planta Med.*, **32**, 154–157 (1977).
16. Budhiraja, R. D. and Sudhir, S. *J. Sci. Ind. Res.*, **46**, 488–491 (1987).
17. Chadha, Y. R. *The wealth of India* Publications and Informations Directorate, CSIR, New Delhi (1976).
18. Chattopadhyay, P., Mahaur, K., Saha, S. K., Singh, L., Shukla, G., and Wahi, A. K. *Indian J. Nat. Prod.*, **23**, 8–12 (2007).
19. Chauhan, A., Sharma, P. K., Srivastava, P., Kumar, N., and Dudhe, R. Plants Having Potential Antidiabetic Activity, A Review. *Dudhe Der Pharmacia Lettre*, **2**, 369–387 (2010).
20. Choudhary, M. I., Dur-e-Shahwar, D., Parveen, Z., Jabbar, A., Ali, I., and Atta-ur-Rahman. *Phytochemistry.*, **40**, 1243–1246 (1995).
21. Chowdhury, K. and Neogy, R. K. *Biochem. Pharmacol.*, **24**, 919–920 (1975).
22. Dash, B. and Sharma. B. K. *Charak Samhita*, Chaukhamba Sanskrit series Office, Varanasi, India (2001).
23. Dymock, W., Warden, C. J. H., and Hooper, D. *'Pharmacographia indica'*; Reprinted by Institute of Health and Tibbi Research, Karachi, Pakistan (1972).
24. Gadro, A. Y., Uchi, D. A. Rege, N. N., and Daha, S. A. *Indian J. Pharmacol.*, **33**, 124–145 (2001).
25. Gaind, K. N. and Budhiraja, R. D. *Indian J. Pharm.*, **29**, 185–186 (1967).
26. Jung, M., Park, M., Lee, H. C., Kang, Y. H., Kang, E. S., and Kim, S. K. *Curr. Med. Chem.*, **13**, 1203–1218 (2006).
27. Hemalatha, S., Kumar, R., and Kumar, M. *Pharmacog. Rev.*, **2**, 351–358 (2008).
28. Hemalatha, S., Mishra, N., Kumar, M., Singh, P. N., Chansouria, J. P. N., and Mandal, V. *12th Annual national Convention of Indian Society of Pharmacognosy*, Moga, Punjab, OP, **13**, (2008).
29. Hemalatha, S., Sachdeva, N., Wahi, A. K., Singh, P. N., and Chansouria, J. P. N. *Indian J. Nat. Prod.*, **21**, 20–21 (2005).
30. Hemalatha, S., Wahi, A. K., Singh, P. N., and Chansouria, J. P. N. *J. Ethnopharmacol.*, **93**, 261–264 (2004).
31. Hemalatha, S., Wahi, A. K., Singh P. N., and Chansouria, J. P. N. *Phytother. Res.*, **20**, 614–617 (2006).
32. Hoda, Q., Ahmad, S., Akhtar, M., Najmi, A. K., Pillai, K. K., and Ahmad, S. *J. Hum. Exp. Toxicol.*, **29**, 653–658 (2010).
33. Jaiswal, D., Rai, P. K., and Watal, G. *Indian J. Clin. Biochem.*, **24**, 88–93 (2009).

34. Karami, M., Gohari, A. R., and Ebrahimzadeh, M. A. *Pharmacol. Online*, **3**, 166–171 (2006).
35. Khan, M. T. J., Ashraf, M., Tehniyat, S., Bukhtair, M. K., Ashraf, S., and Ahmad, W. *Fitoterapia*. **64**, 367–70 (1993).
36. Kirtikar, K. R. and Basu, B. D. *Indian Medicinal Plants*, M/s Bishen Singh, Mahendra Pal Singh Publication, Dehradun (1993).
37. Kiritikar, K. R. and Basu, B. D. *Indian Medicinal Plants*, International Booksellers and Publishers, Dehradun, India (1999).
38. Kupchan, S. M., Doskotch, R. W., Bollinger, P., Mcphail, A. T., Sim, G. A., and Renauld, J. A. *Am. Chem. Soc.*, **87**, 5805–5806 (1965).
39. Lamba, H. S., Bhargava, C. S., and Bhargava, S. *Indian J. Nat. Prod.*, **27**, 14–18 (2011).
40. Li, W. L, Zheng, H. C., Bukuru, J., and De Kimpe, N. *J. Ethnopharmacol.*, **92**, 1–21 (2004).
41. Malviya, N., Jain, S., and Malviya, S. *Acta Pol. Pharm.*, **67**, 113–118 (2010).
42. Mauryaa, R., Akankshaa., and Jayendraa. *J. Pharm. Pharmcol.*, **62**, 153–160 (2010).
43. Mauryaa, R., Akankshaa., Jayendraa., Singh, A. B., and Srivastava, A. K. *Bioorg. Med. Chem. Lett*, **18**, 6534–6537 (2008).
44. Meenakshi, P., Bhuvaneshwari, R., Rathi, M. A., Thirumoorthi, L., Guravaiah, D. C, Jiji, M. J., and Gopalakrishnan, V. K. *Appl. Biochem. Biotechnol.*, **162**, 1153–1159 (2010).
45. Mesaik, M. A., Haq Zu., Muradb, S., Ismail, Z., Abdullah, N. R., Gill, H. K., Atta-ur-Rahman, Yousaf, M., Siddiqui, R. A., Ahmade, A., and Choudhary, M. I. *Mol. Immunol.*, **43**, 1855–1863 (2006).
46. Mishra, S. and Dubey, S. D. *Thesis on Doctor of Philosophy in Dravaguna*, Department of Dravaguna, Institute of Medical Sciences, Banaras Hindu University, Varanasi-221005, India (2008).
47. Mohan, R., Hammers, H. J., Bargagna-Mohan, P., Zhan, X. H., Herbstritt, C. J., Ruiz, A., Zhang, L., Hanson, A. D., Conner, B. P., Rougas, J., and Pribluda, V. S. *Angiogenesis.*, **7**, 115–122 (2004).
48. Neogi, P., Kawai, M., Butsugan, Y., Mori, Y., and Suzuki, M. *Bull. Chem. Soc. Jpn.*, **61**, 4479–4481 (1988).
49. Nur-e-Alam, M., Yousaf, M., Qureshi, S., Baig, I., Nasim, S. Atta-ur-Rahman, and Choudhary, M. I. *Helv. Chim. Acta.*, **86**, 607–614 (2003).
50. Pareek, H., Sharma, S., Khajja, B. S., Jain, K., and Jain, G. C. BMC Complement. *Altern. Med.*, **9**, 48 (2009).
51. Prasad, S. K., Kumar, R., Patel, D. K., and Hemalatha, S. *Pharm. Biol.*, **48**, 1397–1404 (2010a).
52. Prasad, S. K., Singh, P.N., Wahi, A.K., and Hemalatha, S. *Pharmacog. J.*, **2**, 386–394 (2010b).
53. Rajurkar, S. M., Thakre, P. N., and Waddukar, S. G. 53rd Indian pharmaceutical congress. New Delhi CP, **38**, 215 (2001).
54. Sankara, S. S., Sethi, P. D., Glotter, E., Kirson, I., and Lavie, D. *Phytochemistry.*, **10**, 685–688 (1971).
55. Sattar, A., Ghanai, M. Y., and Shafiq, K. A. *Pakistan J. Sci. Ind. R.*, **31**, 139–141 (1988).

56. Saxena, A. and Vikram, N. K. J. *Altern. Complement. Med.*,**10**, 369–378 (2004).
57. Shohat, B. and Joshua, H. *Int. J. Cancer.*, **8**, 487–496 (1971).
58. Shohat, B., Kirson, I., and Lavie, D. *Biomedicine.*, **28**, 18–24 (1978).
59. Subramanian, S. and Sethi, P. D. *Current Science.*, **38**, 267–268 (1969).
60. Sy, G. Y., Cissé, A., Nongonierma, R. B., Sarr, M., Mbodj, N. A., and Faye, B. J *Ethnopharmacol.*, **98**, 171–175 (2005).
61. Vincent, V. V., David, L., Budhiraja, R. D., Sharan, S., and Garg, K. N. *Phytochemistry.*, **22**, 2253–2257 (1983).
62. Weniger, B., Lagnika, L., Vonthron-Sénécheau, C., Adjobimey, T., Gbenou, J., Moudachirou, M., Brun, R., Anton, R., and Sanni, A. J. *Ethnopharmacol.*, **90**, 279–284 (2004).
63. Waxler, N. E. *Sac. Sci. Med.*, **27**, 531–544.

CHAPTER 3

EVALUATION OF TOTAL PHENOLICS AND FREE RADICAL QUENCHING ACTIVITY OF *GLYCOSMIS PENTAPHYLLA* (RETZ.) A. DC.

RAHUL CHANDRAN and THANGARAJ PARIMELAZHAGAN

CONTENTS

ABSTRACT

India is rich in biodiversity, ethnicity, geography, languages, arts, and culture. Indian traditional system of medicines like Ayurveda, *Siddha*, and ethnomedicine offer much useful, effective and simple herbal medicine. *Glycosmis pentaphylla,* of the family rubiaceae is used against cough, rheumatism, anemia and jaundice. The leaves of this plant are used in the treatment of fever, skin, and liver complaints. Glycosine, arborine, arborinine, glycerine, and glycosamine are some of the major alkaloids found in leaves. *Glycosmis pentaphylla* leaf extract was obtained by boiling the leaves in distilled water for 24 hr. The extract was dried and estimated for its phenolic, tannin, and flavonoid contents. Further, antioxidant property was measured by 2, 2-diphenyl-1-picrylhydrazyl (DPPH), 2, 2'-azino-bis ($ABTS^+$), metal chelating, ferric reducing ability of plasma (FRAP), and phosphomolybdeum assays. The total phenolic, tannin, and flavonoid content were found in moderate amount. All the assays proved to have reasonable radical scavenging activity when compared to standards. Hence, further research is going on in the laboratory to figure out the mechanism of action and compounds responsible for having antioxidant property by molecular and analytical tools.

3.1 INTRODUCTION

The free radicals are chemically active atoms that have a charge due to an excess or deficient number of electrons (Shetti et al., 2009). These unpaired electrons are very much reactive with adjacent molecules such as lipids, proteins, and carbohydrates that can cause cellular damage (Kuhn, 2003). Free radicals containing oxygen, known as reactive oxygen species (ROS) are the most biologically significant. They and other ROS are derived either from normal essential metabolic processes in the human body or from external sources such as exposure to X-Rays, ozone, cigarette smoking, air pollutants, and industrial chemicals. As these free radicals have one or more unpaired electrons, they are highly unstable and undergo chemical reactions either to grab or donate electrons, thereby causing damage to proteins, cells, and deoxyribonucleic acid (DNA) (Shetti et al., 2009). Increasing evidence in both experimental and clinical studies suggests that oxidative stress plays a major role in the pathogenesis of both types of diabetes mellitus. Free radicals are formed disproportionately in diabetes by glucose oxidation, nonenzymatic glycation of proteins, and the subsequent oxidative degradation of glycated proteins. Abnormally high levels of free radicals and the simultaneous decline of antioxidant defense mechanisms can lead to damage of cellular organelles and enzymes, increased lipid peroxidation, and development of insulin resistance. These consequences of oxidative stress can promote the development of complications of diabetes mellitus (Maritim et al., 2003).

However, the presence of free radicals within the body can also have significant role in the development and progression of many disease processes like congestive heart failure, hypertension, cerebrovascular accidents, and diabetic complications (Chen et al., 2002). The degradation due to oxidative reactions can affect all biomolecules but mostly lipids, carbohydrates, and proteins (Hinnerburg et al., 2006). The oxidative reactions also generate ROS that are linked to carcinogenesis, inflammation, ageing, and cardiovascular disorders (Raza et al., 2009). Both natural and synthetic antioxidants are available. Antioxidants are substances which are capable of counteracting the damaging effects of oxidation in body tissues. The synthetic antioxidants like Butylated hydroxyl anisole (BHA) and butylated hydroxyl toluene (BHT) have been restricted in foods, as they are suspected to be carcinogenic (Madhavi and Salunkhe, 1995). So, the interest is highly focused on searching plant based antioxidants because of their therapeutic performance and low toxicity.

Glycosmis pentaphylla, or "orange berry" as it is commonly known, is an obscure berry that is akin to citrus and grows in the tropics of Asia and Australia. Glycosine, arborine, arborinine, glycerine, and glycosamine are some of the major alkaloids found in leaves. Leaf juice of the plant is given with sugar in empty stomach in the morning to eradicate ascaris. Young leaves along with the leaf juice of "*Ananas sativus*" are also given in the treatment of ascaris. Leaves juice is also given in fever and liver complaints. Paste of leaves with ginger is used in eczema and skin affections. As with many fruits and vegetables, this obscure plant boasts some medicinal uses that can be extremely beneficial to human health. However, before taking any herbal supplement, it is important to understand its known effects and the claims about its benefits.

Arborine

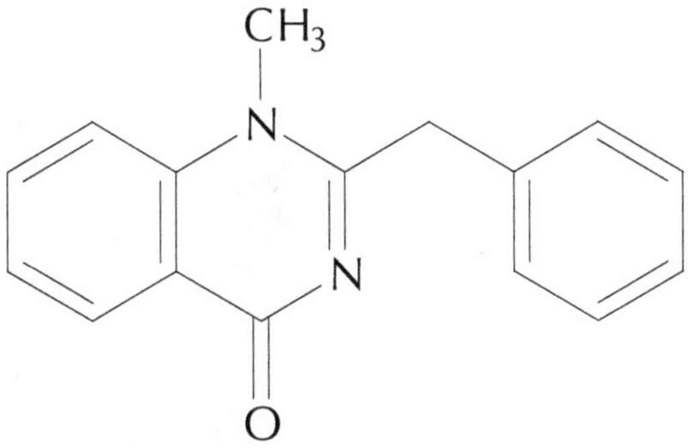

CH_3 N N O

Glucosamine

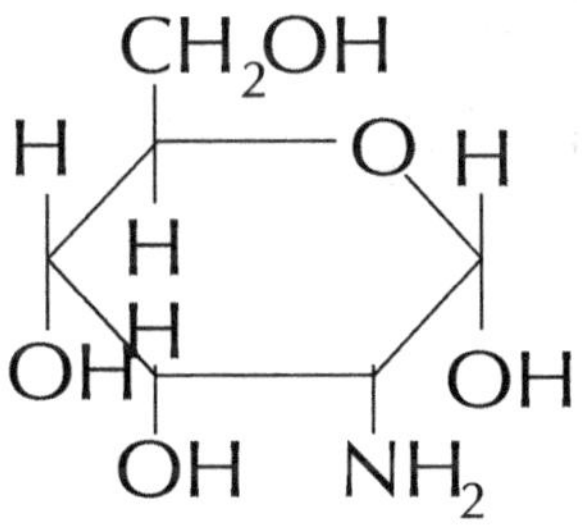

CH_2OH H O H H H OH OH OH NH_2

Glycerine

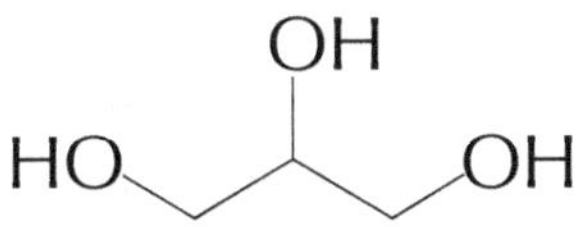

OH HO OH

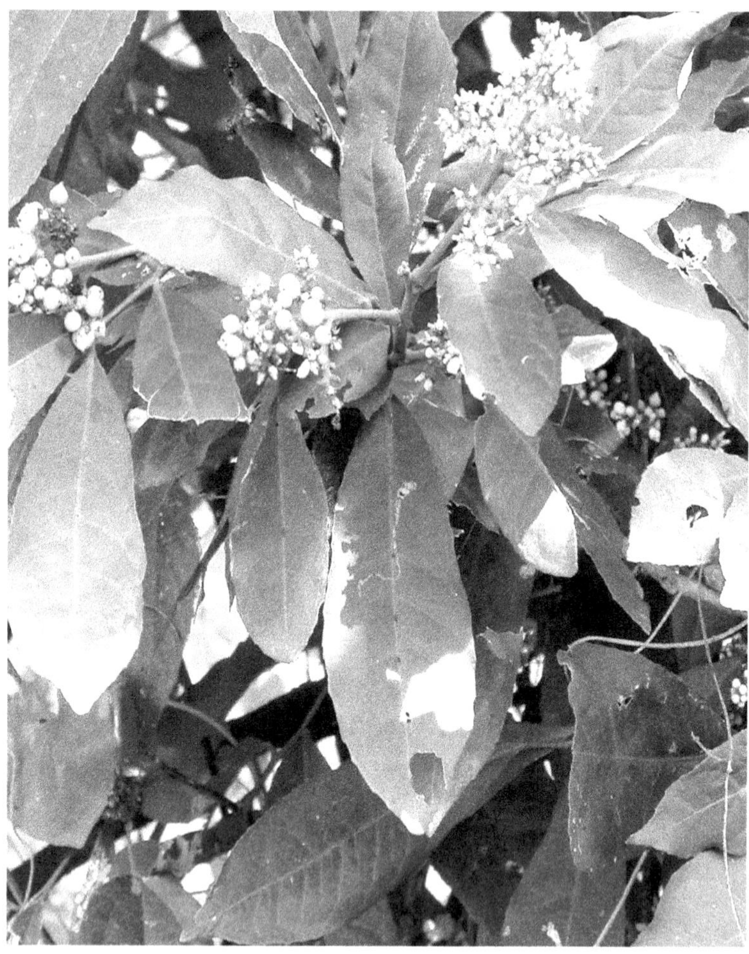

FIGURE 1 Plant profile: *G. pentaphylla*.

Systematic position

Division	:	Angiosperms
Class	:	Dicotyledons
Order	:	Sapindales
Family	:	Rutaceae
Genus	:	*Glycosmis*
Species	:	*Glycosmis pentaphylla* (Retz.) A. Dc

3.2 MATERIALS AND METHODS

3.2.1 COLLECTION OF PLANT MATERIALS

Glycosmis pentaphylla were collected from Nilamboor, Malapuram district during the month of May–June 2011. The collected plant material was identified and their authenticity was confirmed by comparing the voucher specimen at the herbarium of Botanical survey of India, Southern circle, Coimbatore, Tamil Nadu. Freshly collected plant material was cleaned to remove adhering dust.

3.2.2 CHEMICALS

Potassium ferricyanide, ferric chloride, DPPH, potassium persulfate, ABTS, 6-hydroxy-2,5,7,8-tetramethylchroman-2-carboxylic acid (Trolox), ferrous chloride, ammonium thiocyanate, 2,4,6-tripyridyl-*s*-triazine (TPTZ), polyvinyl polypyrrolidone (PVPP), ferrous ammonium sulfate, ethylenediamine tetracetic acid (EDTA) disodium salt, nitroblue tetrazolium (NBT), BHT were obtained from Himedia (Mumbai, Maharashtra, India), Merck (Hyderabad, Andhra Pradesh, India), and Sigma (Thane, Maharashtra, India). All other reagents used were of analytical grade.

3.2.3 SUCCESSIVE SOLVENT EXTRACTION

The fresh leaves were boiled in distilled water for nearly 24 hr to extract the contents by decoction method. The contents were filtered and dried in water bath. The extract thus obtained was used directly for the estimation of total phenolics and assessment of antioxidant potential through various biochemical assays.

3.2.4 DETERMINATION OF TOTAL PHENOLICS AND TANNINS

The total phenol content was determined according to the method described by Siddhuraju and Becker, 2003. Triplicate concentration of leaf extract (2 mg/2 mL) was taken in the test tubes and made up to the volume of 1 mL with distilled water. Then 0.5 mL of Folin–Ciocalteu reagent (1:1 with water) and 2.5 mL of sodium carbonate solution (20%) were added sequentially in each tube. Soon after vortexing the reaction mixture, the test tubes were placed in dark for 40 min and the absorbance was recorded at 725 nm against blank. Reaction mixture without plant extract was taken as blank. The analysis was performed in triplicate and the results were expressed in gallic acid equivalents.

Using the same extract the tannins were estimated after treatment with polyvinyl polypyrrolidine (PVPP) Sidduraju and Manian, 2009. 100 mg of PVPP was weighed into a 100 × 12 mm test tube and to this 500 μL distilled water and then 500 μL of the sample extract was added. The content was vortexed and kept in the test tube at 4°C for 15 min. Then the sample was centrifuged at 4000 rpm for 10 min at room temperature and the supernatant was collected. This supernatant has only simple phenolics other than the tannins (the tannins would have been precipitated along with the PVPP). The phenolic content of the supernatant was measured and expressed as the content of non-tannin phenolics. The tannin content of the sample was calculated as follows:

Tannin (%) = Total phenolics (%) – Non-tannin phenolics (%)

3.2.5 ESTIMATION OF TOTAL FLAVONOIDS

The flavonoid content of the extract was quantified as it acts as major antioxidant in plants, reducing oxidative stress. The content was estimated as per described by Zhishen et al., 1999. Initially, the plant extract was taken in different test tubes. To each extracts 2 mL of distilled water was added. Then, 150 μL of $NaNO_2$ was added to all the test tubes followed by incubation at room temperature for 6 min. After incubation 150 μL of $AlCl_3$ (10%) was added to all the test tubes. The test tubes were incubated for 6 min at room temperature. Then 2 mL of 4% NaOH was added to all the test tubes which were made up to 5 mL using distilled water. The contents in all the test tubes were vortexed well and they were allowed to stand for 15 min at room temperature. The pink color developed due to the presence of flavonoids was read spectrophotometrically at 510 nm. The amount of flavonoid was calculated in rutin equivalents.

3.2.6 *IN VITRO* ANTIOXIDANT STUDIES

RADICAL SCAVENGING ACTIVITY USING DPPH METHOD

The antioxidant activity of the extract was determined in terms of hydrogen donating or radical scavenging ability, using the stable radical DPPH, according to the method of Blois, 1958. The extract at various concentrations (100–300 μL) was added to 5 mL of 0.1 mM methonolic solution of $DPPH^{\cdot}$ and allowed to stand for 20 min at 27°C. The absorbance of the sample was measured at 517 nm. Methanol was served as blank and solution without extract served as control. The mixture of methanol, DPPH, and standard (BHT, BHA, quercetin, and α-tocopherol) served as positive control. Radical scavenging activity was expressed in IC_{50} of the extracts.

TOTAL ANTIOXIDANT ACTIVITY (TAA) BY 2, 2′-AZINOBIS (3-ETHYLEBENZOTHIOZOLINE-6-SULPHONIC ACID) (ABTS□+) ASSAY

The TAA of the extract was measured by ABTS radical cation decolorization assay according to the method of Re et al., 1999 described by Siddhuraju and Manian, 2007. The $ABTS^{+}$ was produced by reacting 7 mm $ABTS^{+}$ aqueous solution with 2.4 mm potassium persulphate in the dark for 12–16 hr at room temperature. Prior to assay, this solution was diluted in ethanol (about 1:89 v/v) and equilibrated at 30°C to give an absorbance at 734 nm of 0.7 ± 0.02. The stock solution of the sample extracts were diluted such that after addition of different aliquots into the assay, they produced between 20–80% inhibitions of the blank (ethanol) absorbance. After the addition of 1 mL of diluted $ABTS^{+}$ solution to different concentration of sample or trolox standards (final concentration 0–15 μM) in ethanol, absorbance was measured at 30°C exactly 30 min after initial mixing. Appropriate solvent blanks were also run in each assay. Triplicate determinations were made at each dilution of the standard, at 734 nm and it was plotted as a function of trolox concentration. The unit of TAA is defined as the concentration of trolox having equivalent antioxidant activity expressed as μMol/g.

FERRIC REDUCING ANTIOXIDANT POWER (FRAP) ASSAY

The antioxidant capacities of phenolic extracts of samples were estimated according to the procedure described by Pulido et al., 2000. FRAP reagent (900 μL), prepared freshly and incubated at 37°C, was mixed with 90 μL of distilled water and 50 μL of test sample or distilled water (for the reagent blank). The test sample and reagent blank were incubated at 37°C for 30 min in a water bath. The final dilution of the test sample in the reaction mixture was 1/34. The FRAP reagent contained 2.5 mL of 20 mmol/L TPTZ (2, 4, 6-tripyridyl-*s*-triazine) solution in 40 mmol/l HCl plus 2.5 mL of 20 mmol/L $FeCl_3 \cdot 6H_2O$ and 25 mL of 0.3 mol/L acetate buffer (pH 3.6) described by Siddhuraju and Becker. At the end of incubation, the absorbance readings were taken immediately at 593 nm. The FRAP value is expressed as mmol Fe (II) equivalent/mg extract.

METAL CHELATING ACTIVITY

The chelating of ferrous ions by *G. pentaphylla* extract was estimated by the method of Dinis et al., 1994. Briefly, 50 μL of 2 mm $FeCl_2$ was added to 1 mL of triplicate concentration of the extract. The reaction was initiated by the addition of 0.2 mL of 5 mm ferrozine solution. The mixture was vigorously shaken and left to stand at room temperature for 10 min. The absorbance of the solution was thereafter measured at 562 nm against deionized water which was used as blank. The BHT was taken as standard. All the reagents without addition of sample extract were used as negative control. The percentage inhibition of ferrozine Fe^{2+} complex formation was calculated.

PHOSPHOMOLYBDENUM ASSAY

The antioxidant activity of samples was evaluated by the phosphomolybdenum method (Prieto et al., 1999). An aliquot of 50 μL of sample solution (1 mm in dimethyl sulphoxide) was combined in a 4 mL vial with 1 mL of reagent solution (0.6 M sulfuric acid, 28 mM sodium phosphate and 4 mM ammonium molybdate). The vials were capped and incubated in a water bath at 95°C for 90 min. After the samples had cooled to room temperature, the absorbance of the mixture was measured at 765 nm against a blank. The results reported are mean values expressed as grams of ascorbic acid equivalents per gram sample ascorbic acid equivalent antioxidant capacity (AEAC).

STATISTICAL ANALYSIS

All experiments were repeated at least three times. Results were reported as Mean ± SE. The statistical significance between antioxidant activity values of the extract was evaluated with one way ANOVA followed by Holm–Sidak test.

3.3 DISCUSSION AND RESULTS

3.3.1 TOTAL PHENOLICS, TANNINS, AND FLAVONOIDS.

In Table 1, phenolic of the leaf decoction was found to be 7.31 g GAE/100 g extract and 3.56 g GAE/100 g tannin content. The estimation of total flavonoid content revealed the presence of 4.8 g RE/100g extract. The polyphenolic contents of the extract appear to function as good electron and hydrogen atom donor and therefore should be able to terminate radical chain reaction by converting free radical and reactive oxygen species to more stable products. It is important to examine the correlation between the content of total polyphenols and the antioxidant potential because some authors have reported that there is no correlation between the content of these main antioxidant compounds and the radical scavenging activity (Yu et al., 2002). Hence, presence of phenols and flavonols supports that *G. pentaphylla* and can have antioxidant and other medicinal property.

3.3.2 RADICAL SCAVENGING ACTIVITY USING DPPH METHOD

The free radical scavenging activity of the leaves *G. pentaphylla* were estimated by comparing with standards such as BHT, BHA, quercetin, and rutin and the result is shown in Figure 2 importantly IC_{50} value of extract was also calculated to determine the amount of extract needed to quench 50% of radicals. A lower value of IC_{50} indicates a higher antioxidant activity. The extract of leaf registered moderate DPPH radical scavenging activity (IC_{50} 182 21) when compared to standards. Eventhough, the radical scavenging activity shown by the extract was low, when compare to synthetic antioxidants like BHT and BHA, coming to the point of safety, it can be prescribed as a safe antioxidant source, as the synthetic antioxidants are reported to pose certain side effects.

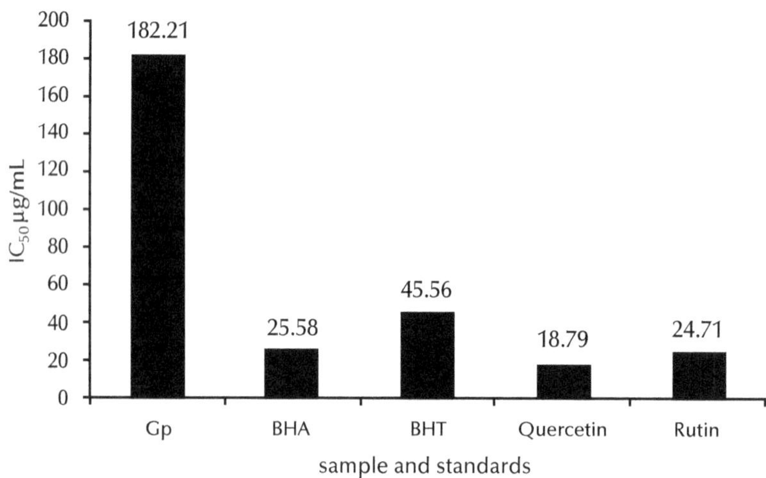

FIGURE 2 The DPPH radical scavenging property of *G. pentaphylla.*

GP – G. pentaphylla, BHT – Butylated Hydroxy Toluene, and BHA – Butylated Hydroxy Anisole

3.3.3 TAA BY 2, 2′-AZINOBIS (3-ETHYLEBENZOTHIOZOLINE-6-SULFONIC ACID) ($ABTS^+$) ASSAY

The result of TAA extract is given in the Table 1. The extract of *G. pentaphylla* showed a good ability to scavenge ABTS radicals (893.02 µmoles/g extract). Hagerman et al., 1998 have reported that the high molecular weight phenolics (tannins) have more ability to quench free radicals ($ABTS^+$). The TAA of the extract will support the total phenolic content in the leaves which seems to be efficient enough for functioning as a potential nutraceuticals.

3.3.4 FERRIC REDUCING ANTIOXIDANT POWER (FRAP) ASSAY

The results presented in Table 1, shows that the ferric reducing capacity of decoction extract is 489.7 mM/mg extract. The FRAP assay measures the antioxidant effect of any substances in the reaction medium as reducing ability. Inactivation of oxidants by such reductant can be described as redox reactions where oxidation by antioxidants reduces reactive species. Result shown by the leaf extract of *G. pentaphylla* proves to be an efficient hydrogen donor to make the free radical a stable one.

3.3.5 METAL CHELATING ACTIVITY

The Fe^{2+} chelating activity of extracts are shown in Figure 3. A moderate chelation was observed in the extract (23.43%). The results are comparably low to that of standard BHT (92%). The result of standard was significant ($P< 0.01$) over the extract ($P< 0.05$). The least activity of extracts may be because of the interference of other metal ions in the extract or reaction mixture. Iron is an essential element which is necessary for transport of oxygen molecule through blood. But under certain stress conditions these iron act as harmful free radical which will catalyze oxidative change in lipid, protein, and other cellular components (Decker and Hultin, 1992) which are needed to be scavenged using efficient antioxidants. Metal chelating ability was significant as they reduce the concentration of catalyzing transition metal in lipid peroxidation (Duh et al., 1999).

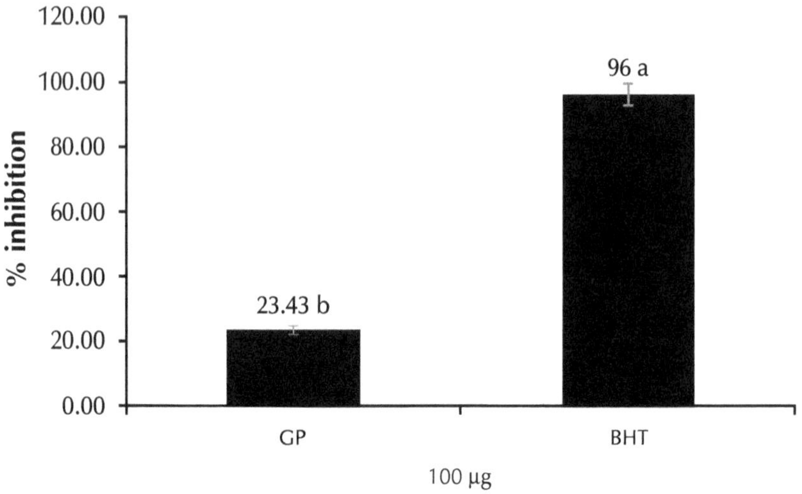

FIGURE 3 Metal chelating activity of *G. pentaphylla.*

Data expressed as mean ± standard deviation. a-P< 0.01, b-P< 0.05
GP – *G. pentaphylla,* BHT – Butylated Hydroxy Toluene

3.3.6 PHOSPHOMOLYBDENUM ASSAY

The decoction extract of *G. pentaphylla* (19.87 g AA equiv/ 100 g extract) depicted good AAE content. The results were calculated in equivalents to ascorbic acid and are shown in Table 1. The experimental study was done to compare and evaluated for the capacity to reduce Mo (VI) to Mo (V) by the antioxidant compound present in the sample. This reduction ability was relatively shown by the active extract of *G. pentaphylla.* The assay is successfully used to quantify vitamin E in seed and being simple and independent of other antioxidant assays commonly employed, it was decided to extend its application to plant extract (Prieto et al., 1999). Hence, the estimation of Mo reduction activity by *G. pentaphylla* became an essential report of having antioxidant potential.

TABLE 1 Total Phenolics, Tannins, Flavonoids, ABTS$^+$, FRAP, and Phosphomolybdenum properties of *G. pentaphylla*

Glycosmis pentaphylla	Phenolics G GAE/100 g extract	Tannins G GAE/100 g extract	Flavonoid G RE/100 g extract	ABTS µ M tro-lox equi/g extract	FRAP mM Fe II/g extract	Phosphomolybdenum gAA equi/100g extract
Decoction extract	7.31 ± 0.08	3.56 ± 0.03	4.8 ± 0.089	893.02 ± 13.28	489.7 ± 43.60	19.87 ± 4.5

Data expressed as mean ± standard deviation.

3.4 CONCLUSION

The decoction method was followed to extract plant components traditionally and is still being used as an effective way to treat various ailments. Hence an attempt has been made to screen the antioxidant potential of the decoction extract of *G. pentaphylla*. The study showed moderate free radical scavenging property of the extract but well acceptable when being shown by a natural product. Extensive *in vivo* studies has also been made to prove the relationship of free radical defense and diabetic complications. Hence, further studies are needed to examine the exact mechanism behind these relationships and its action.

KEYWORDS

- **Antioxidants**
- **Decoction extract**
- **Free radical**
- **Glycosmis pentaphylla**

ACKNOWLEDGMENT

The authors are thankful to Department of Science and Technology, Govt. of India and INSPIRE program for providing financial support for carrying out the work.

REFERENCES

1. Blois, M. S. Antioxidants determination by the use of a stable free radical. *Nature*, **4617**, 1199–1200 (1958).
2. Chen, J., He, J., Hamm, L., Vatuman, V., and Whelton, P. K. Serum antioxidant vitamin and blood pressure in the United States population. *Hypertension* (2002).
3. Decker, E. and Hultin, H.O. Lipid peroxidation in muscle foods via redox iron. In a Lipid oxidation in food (Chapter 3), J. St. Angelo (Ed.), ACS symposium series 500m. Washington, DC, *J. Am. Chem. Soc.* (1992).
4. Dinis, T. C. P., Madeira, V. M. C., and Almeida, L. M. Action of phenolic derivatives (acetoaminophen, salycilate and 5-aminosalycilate) as inhibitors of membrane lipid peroxidation and as peroxyl radical scavengers. *Arch. Biochem. Biophys*, **315**, 161–169 (1994).
5. Duh, P. D., Tu Y. Y., and Yen, G. C. Antioxidant activity of water extract of harng Jyur (*Chrysanthemum morifolium* Ramat). *Lebensmittel-Wissenschaft Und technologie*, **32**, 296–277 (1999).
6. Hagerman, A. E., Reidl, K. M., Jones, G. A., Sovic K. N., Ritcard, N. T., Hartzfield, P. W., et al. High molecular weight polyphenolics (tannins) as biological antioxidants. *J. Agric. Food Chem*, **46**, 1887–1892 (1998).
7. Hinnerburg, I., Dorman, H. J. D., and Hiltunen, R. Antioxidant activities of extracts from selected culinary herbs and spices. *Food chemistry*, **97**, 122–129 (2006).
8. Kuhn, M. A. Oxygen free radicals and antioxidants, *American journal of nutrition*, **103**(4), 58–62 (2003).
9. Madhavi, D. L. and Salunkhe, D. K. *Toxicological Aspects of Food Antioxidants. In Food Antioxidants.* D. L. Madavi, S. S. Deshpande, and D. K. Salunkhe, (Eds). Dekker, New York. 267 (1995).
10. Maritim, A. C., Sanders, R. A., and Watkins J. B. Diabetes, Oxidative Stress, and Antioxidants: A Review. *J Biochem Molecular Toxicology*, **17**(1), 25–38 (2003).
11. Prieto, P., Pineda, M., and Aguilar, M. Spectophotometric quantitative of antioxidant capacity through the formation of a phosphomolybdenum complex: Specific application to the determination of vitamin E. *Analyt. Biochem*, **269**, 337–341 (1999).
12. Pulido, R., Bravo, L., and Sauro-Calixto, F. Antioxidant activity of dietary polyphenols as determined by a modified ferric reducing/antioxidant power assay. *J. Agric. Food Chem*, **48**, 3396–3402 (2000).

13. Raza, S. A., Rashid, A., William, J., Najaf, S., and Arshad, M. *Effect of synthetic antioxidant on shelf life of locally manufactured butter known as Makhan in Pakistan Biharean Biologist.* **3**(2), 91 (2009).
14. Re, R., Pellegrini, N., Proteggente, A., Pannala, A., Yang, M., and Rice-Evans, C. Antioxidant activity applying an improved ABTS radical cation decolorization assay. *Free Radic. Biol. Med,* **26**, 1231–1237 (1999).
15. Shetti, A., Kelushar, V., and Agarwal, A. Antioxidants; Enhancing Oral and General Health. *Journal of Indian academy of oral medicine and radiology*, **21**(1) (2009).
16. Siddhuraju, P. and Becker, K. Studies on antioxidant activities of Mucuna seed (*Mucuna pruriens* var. utilis) extracts and certain non-protein amino/imino acids through in vitro models. *J. Sci. Food Agric*, **83**, 1517–1524 (2003).
17. Siddhuraju, R. and Manian, S. The antioxidant activity and free radical scavenging capacity of dietary phenolic extracts from horse gram (*Macrotyloma uniflorum* (Lam.) Verdc.) seeds. *Food Chem*, **105**, 950–958 (2007).
18. Yu, L., Haley, S., Perret, J., Harris, M., Wilson, J., and Qian, M. Free radical scavenging properties of wheat extracts. *J. Agric. Food Chem*, **50**, 1619–1624 (2002).
19. Zhishen, J., Mengecheng, T., and Jianming, W. The determination of flavonoid contents on mulberry and their scavenging effects on superoxide radical. *Food Chem,* **64,** 555–559 (1999).

CHAPTER 4

ANTIOXIDANT, ANTIDIABETIC, AND CHEMICAL COMPOSITION OF *SYZYGIUM AQUEUM* LEAF EXTRACTS

UMA D. PALANISAMY and THAMILVAANI MANAHARAN

CONTENTS

ABSTRACT

The various parts of *Syzygium aqueum (S. aqueum)* has been used in traditional medicine. In this study, the leaf extracts have been shown to have significant compositions of phenolic compounds, protective activity against free radicals as well as having lipid peroxidation inhibition activity and low pro oxidant capability. This investigation also revealed its effectiveness in inhibiting the carbohydrate hydrolyzing enzymes, α-glucosidase and α-amylase at more significant levels than the drug acarbose. In addition, it was able to inhibit the key enzyme in polyol pathway, aldose reductase (AR) and prevent the advanced glycation end-products (AGEs) formation. We also found that non-toxic concentrations of *S. aqueum* leaf extract was able to induce differentiation in 3T3-L1 pre-adipocytes, enhance fluorescent deoxyglucose analog (2-NBDG) uptake into mature adipocytes in the absence and presence of insulin and was able to increase adiponectin secretion. In subacute toxicity studies, where leaf extract were administered to rats for 14 days did not result in death or show any adverse effects. No significant differences in body weight or relative organ weight and no gross or microscopic abnormalities were observed. Furthermore, all biochemical tests performed on the sera of the experimental animals was in the range of the normal control groups. In addition, the elemental content in the extract was far below the permissible level for nutraceuticals. Thus, the standardized ethanolic extract of *S. aqueum* leaf can be considered devoid of any toxic risk. Six flavonoid compounds, 4-hydroxybenzaldehyde (1), myricetin-3-*O*-rhamnoside (2), europetin-3-*O*-rhamnoside (3), phloretin (4), myrigalone-G (5) and myrigalone-B,and (6), were isolated from the ethanolic extract of *S. aqueum* leaf. The results strongly suggest the antioxidant and antidiabetic potential of *S. aqueum* leaf extract.

4.1 INTRODUCTION

The diabetes mellitus is defined by the American Diabetic Association (ADA, 2008) as "a metabolic disease characterized by hyperglycemia resulting from defect in insulin action, insulin secretion or both". Diabetes can be classified into type 1 diabetes, insulin dependent diabetes mellitus (IDDM) and type 2 diabetes, non-insulin dependent diabetes mellitus (NI-DDM). More than 90% cases of diabetes fall into type 2 diabetes. Type 2 diabetes is a major and growing public health problem throughout the world. In the year 2000 type 2 diabetes prevalence was estimated in 180 million people worldwide and this number is expected to double in 2030 (WHO, 2008). Insulin-resistance is a characteristic feature in type 2 diabetes and several drugs to increase the insulin sensitivity are currently being used. There is a great interest in the development of new drugs to prevent this disease and to evaluate natural products in experimental studies (Liu *et al*., 2004).

During onset and development of type 2 diabetes, carbohydrate and lipid metabolism is affected by improper glucose metabolism, which leads to elevated postprandial blood glucose levels (Chang et al., 2002). The postprandial hyperglycemia happens due to hydrolysis of starch by pancreatic α-amylase and uptake of glucose by intestinal α-glucosidase (Gray, 1995). One of the therapeutic approaches to decrease postprandial hyperglycemia is by retarding absorption of glucose through inhibition of carbohydrate hydrolyzing enzymes like α-glucosidase and α-amylase in the digestive tract.

The α-glucosidase inhibitors decrease the absorption of carbohydrate from the intestine, which causes a slower and lower rise in blood glucose, especially right after meals.The commercialized α-glucosidase inhibitors; acarbose, miglitol, and voglibose have been used for type 2 diabetes management (De Fronzo, 1999). The α-amylase inhibitors known as 'starch blockers', slows down the carbohydrate breaking down process prior to absorption. Thus inhibition of α-amylase reduces the postprandial hyperglycemia in diabetes.

During chronic hyperglycemia, excessive glucose uptake in tissues affects the key enzyme AR in the polyol pathway. This results in the reduction of various sugars to sugar alcohols, such as glucose to sorbitol, followed by nicotinamide adenine dinucleotide (NADH)-dependent sorbitol-dehydrogenase catalysed fructose production. Increased fructose formation leads to reactive oxygen species (ROS) formation (Kaneko et al., 2005). In addition, sorbitol and its metabolites accumulates in the nerves, retina, lens, and kidneys due to their poor penetration across membranes and inefficient metabolism, results in development of diabetic complications, including retinopathy, neuropathy, nephropathy, and cataracts (Kawanishi et al., 2003; Kador et al., 1980; Fuente et al., 2003).

The prolonged hyperglycemia also results in the formation of AGEs in body tissues. This complex and fluorescent AGEs molecules thus formed during the Maillard reaction can lead to protein cross-linking and contribute to the development and progression of several diabetic complications such as peripheral neuropathy, cataracts, impaired wound healing, vascular damage, arterial wall stiffening and decreased myocardial compliance (Thomas et al., 2005; Wada and Yagihashi, 2005). Previously, it has been reported that long standing hyperglycemia with diabetes mellitus leads to the formation of AGEs which are involved in the generation of ROS and causes oxidative damage (Mohamed et al., 1999). Therefore, the inhibition of AR and AGEs is yet another mode of diabetes treatment not dependent on the control of blood glucose level, and would be used in the prevention or reduction of certain diabetic complications (Jung et al., 2008; Tsuji-Naito et al., 2009).

Plants have been utilized as important sources of medicinal drugs and health products since ancient days. Plants have been suggested as a rich antioxidant, as yet unexplored source of potentially useful antidiabetic drugs.There are more than 200 pure compounds from plants that have been reported to show blood glucose lowering activity (Marles and Farnsworth, 1994). The recent scientific investigations have confirmed the efficacy of many of these preparations, some of which are remarkably effective. Some such examples include; Mangiferin (leaf extract) has some pharmacological functions in altering the oxidative mechanisms (Sanchez et al., 2000) and has also been found to be effective in NIDDM (Ichiki et al., 1998); Rosmarinic acid, a phenolic antioxidant has the ability to inhibit porcine pancreatic α-amylase activity (McCue et al., 2004) *Pycnogenol* (pine bark extract), found to be effectively inhibit α-glucosidase and used to treat NIDDM (Angelika and Petra, 2007); *Phaseolamin* in white kidney bean (Maurizio et al., 2008), shows α-amylase inhibitory activity and also promoting weight loss, Genistein in soybean (Lee *et al.*, 2001) and flavonoids from *cichorium glandulosum* seeds (Yao *et al.*, 2013) are potent α-glucosidase inhibitors and have the potential to decrease post prandial hyperglycemia; *Gymnema* (Moghaddama, 2005) and

Alternanthera paronychioides extract (Wu et al., 2013) improves the ability of insulin to lower blood sugar in both type 1 and type 2 diabetes; *Vitis vinifera* seeds (Pinent et al., 2004), experimental and clinical studies have demonstrated the blood glucose lowering activity and the seeds contains the flavonoids, epicatechin, catechin, and epicatechin gallate.

Adipocytes are emerging as a potential therapeutic target for type 2 diabetes, obesity, and cardiovascular diseases (Hassan et al., 2007; Tsuduki et al., 2013). Adipogenesis on the other hand, is a complex process of cell differentiation by which pre-adipocytes become adipocytes. Peroxisome proliferator-activated receptor gamma (PPARγ) expression during differentiation is an important nuclear hormone receptor in adipocytes (Lio et al., 2010). During, the adipogenesis process, adipocytes express and secrete numerous bioactive substances called adipokines (Diezand Iglesias, 2003). Among these, adiponectin is an adipocyte derived insulin-sensitizing hormone with antidiabetic, anti-inflammatory, and antiatherosclerotic properties (Xu et al., 2009). The pharmacological intervention aimed at elevating adiponectin production in adipocytes might hold promise for the treatment and/or prevention of obesity and type 2 diabetes (Spranger et al., 2003).

Besides this, insulin-stimulated glucose uptake in adipocytes also plays an essential role in glucose homeostasis. Insulin lowers the concentration of glucose in the blood; failure to do so causes the rapid onset symptoms of diabetes. Insulin's ability to lower blood glucose levels is partly explained by an increase in the transport of glucose into muscle and adipose tissue (Gustavsson et al., 1996). The mechanism involves an insulin-triggered re-localization of glucose transporter type 4 (GLUT4). In adipocytes GLUT4 is highly expressed and insulin stimulates glucose uptake in adipocytes by rapidly trans-locating GLUT4 from intracellular stores to the plasma membrane (Choi et al., 2009).

The oral antidiabetic drugs like thiazolidinediones (TZDs) display undesirable side effects and fail to control the glycemic level effectively (Park et al., 2008). Therefore, recent attention has been focused on plant extract and plant derived compounds to treat diabetes. The numerous studies have been established on the ability of plants to enhance adipogenesis, stimulate glucose uptake and increase adiponectin secretion in adipocytes for the management of type 2 diabetes. Some such examples include;

Phloretin (apple extract); enhances adipocyte differentiation and adiponectin expression in 3T3-L1 cells (Hassan et al., 2007), Chlorogenic acid; from *Cecropia obtusifolia bertol* is a phenolic antioxidant which stimulate glucose uptake in both insulin-sensitive and insulin-resistant adipocytes (Alonso-Castro et al., 2008), Magnolol; from *Magnolia officinalis* bark found to have anti-inflammatory properties (Lo et al., 1994) and also enhance adipogenesis and glucose uptake in 3T3-L1 cells (Choi et al., 2009), Brazalian red propolis (resin); used as dietary supplementation in the management of type 2 diabetes and promote adipocyte differentiation through PPARγ activation (Lio et al., 2010), *Momodica charantia* (fruit); shown to have hypoglycemic effects in diabetic patients (Tongia et al., 2004) and also increase glucose uptake and adiponectin secretion in 3T3-L1 cells (Roffey et al., 2007).

The Malaysian rainforest store plenty of plant species which are important sources of traditional medicine. Approximately, 16% from about 10,000 species of higher plants and 2000 species of lower plants were identified to be used as herbal medicines (Lattif et al., 1984). In Peninsular Malaysia, some plants in particular; *Carica papaya* (pucuk betik), *Cosmos caudatus* (ulam raja), *Orthosiphon stamineus* (misai kucing), *Momordica charantia* (peria), and *Andrographis paniculate* (hempedu bumi) have been consumed as dietary supplementation to treat diabetes. Obviously, there are still a great number of unexplored plants that have high potential to be developed as antidiabetic drugs. Appropriate use of medicinal plants in dietary supplementation is very important in the maintenance of health (Wang et al., 2007). There are many studies have been reported on harmful effects from improper use of medicinal plants (Kao et al., 1992; Tai et al., 1992; Vanherweghem et al., 1993). Selective Malaysian plants have been reported, safe to be used as a medicinal plant because its do not contain heavy metals or are at permissible levels and also being non-cytotoxic at high concentration (Ling et al., 2010). There fore, further *in vitro* and *in vivo* investigations on toxicity are vital before it is used as a medicinal plant (Jung et al., 2010; Wang et al., 2011).

There is yet no systematic information concerning the profile of *S.aqueum* with regards to its antioxidant and antihyperglycemic activities. The purpose of this study is to contribute to the important body of knowledge about this plant in the management of type 2 diabetes. The general research approach was to initially screen the plant extract for its antioxidant properties, followed by the antihyperglycemic screen;α-glucosidase, α-amylase, aldol reductase,and advanced glycation endproducts inhibition activity. Eventually the mechanistic studies using adipocytes to measure the extracts effectiveness in adipogenesis, glucose uptake and adiponectin secretion. In order to ensure the extracts safety for consumption its heavy metal content and *in vivo* subacute toxicity in rat models was also evaluated. A bioassay-guided fractionation approach was also attempted to identify the active compounds in the extract.

4.2 METHODOLOGY

4.2.1 PLANT COLLECTION AND EXTRACTION

The leaves were obtained from Kuala Lumpur, Malaysia. They were harvested and collected from January to March, 2009. The leaves were authenticated at the Herbarium of the Forest Research Institute of Malaysia (FRIM). The extraction was carried out at Standards and Industrial Research Institute of Malaysia (SIRIM) Berhad, Shah Alam, Malaysia. The leaves were washed with copious amounts of water and distilled water. These were then allowed to air dry at room temperature for 2–3 hr. Following this the leaves were placed in a circulating oven at 40°C, until completely dry. The dried plants were powdered using a Fritsch dry miller. Ethanol (analytical grade) at 1:10 (w/v) concentrations was added to the powdered leaves. Ethanolic extraction was carried out at room temperature and was left for shaking for 24 hr in an orbital shaker. The suspension obtained was filtered using a 114 Whatman filter paper and the filtrate collected. The ethanol filtrate was concentrated using a rotary evaporator at 40°C.

4.2.2 ANTIOXIDANT ASSAYS

Three different free radical scavenging (FRS) assays: 2,2-diphenyl-1-picrylhydrazyl (DPPH), 2,2′-azino-bis-3-ethylbenzthiazoline-6-sulphonic acid (ABTS), and galvinoxyl scavenging activity and the lipid peroxidation inhibition assay were performed according to Ling et al. (2009).

4.2.3 DETERMINATION OF TOTAL PHENOLIC CONTENT (TPC)

Total phenolics were determined using the Folin–Ciocalteu method described by Miliauskas et al. (2005). This assay is based on a colorimetric oxidation and reduction reaction. First, 1mL aliquots of the extracts were added to 5mL of Folin–Ciocalteu reagent. After 3 min, 4mL of 7.5% Na_2CO_3 solution in water was added to the mixture and the content was thoroughly mixed. The absorbance at 765nm was read after 1 hr. Blank consisted of Folin-Ciocalteu reagent (5 mL), ethanol/ distilled water (1 mL) and 7.5% Na_2CO_3 solution (4 mL). A linear dose–response regression curve was generated using absorbance reading of gallic acid at the wavelength of 765 nm. The calibration curve using gallic acid was obtained in the same manner as above except that the absorbance was read after 30 min. Results were expressed as milligrams of gallic acid equivalent per gram of dry weight (mg GAE/g) of extracts. Total content of phenolic compounds in the plant extracts was calculated using this formula:

$C = A/B$

A = the equivalent concentration of gallic acid established from calibration curve (mg)

B = the dry weight of extract (g).

C = expressed as mg GAE/g dry weight of the extract

4.2.4 PRO-OXIDANT ASSAY

Pro-oxidant and antioxidant effects are attributable to the balance of two activities: free radical-scavenging activity and reducing power on iron ions. In a Fenton reaction, Fe^{2+} reacts with H_2O_2, resulting in the production of hydroxyl radical, which is considered to be the most harmful radical to biomolecules. In the Fenton reaction, Fe^{2+} is oxidized to Fe^{3+}. Many reductants such as ascorbic acid can reduce the oxidized form of iron (Fe^{3+}) to reduced form (Fe^{2+}). This reaction could enhance the generation of hydroxyl radicals. The predomination of reducing power (on iron ions) over the free radical scavenging activity results in the pro-oxidant effect. Reducing power of iron ion was measured according to the method of Tian and Hua, (2005) where 500 μL of the extract and 50 μL of 1% potassium ferricyanate [K_3Fe (CN_6)] were incubated at 50°C for 20 min. An equal volume of 10% trichloroacetic acid was then added, and mixture was centrifuged at 3000 g for 10 min. The upper layer of the solution (1 mL) was mixed with 1 mL of distilled water and 0.2 mL of 0.1% ferric chloride ($FeCl_3$), and its absorbance was recorded at 700 nm. Ethanol or distilled water was used as negative control, whereas Vitamin C and Emblica™ (a commercial antioxidant with very low pro-oxidant activity) was used as positive controls. Results are expressed in comparison with positive controls at concentration ranging from 0.1 to 0.5 mg/mL.

4.2.5 α-GLUCOSIDASE INHIBITION ASSAY

The α-glucosidase inhibition assay was performed, using the modified method of Liu et al. (2004), on 96 well plates. The α-glucosidase from *S. cerevisiae* (0.4 U/mL) was dissolved in phosphate buffer pH 6.8 supplemented with 0.2% bovine serum albumin (BSA). In the assay, 20 μL of various dilutions of the leaf extract, 0.4 U/mLof the enzyme, 20 μL of dithiothreitol (DTT) (1 mM) and 20 μLof substrate 4- nitrophenyl-α-D-glucopyranoside (PNPG) was added with 0.1 M sodium phosphate buffer pH 6.8 and incubated at 37˚C for 15 min. The reaction was stopped with 80 μl of 0.2 M sodium carbonate and the yellow color of PNPG was determined at 400 nm on a Cary 50 Bio UV–visible spectrophotometer (Varian, Inc., Palo Alto, CA). All measurements were performed in triplicates. Acarbose was used as the positive control while absence of any inhibitor was the negative control. Appropriate blanks; sample blank: sample without the enzyme; blank: without sample and enzyme were used to exclude sample color and background absorbance. The percentage inhibition was calculated as follows:

%Inhibition = [Acontrol – Asample/Acontrol] × 100%

A = absorbance

The activity of the plant extracts were assessed by plotting percentage inhibition against a range of plant extracts concentrations. EC_{50} value (effective concentration with 50% inhibition) was thus determined and expressed as means ± SEM of the triplicate measurements.

4.2.6 α-AMYLASE INHIBITION ASSAY

The α-amylase inhibition assay was performed using the modified method of Liu et al. (2004), on 96 well plates. Porcine pancreatic α-amylase (Sigma Type IV-B) was dissolved in ice-cold distilled water to give a concentration of 2 U/mL. Potato soluble starch solution (1%) was prepared in 20 mM phosphate buffer pH 6.9. The dextrose and sodium chloride (DNS) solution was prepared with 1 g DNS, 30g sodium potassium tartrate dehydrate and 2 M NaOH in 100 mL solution. In the assay, 80 μL of various dilutions of the leaf extract and 40 μL of amylase enzyme were added and incubated at room temperature for 10 min. After which 40 μL of starch was added and incubated at 37°C for 10 min. Finally, 80 μL of DNS solution was added and solution incubated in a water bath at 95°C for 10 min, to detect the reducing sugar which will change the DNS from orange to brick red color. The absorbance was measured at 540 nm on a Cary 50 Bio UV–visible spectrophotometer (Varian, Inc., Palo Alto, CA). All measurements were performed in triplicates. Acarbose was used as the positive control. Appropriate blanks as described were used. The percentage inhibition and EC_{50} value was determined as described in section 4.2.5.

4.2.7 AR INHIBITORY ACTIVITY

The activities of recombinant human aldol reductase (AR) were measured according to the procedure of Nishimura et al. (1991). The reaction solution consisted of 870 μL 100 mM sodium phosphate buffer (pH 6.2), 10 μL AR enzyme (0.2 U/mL), 50 μL 3 mM nicotinamide adenine dinucleotide phosphate (NADPH), 20 μL extract (dissolved in ethanol), and 50 μL of 5 mM DL-glyceraldehyde as the substrate. The reaction mixture was incubated at 25°C for 3 min and AR activity was determined by measuring the decrease in NADPH absorption at 340 nm over a 10 min period. Quercetin was used as the positive control, while negative control was the assay performed without the sample. The percentage inhibition was calculated as follows:

$$\%\text{Inhibition} = [A_{control/min} - A_{sample/min} / A_{control/min}] \times 100\%$$

$A_{control/min}$ = the reduction of absorbance for 10 min with buffer and substrate, respectively.

$A_{sample/min}$ = the reduction of absorbance for 10 min with the test sample and substrate,respectively.

EC_{50} value was determined as described.

4.2.8 AGE'S FORMATION INHIBITORY ACTIVITY

The inhibitory effect of *S. aqueum* extracts on the Maillard reaction was carried out by measuring the fluorescent AGE molecules according to Matsuura et al. (2002). The reaction mixture consisted of 4 mg BSA in 400 μL 50 mM sodium phosphate buffer (pH 7.4), 80 μL 1M glucose, and 20 μL 1 mg/mL extracts (dissolved in ethanol). The reaction solution (500 μL) was incubated at 80°C for 0, 1, 3, 5, and 7 days while the negative control was kept at 4°C. Green tea (1 mg/mL) was used as the positive control in the AGE assay. After the incubation period, the reaction was stopped with the addition of 25 μL 100% Trichloroacetic acid (TCA) followed by centrifugation at 15000 rpm for 10 min. The AGE-BSA precipitate thus formed was dissolved in 1 mL phosphate buffer saline (PBS) (pH 10) and its fluorescence intensity determined with excitation and emission wavelengths at 385 nm and 415 nm, respectively on a Tecan fluorescence reader (Mannedorf, Switzerland). The inhibition percentage was calculated as described above. The inhibitory activity of the leaf extract was determined by plotting the % inhibition (fluorescence intensity) against a range of incubation time (days).

4.2.9 MTT VIABILITY ASSAY

Cell viability was assessed by the 3, (4-5-dimethylthiazol-2-yl)-2,5-diphenyl tetrazolium (MTT) viability assay (Popovich et al., 2010). The 3T3-L1 cells were seeded in 96-well plates (3000 cells/well) and allowed to adhere overnight. After 24 hr, culture media containing *S. aqueum* leaf extract (1-100 μg/ml) was added to each well. The control culture was treated in basal medium (Dulbecco's modified Eagle's medium (DMEM) with 10% fetal calf serum (FBS) and 0.1 % dimethyl sulfoxide (DMSO)). The cells were incubated for 48 hr at 37°C in a humidified atmosphere of 5% CO_2. After 48 hr, the culture medium and test samples were replaced with 20 μl of MTT (1 mg/ml) and incubated in the dark for 2 hr. Formazan crystals were formed and solubilized using 0.02 M HCl in 10% sodium dodecyl sulfate (SDS). Absorbance was measured using a microplate reader (Bio-Rad, MA, USA) at 570 nm. Cell viability (%) was calculated as:

[(mean A sample – mean A blank)/mean A control] x 100

A= absorbance

4.2.10 3T3-L1 PRE-ADIPOCYTE DIFFERENTIATION

Pre-adipocyte differentiation assay was assessed according to the modified method of Alonso-Castro et al.(2008). The 3T3-L1 pre-adipocytes were plated into 24-well plate at approximately 3×10^4 cells/well. The cells were incubated until 90% confluence and maintained in DMEM supplemented with 10% FBS, 1% penicillin and 1% hepes buffer at 37°C under a humidified 5% CO_2 atmosphere. In order to initiate differentiation of pre-adipocyte into adipocytes, at 2 days after 90% confluence (defined as day 0), cells were incubated in differentiation initiation medium (DIM) containing 0.5 mM 3-isobutyl-1-methylxanthine (IBMX) and 0.25 μM dexamethasone (DEX) in DMEM containing 10% FBS. After 2 days (defined as day 3), the culture media was changed to the differentiation progression medium (DPM) containing 100 nM insulin and 10% FBS in DMEM. After 2 days (defined as day 5), the medium was replaced again with fresh DMEM with/without insulin (100 nM), and the replacement of fresh medium every 2 days were continued until day 10. To examine the effect of samples in 3T3-L1 pre-adipocyte differentiation, the cells were treated (from day 0) with *S. aqueum* leaf extract (0.04-5 μg/mL) at indicated concentrations for the entire 10 days. The concentrations of samples used in this assay were determined to be non-cytotoxic to the 3T3-L1 cells, as established in the MTT viability assay. The control cultures were treated in basal medium (DMEM with 10 % FBS and 0.1 % DMSO) and insulin (100 nM). The cells treated with rosiglitazone served as positive control. On day 10, the adipocytes were washed three times with (PBS) and fixed with 10% formalin in PBS for 1 hr. Each well was washed with PBS three times and stained with 200 μl of 60% oil-red-O solution for 30 min. The cells were again washed once with PBS and allowed to air dry. The cells were photographed using an Olympus CKX41 inverted microscope. Lipid and oil-red-O were extracted using 100% isopropanol and the absorbance was measured using a spectrophotometer (Bio-Rad, MA, USA) at a wavelength of 520 nm.

4.2.11 2-NBDG UPTAKE IN 3T3-L1 ADIPOCYTES

Glucose uptake into 3T3-L1 adipocytes was measured according to the modified method of Alonso-Castro et al. (2008). Mature adipocytes, differentiated on 24-well fluorescence plates (Thermo Scientific, USA) were incubated for 48 hr with plain DMEM medium (serum and glucose free), 80 μM of the fluorescent glucose analog 2-NBDG and added with *S. aqueum* leaf extract (0.04–5 μg/ml) at indicated concentrations, with/without insulin (100 nM). The control cultures were treated in basal medium (DMEM with 10% FBS and 0.1% DMSO) and insulin (100 nM). The cells treated with rosiglitazone served as positive control. After incubation, cultures were washed out of free 2-NBDG using PBS. The fluorescence retained in cell monolayers was measured with a fluorescence microplate reader (Perkin Elmer, Boston, MA, USA), set at an excitation wavelength of 485 nm and emission wavelength of 535 nm, using the software Workout 5.0.

4.2.12 ADIPONECTIN QUANTIFICATION

Adiponectin secreted by the 3T3-L1 adipocytes was measured using a Quantikine enzyme-linked immunosorbent assay (ELISA) Mouse Adiponectin Immunoassay kit (SPI Bio, Belin Pharma, France). The culture medium tested for adiponectin level was collected at 48 hr of treatment period with *S. aqueum* leaf extracts (0.04–5 μg/mL), after differentiation induction with insulin (100 nM). The basal medium (DMEM with 10% FBS and 0.1 % DMSO) and insulin (100 nM) served as control. Culture medium treated with rosiglitazone served as positive control. The culture medium was centrifuged for 10 min at 1500 rpm and the supernatants were used in the assay. The concentration of adiponectin secreted in the cell culture supernatant was determined according to the method recommended by the manufacturer. A reference curve was obtained in the range of mouse adiponectin standard from 5–150 ng/mL.

4.2.13 TOXICITY EVALUATION

HEAVY METAL CONTENT DETERMINATION

Lead, arsenic, and mercury content of the powderized leaf of *S. aqueum* was determined against international standards, inductively coupled plasma — optical emission spectrometry (ICP-OES) for the determination of arsenic and lead, and atomic absorption spectroscopy (AAS) for the determination of mercury.

ACUTE TOXICITY STUDY

The acute toxicity study was conducted according to the organization of economic co-operation and development (OECD) guideline 420, (2001a). A dose limit of 2000 mg/kg of the standardized ethanolic extract of *S. aqueum* leaf was used in five healthy male sprague dawley (SD) rat (160–200g). Prior to dosing with the extract, the rats were fasted overnight from food, but were allowed free access to water. Then, a single dose of 2000 mg/kg was administered to all the rats in the treatment group. The rats in the control group did not receive any extract. The rats were observed for mortality, clinical signs, behaviors (unusual aggressiveness, unusual vocalisation, restlessness, sedation, and somnolence); movements (twitch, tremor, ataxia, catatonia, paralysis, convulsion, fasciculation, prostration, and unusual locomotion); convulsion (clonic, tonic, tonic–clonic, asphyxia, and opisthotonus) for the first 2 hr and then hourly for 5 hr and, finally periodically until 24 hr. All of the experimental animals were maintained under close observation for 7 days. The LD_{50} was predicted to be above 2000 mg/kg if three or more rats survived.

SUBACUTE TOXICITY STUDY

The subacute toxicity study was also evaluated according to the OECD guideline 407, (2001b). Fifteen male SD rats were divided randomly into five groups (3 rats per group). Rats in group one received a dose of 50 mg/kg (0.3 mL) of standardized ethanolic extract of *S. aqueum* leaf while rats group two, three and four received the same volume of extracts corresponding to 300, 900 and 2000 mg/kg, respectively. Rats in group five served as the control group and they received 0.3 ml of vehicle (olive oil). Toxic manifestations and mortality were monitored daily for 14 days. The body weight as well as food and water consumption of all the animals were recorded daily. On day 14, all the rats were anaesthetized using dimethyl ether and blood samples were collected *via* cardiac puncture for biochemical analyses. Following this, the rats were sacrificed by clavicle dislocation. Serum was obtained from the clotted blood *via* centrifugation (5000 rpm for 15 min) and stored at –80°C prior to analysis. The serum samples were analyzed for determination of alanine aminotransferase (ALT), alkaline phosphate (ALP), creatinine, urea and total protein. Their vital organs (heart, liver, kidney and pancreas) were harvested and cleaned with saline, weighed and preserved in 10% formalin for histopathological analyses. Each organ to body weight ratio (relative organ weight) was calculated as (weight of organ/body weight of rat on day of sacrifice) × 100% (Mohamed et al., 2011). Small blocks of tissues were taken from the organs harvested from the rats and processed using an automated tissue processor. After processing, the paraffin embedded tissues were sectioned to a thickness of 6 μM using a rotary microtome and dried overnight in an oven at 37°C. The sections were stained with Hematoxylin and Eosin (H and E) and examined microscopically for signs of toxicity.

4.2.14 ISOLATION AND IDENTIFICATION OF ACTIVE COMPOUNDS FROM S. AQUEUM LEAF

The leaf extract (0.8 g) dissolved in absolute ethanol was subjected into a Gilson Preparative high-performance liquid chromatography (HPLC) GX-281/322/156 (Middleton, Wisconsin) using a Waters Xterra Prep RP18 on-board diagnostics (OBD) (19 × 50 mm, 5 μm) (Milford, USA) and the active compounds were detected with a UV detector (210 and 254 nm). The mobile phases consisted of 0.1% formic acid in acetonitrile and 0.1% formic acid in water. The flow rate was 12 mL/min with an injection volume of 3 mL at 40°C. The solvent gradient consisted of 0–10% acetonitrile for 10 min, 10–85% acetonitrile for 70 min, and finally 100% acetonitrile for 5 min to recondition the column. 40 fractions were collected and analyzed for its α-glucosidase and α-amylase activity. The active fractions were then analyzed on a Shidmazu Prominence UFLC-LCMS-IT-TOF (Kyoto, Japan).

The analysis was performed in both the positive and negative modes. The capillary temperature was 250°C; voltage was 1.65 kV and nitrogen gas was used as the sheath gas. A mass range of 200–2000 m/z was scanned in both positive and negative full ion monitoring mode. The compounds were monitored by measuring absorbance at 254 nm and separated using a Waters Xterra MS C18 (2.5 × 20 mm, 2.5 μm) IS (Milford, USA) column eluted with 0.1% formic acid in acetonitrile and 0.1% formic acid in water. The solvent gradient consisted of 0–10% acetonitrile for 3 min, 10–40% acetonitrile for 10 min, and finally 100% acetonitrile for 5 min to reconditioning the column. The flow rate was 0.5 mL/min with an injection volume of 10 uL at 40°C. The active compounds were characterized by 1H and 13C NMR spectra using a Jeol ECA 400 (400 MHz) NMR spectrometer (Jeol Ltd, USA).

4.3 DISCUSSION AND RESULTS

4.3.1 TAXONOMIC CLASSIFICATION OF S. AQUEUM

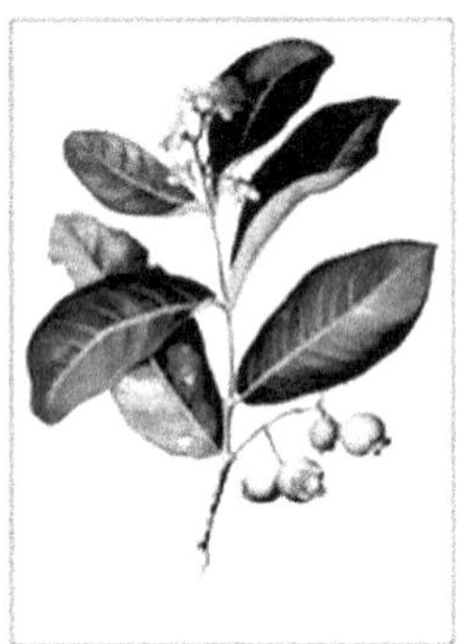

Source: Blanco, 1880

Name	***Syzygium aqueum***
Local names	Water jambu, Rose apple, watery apple
Synonyms	Eugenia aqua
Division	Magnoliophyta Magnoliophytina
Class	Magnoliatae Rosidae Cornanae
Order	Myrtales Myrtineae
Family	Myrtaceae
Genus	*Syzygium*
Species	*Syzygium aqueum* (Burm.f.) Alston

4.3.2 ANTIOXIDANT ACTIVITY

The extracts were evaluated for its DPPH, galvinoxyl and ABTS scavenging ability and its activity is as shown in Table 1. As observed in Table 1, the leaves of *S. aqueum* displayed almost similar free radicals scavenging (FRS) ability to grape seed extract. Among the three FRS assays, the

ABTS assay was observed to show the lowest IC_{50}value indicating its sensitivity over the other assays. Although, the ABTS assay showed the highest sensitivity compared to DPPH and galvinoxyl assays, the DPPH assay isfavored owing to its ease of use and reproducibility. The leaf extract also displayed high total phenolic content (TPC) compared to the grape seed extract (Table 1). A strong correlation between the FRS activity and TPC of *S. aqueum* and grape seed extracts was evident in that higher TPC corresponded to higher FRS activity (Palanisamy et al., 2011).

In addition, *S. aqueum* leaf extract displayed far better lipid peroxidation inhibition activity compared to the grape seed extract (Table 1). It has been shown that treatment with grapeseed extract suppresses lipid peroxidation and reduces hypoxic ischemic brain injury in neonatal rat (Feng et al., 2005). In this chapter, we noticed that the *S. aqueum* leaf extract is a more potent lipid peroxidation inhibitor than the grape seed extract. This could be due to its outstanding FRS ability and high total phenolic content compared to the grape seed extract.

TABLE 1 Free radical scavenging activity, lipid peroxidation inhibition and total phenolic content

	IC_{50} (mg/ml)				IC_{50} (GAE mg/g)
Extracts	**DPPH Scavenging**	**ABTS Scavenging**	**Galvinoxyl Scavenging**	**Lipid Peroxidation Inhibition**	**Total Phenolic Content (TPC)**
Syzygium aqueum leaf	0.21 ± 0.02	0.03 ± 0.002	0.08 ± 0.01	0.04 ± 0.001	497 ± 83
Grape seed@	0.27 ± 0.1	0.04 ± 0.01	0.09 ± 0.03	0.06 ± 0.02	312 ± 67

@ Positive control, Data shown as mean ± SD, n = 3.

4.3.3 PRO-OXIDANT CAPABILITY

A pro-oxidant is defined as a substance that can produce oxygen by-products of metabolism that can cause damage to cells. It is known that vitamin C and other antioxidants at higher concentrations tend to behave like a pro-oxidant (Linget al., 2010). The interaction of vitamin C with 'free' catalytically active metal ions could contribute to oxidative damage through the production of hydroxyl and aloxyl radicals; whether these mechanisms occur *in vivo*, however, is uncertain. Plant extracts with significant antioxidant activity have been marketed for its health benefits. However, their use as dietary supplements should be considered with caution as they could also exhibit pro-oxidant effects (Joubert et al., 2005).

In this, the pro-oxidant capability of *S. aqueum* extract was compared with that of vitamin C and Emblica™ (Figure 1), a commercially available plant extract which is known for its very low pro-oxidant capacity (Xiaoli et al., 2008). As expected, vitamin C showed the highest pro-oxidant activity, induced by transition metals, and the positive control Emblica™ showed the lowest pro-oxidant capacity. Interestingly, *S. aqueum* leafextracts exhibited lower pro-oxidant capacity than vitamin C, and comparable to that of Emblica™ over the range of concentration tested. Suggesting, *S. aqueum* leaf extract could be a good antioxidant with a low pro-oxidant capability.

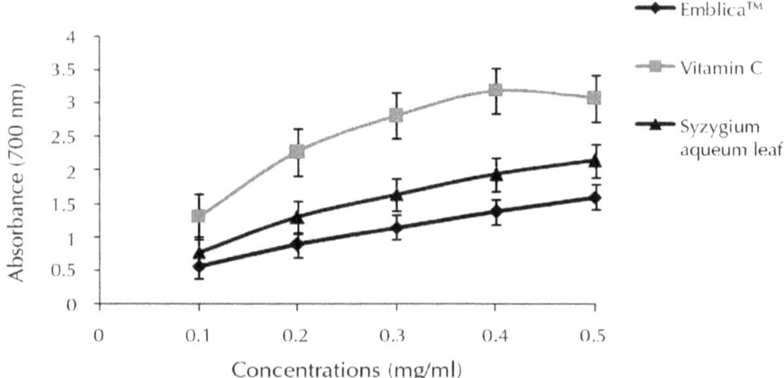

FIGURE 1 Prooxidant capacity of *S. aqueum* leaf extracts compared with vitamin C and Emblica™. Data expressed in mean ± SD, n=3.

4.3.4 ANTIDIABETIC ACTIVITY OF S. AQUEUM LEAF EXTRACT

INHIBITION OF α-GLUCOSIDASE AND α-AMYLASE

α-Glucosidase is one of the glucosidases located in the brush border surface membrane of intestinal cells, and is a key enzyme for carbohydrate digestion.α-Amylases are endoglucanases, which hydrolyze the internal alpha 1,4 glucosidic linkages in starch. These enzymes have been recognized as therapeutic targets for modulation of postprandial hyperglycemia (Shobana *et al.*, 2009). The antiglycemic assays, α-glucosidase and α-amylase, were determined with Acarbose as a positive control. Acarbose(Glucobay) is used in the clinical management of early diabetes (Heo*et al.*, 2009).

It was observed that(Figure 2), the *S.aqueum* leaf extracts were far more effective (*$p<0.05$)in inhibiting the carbohydrate hydrolyzing enzymes, α-glucosidase(EC_{50}= 11 ± 1 μg/mL) and α-amylase (EC_{50}=8 ± 0.2 μg/mL) than the drug acarbose (EC_{50}= 28 ± 1 μg/mL, α-glucosidase; EC_{50}=12± 1 μg/mL, α-amylase).

It has been reported that plant extracts with both antioxidant activity and high total phenolic content exhibited α-glucosidase and α-amylase inhibition activity, *Nephelium lappaceum* rind extracts (Palanisamy et al.,2011), *Peltophorum pterocarpum* leaf extracts (Manaharan et al.,2011), and *Psidium guajava* leaf extracts (Wang et al., 2010).

Antioxidants which predominantly originate from phytochemicals have been reported to play an important role in the treatment of diabetes (Kim et al., 2011). It was thought that the high content of phenolic along with its antioxidant property in *S.aqueum* leaf extracts also contributes to its α-glucosidase and α-amylase inhibition activity.

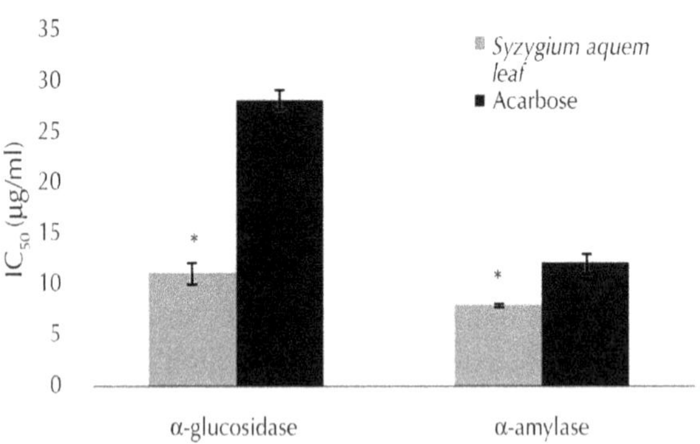

FIGURE 2 α-Glucosidase and α-amylase inhibitory activity of *S. aqueum* leaf extracts. Data expressed in mean ± SD, n = 3. Paired *t*-test showed significant value, *$p<0.05$.

INHIBITION OF AR AND AGE'S FORMATION

The AR and AGEs were widely identified as the major byproducts in glucose pathway which contribute to the development of oxidative stress and progression of diabetes and its related microvascular and macrovascular complications(Baynes, 1991;Baynes and Torpe, 1999). Increased blood glucose level causes the generation of free radicals (Halliwell and Gutteridge,1999) *via* various mechanisms. Interconnection between free radicals and oxidative stress with pathogenesis of diabetes and its complications are well established (Baynes, 1991; Baynes and Torpe, 1999; Jung et al., 2009).Therefore, the inhibition of AR and AGEs is yet another mode of diabetes treatment not dependent on the control of blood glucose level, and would be used in the prevention or reduction of certain diabetic complications (Jung *et al.*, 2008; Tsuji-Naito *et al.*, 2009).

TABLE 2 The AR inhibitory activity of *S. aqueum* leaf extracts and compared with other plant extracts

	IC_{50} (µg/ml)
Extracts	**AR inhibition**
Syzygium aqueum leaf	0.03 ± 0.01

TABLE 2 *(Continued)*

Peltophorum pterocarpum leaf	0.06 ± 0.02[a]
Nephelium lappaceum rind	0.04 ± 0.02[b]
Cirsium maackii leaf	0.54 ± 0.04[c]
Quercetin[@]	1.67 ± 0.02
Quercetin[@]	1.68 ± 0.05[a]
	1.72 ± 0.12[b]

Data shown as mean ± SD, n = 3, [@]Positive control,[a]Manaharan et al. (2011),

[b] Palanisamy et al. (2011), Manaharan et al. (2011),[c] Jung et al. (2009).

In this chapter, the ethanolic extract of *S. aqueum* leaf was seen to inhibit AR activity far better than the pure compound quercetin which was used as the positive control in this assay (Table 2). Quercetin, a phenolic compound, has been used as a positive control in AR inhibition studies (Kawanishi et al., 2003; Manaharan et al., 2011). The *S. aqueum* leaf ethanolic extract was found to be about 55 times more effective than quercetin. We compared the extracts ability to inhibit AR with other plant extracts that have been reported (Table 2). Among the plant extracts reported, *S. aqueum* was seen to exhibit the highest activity. A similar trend was observed with the inhibitory activity of AGEs formation. The high antioxidant *S. aqueum* leaf extracts exhibited higher AGEs inhibition activity compared to green tea throughout the 7day incubation period (Figure 3). The maximum inhibition activity was seen at the indicated incubation time of 7 days, 89% inhibition for ethanolic extract of *S. aqueum* leaf and 45% for green tea. Green tea was used as a positive control in this AGEs inhibition assay. Wu et al. (2009), have reported that epigalocatechingallate from green tea inhibit the glycation process far better than the antiglycation agent, aminoguanidine.

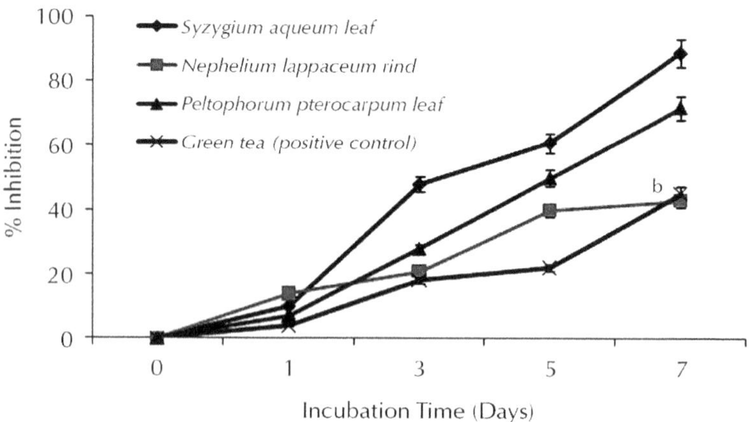

FIGURE 3 Advanced glycation end products (AGEs) inhibitory activity of *S.aqueum* leaf and other plant extracts. Data expressed in mean ± SD, n=3. [a]Manaharan et al. (2011) and [b] Palanisamy, Manaharan et al. (2011).

Figure 3 also compares the AGEs inhibition activity of other plant extracts. Manaharan et al. (2011) reported *P. pterocarpum* leaf extracts ability to inhibit AGEs formation at 7day incubation by about 72%. Palanisamy et al. (2011) observed inhibition of AGEs formation at 7day incubation by ethanolic extracts of *N. lappaceum* rind to be only 43%. A similar study by Wu et al. (2009) reported at 7day incubation period; the inhibition of AGEs formation by guava (*P. guajava* L.) to be only 22.8%. It is therefore concluded that *S. aqueum* leaf ethanolic extract has the highest AGEs formation inhibition activity among the other plant extracts studied. Ho et al. (2010) compared anti-glycation capacities of several herbal infusions with that of green tea and concluded that the amount of phenolic and flavonoid in the infusions highly correlated with their anti-glycation activity. The high phenolic content in *S. aqueum* leaf ethanolic extracts (Palanisamy et al., 2011) may be the reason for its high anti-glycation activity.Flavonoids from plants have been reported (Jung et al., 2009) to have the potential to be developed as therapeutic agents for diabetic complications and oxidative stress-related diseases due to its AR and AGEs inhibition activity.It is envisaged that the high AR and AGEs formation inhibitory activity observed in the *S. aqueum* leaf ethanolic extracts could be due to the presence of particular bio-actives in the crude extract.

4.3.5 VIABILITY OF 3T3-L1 CELLS

The toxic concentration of *S. aqueum* leaf extract was assessed *via* MTT viability assay. There were no significant (p>0.05) differences in viability of 3T3-L1 cells at concentration up to 5 μg/mLfor *S. aqueum* leaf extract compared to the control (Figure 4). The results showed that the viability of 3T3-L1 cells significantly (*p<0.05) decreased at concentration of 10 μg/mLand higher for *S. aqueum* leaf extract compared to the control (Figure 4). A 29% decrease in viability was observed at the highest concentration 75 μg/mLof *S. aqueum* leaf extract. Suggesting that *S. aqueum* leaf extract exerts a toxic effect on 3T3-L1 cells at concentration higher than 75 μg/ml. It was therefore decided that the non-cytotoxic concentrations of 0.04–5 μg/ml of the *S. aqueum* leaf extract will be used in the following experiments.

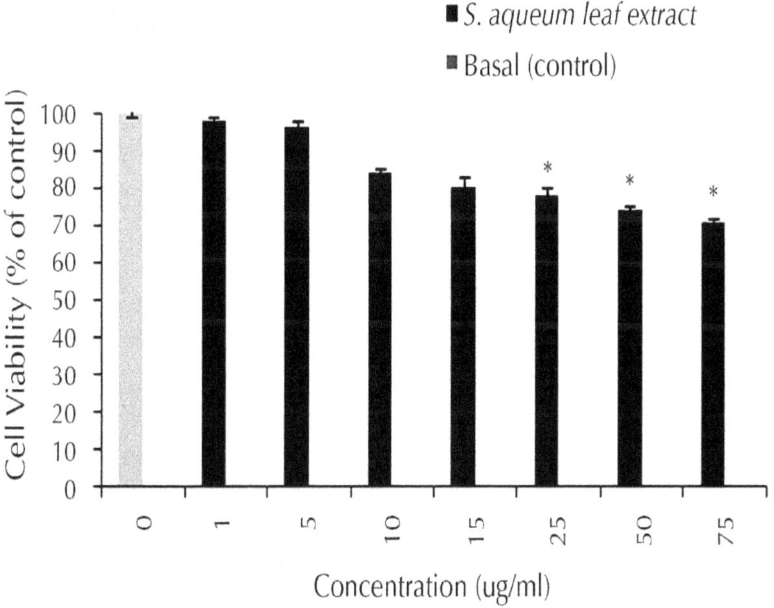

FIGURE 4 The MTT cell viability of *S. aqueum* leaf extracts. Cultures in basal medium served as control. Data expressed in mean ± SD, n = 3. One way ANOVA, Tukey's post hoc test showed significant value, *p<0.05.

4.3.6 DIFFERENTIATION OF 3T3-L1 PRE-ADIPOCYTES

Adipogenesis is a process where the pre-adipocytes undergo growth arrest and subsequent terminal differentiation into mature adipocytes.This is accompanied by a dramatic increase in expression of adipocyte genes including adipocyte fatty acid binding protein and lipid-metabolizing enzymes. Activation of PPARγ by its ligands is a key process for adipocyte differentiation (Bouaboula et al., 2005).Current understanding of adipogenesis is based on 3T3-L1 cells. As pre-adipocytes, 3T3-L1 cells resemble fibroblasts and replicate in culture medium until they form a confluent monolayer. Subsequent stimulation with IBMX, DEX and insulin (as mentioned in methodology section) prompt these cells to express adipocyte-specific genes includingPPARγ (Chien et al., 2005). In this, we assessed the ability of *S. aqueum* leaf extract to induce 3T3-L1 pre-adipocytes differentiation into adipocytes in order to obtain biological evidence that *S. aqueum* leaf extract and its bioactive compounds are activators of PPARγ. However, this can only be further confirmed *via* PPARγ expressionstudies on adipocytes.

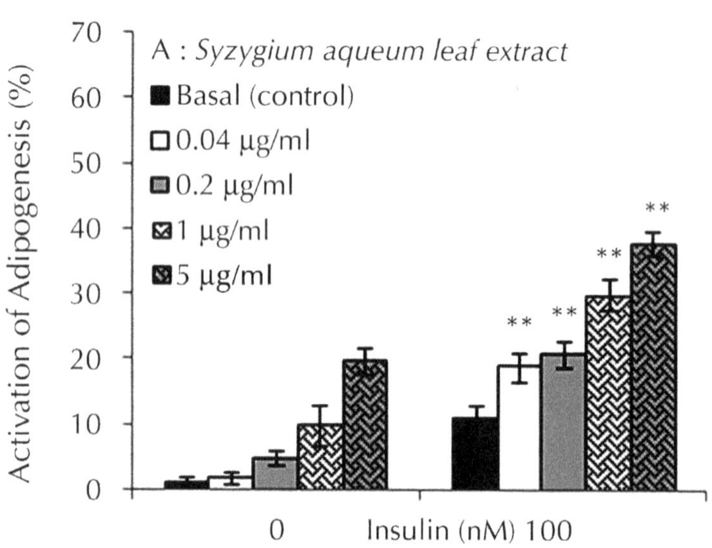

FIGURE 5 *(Continued)*

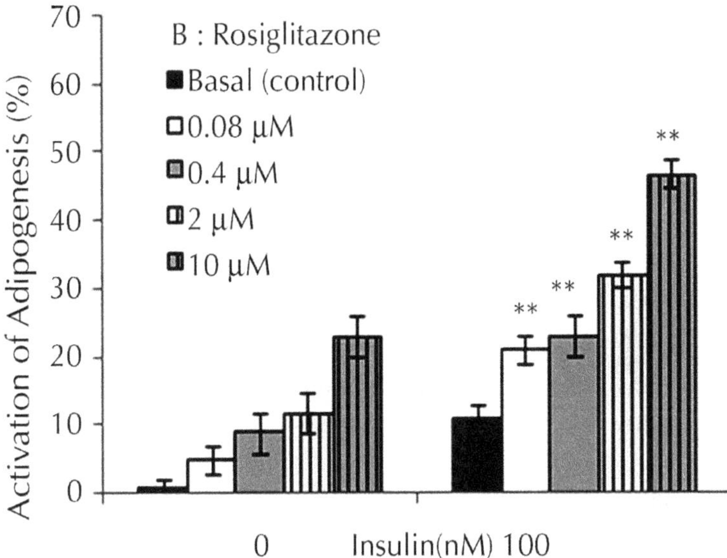

FIGURE 5 The *S. aqueum* leaf extracts (A) ability to enhance adipogenesis in 3T3-L1 pre-adipocytes in the absence(0 nM) and presence of insulin (100 nM) at indicated concentrations of 0.04-5 μg/ml. Cultures in basal medium and insulin served as control. Cells treated with rosiglitazone (B) at indicated concentrations of 0.08–10 μM, served as positive control. Data expressed in mean ± SD, n = 3. Student paired *t*-test showed significant value, **p<0.005.

It was observed that *S. aqueum* leaf extract enhance adipogenesis in the absence and presence of insulin. The results also showed that *S. aqueum* leaf extract enhances adipogenesis in the absence of insulin in a dose-dependent manner and can be said to have insulin-like activity (Figure 5(A)). An 18 % increase in the activation of adipogenesis was observed compared to the control at the highest concentration of 5 μg/mL for the *S. aqueum* leaf extract without insulin. In addition, the leaf extract with insulin (100 nM) displayed a significant (**p<0.005) increase in adipogenesis compared to the extracts without insulin in all the concentrations tested (Figure 5(A)).Overall, it was observed that *S. aqueum* leaf extract and its six bioactive compounds activate adipogenesis (without insulin) and at the same time sensitizes insulin (with insulin) in a dose-dependent manner similar to that observed with rosiglitazone (Figure 5(B)). Rosiglitazone, a

TZDs family of drugs acts primarily by increasing insulin sensitivity through activation of PPARγ (Christensen *et al.*, 2009). Previously, Hassan et al. (2007) reported phloretin's ability to enhance adipogenesis in 3T3-L1 cells by transcriptional activity of PPARγ. The results suggest that these compounds may have the ability to increase insulin sensitivity by activation of PPARγ.

4.3.7 2-NBDG UPTAKE IN 3T3-L1 ADIPOCYTES

The occurrence of type 2 diabetes mellitus is primarily related to the inability of glucose transportation into tissues due to defects ininsulin action, a phenomenon known as insulin resistance. Insulin induces glucose uptake in adipocytes by binding to insulin receptor proteins within the cell leading to the translocation of GLUT 4 to the cell surface (Rathi et al., 2002). Resistance to this effect causes increase in blood glucose level, a condition known as hyperglycemia (De Fronzo et al., 1992).We confirmed the insulin-like and insulin-sensitizes properties of *S. aqueum* leaf extract and its six bioactive compounds in experiments showing the stimulation of 2-NBDG uptake into adipocytes.

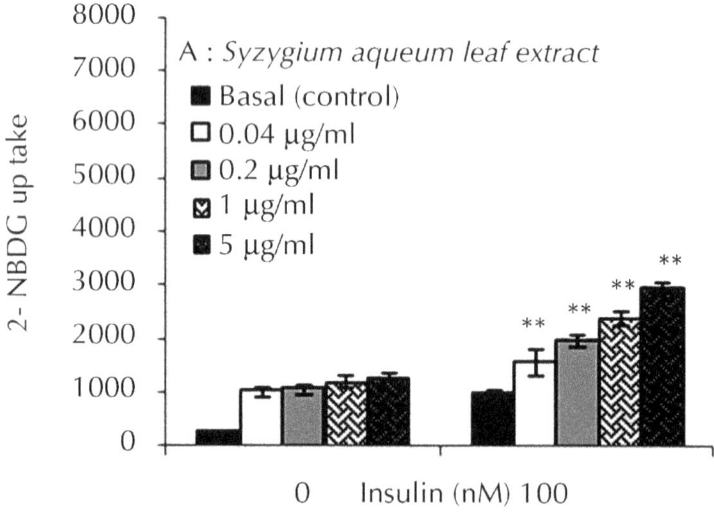

FIGURE 6 *(Continued)*

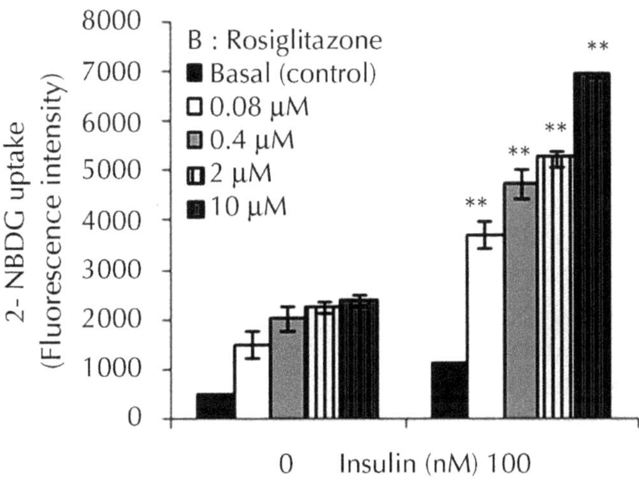

FIGURE 6 The *S. aqueum* leaf extracts (A) ability to stimulate 2-NBDG uptake in 3T3-L1 adipocytes in the absence (0 nM) and presence of insulin (100 nM) at indicated concentrations of 0.04–5 μg/ml. Cultures in basal medium and insulin served as control. Cells treated with rosiglitazone (B) at indicated concentrations of 0.08-10 μM, served as positive control. Data expressed in mean ± SD, n = 3. Student paired *t*-test showed significant value, **p<0.005.

It was noted that, *S. aqueum* leaf extract without insulin stimulates 2-NBDG uptake far better than control (Figure 6(A)) and can be said to have insulin-like activity from concentrations as low as 0.04μg/mL. Recently, Jamun (*Syzygium cumini*) extract at concentration of 100 μg/mL has shown an increase in glucose uptake compared to the control (Kaur et al., 2011). In parallel experiments, the effect of *S. aqueum* leaf extract on 2-NBDG uptake into adipocytes was also assayed in the presence of insulin (100 nM). *S. aqueum* leaf extract with insulin displayed a significant (**p<0.005) increase in glucose uptake dose-dependently compared to the extracts without insulin (Figure 6(A)).Generally, we observed that the leaf extract stimulate 2-NBDG uptake far more efficiently in the presence of insulin (100 nM) than in the absence of insulin in all the concentrations tested (Figure 6(A)) as similar to that observed with rosiglitazone (Figure 6(B)).It has been shown that plant extracts have the ability to stimulate glucose uptake far better in the presence of insulin than in the absence of insulin (Kang and Kim, 2004; Alonso-Castro et al., 2008).

4.3.8 INCREASE IN ADIPONECTIN SECRETION

Adiponectin, also referred as Acrp30, AdipoQ, and GBP-28, is a 244 amino acid protein, which is physiologically active and highly expressed in adipocytes (Tsaoet al.,2002). Adiponectin increases insulin sensitivity by stimulating fatty acid oxidation, decreases plasma triglycerides and improves glucose metabolism (Leeet al., 2009).Therefore, adiponectin is regarded as being a crucial tool for the diagnoses of type 2 diabetes mellitus (Lee et al.,2009).

We evaluated the effect of *S. aqueum* leaf extract on adiponetin secretion in adipocytes. It was noted that, *S. aqueum* leaf extract in the presence of insulin (100 nM) increase adiponectin concentration dose-dependently and far better than basal (control) and insulin alone (Figure 7).The *S. aqueum* leaf extract's ability to increase adiponectin secretion in adipocytes was comparable to the rosiglitazone (Figure 7). This finding suggests that *S. aqueum* leaf extract has the potential to retard the development of diseases in insulin resistance states such as obesity and type 2 diabetes mellitus by increasing adiponectin secretion.

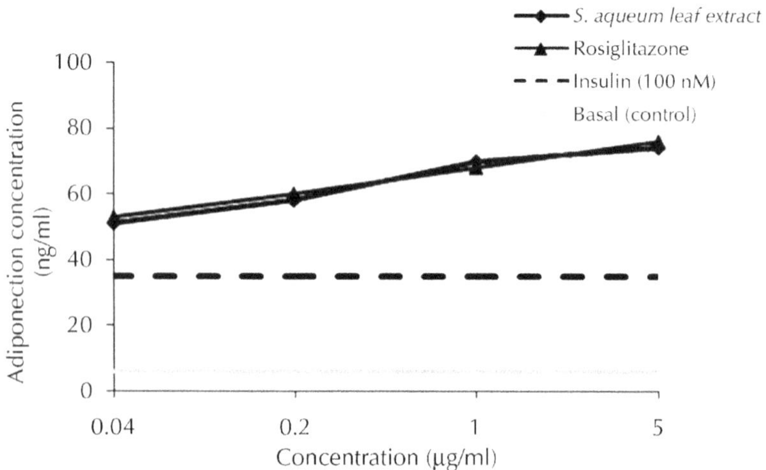

FIGURE 7 Quantification of adiponectin secreted in 3T3-L1 cell culture medium added with *S. aqueum* leaf extract at indicated concentrations 0.04–5 μg/ml. Cultures in basal medium and insulin served as control. Rosiglitazone served as positive control. Data expressed in mean ± SD, n = 3.

4.2.9 TOXICITY EVALUATION OF S.AQUEUM LEAF EXTRACT

DETERMINATION OF HEAVY METAL CONTENT

In the use of plant extracts for nutraceuticals industries, it is deemed important to ensure the safety efficacy of *S. aqueum* extracts. Therefore in this Study, the lead, arsenic, and mercury content of powdered *S. aqueum* was determined against international standards using the ICP-OES for the determination of arsenic and lead, and AAS for the determination of mercury. Table 3 shows the levels of the aforementioned heavy metals in powdered *S. aqueum* were 0.21 < 0.01 and <0.02 ppm, respectively, which is far below the permissible levels for nutraceuticals (10, 5, and 0.5, respectively). This study supports the use of *S. aqueum* extract as a possible nutraceutical product (Ling et al., 2010).

TABLE 3 Heavy metal content in *S. aqueum* leaf powder

Heavy metal (ppm)	*S. aqueum* leaf	Permissible level for nutraceutical[@]
Lead	0.21	10
Arsenic	< 0.01	5
Mercury	< 0.02	0.5

[@](Ling et al.,2010)

SUBACUTE TOXICITY EVALUATION

Medicinal plant sare presumed to be safe without any compromising health effects (Harizal *et al.*, 2010; Hor *et al.*, 2011). However, appropriate use of medicinal plants in dietary supplementation is very important in the maintenance of health (Wang et al., 2007). Till now, there are many reports citing the harmful effects of improper use of medicinal plants (Kao et al.,

1992; Tai et al., 1992; Vanherweghem et al., 1993). The ethanolic extract of *S. aqueum* leaf is safe to be used as a medicinal plant because it does not contain heavy metals and also being non-cytotoxic at high concentration (Ling et al., 2010). We further evaluate the subacute toxicity effect of standardized ethanolic extract of *S. aqueum* leaf using *invivo* model.

The subacute toxicity for 14 days has been advocated as a fundamental test to assess safety, and has been used in many safety assessment studies (Konan and Bacchi, 2007; Asare et al., 2011; Mohamed et al., 2011). In this 14 day period of subacute toxicity evaluation, rats were given standardized ethanolic extract of *S. aqueum* leaf at doses of 50, 300, 900, and 2000 mg/kg showed no mortality and all rats did not produce any symptom of toxicity. On the other hand, in all the doses tested, the standardized ethanolic extract of *S. aqueum* leaf did not affect the body weight of the rats (Figure 8) and caused no significant changes in their food and water consumption (Figure 9). The treated rats body weight is as comparable as the control group (Figure 8). The increase of body weight is may be due to the process of body fat accumulation (Harizal et al., 2010). The food and water consumption of the treated rat group also showed a similar trend as the control group (Figure 9). Utilization of food and water exhibited normal metabolism in the animals (Mukinda and Syce, 2007) and this suggests that the repeated dose of standardized ethanolic extract of *S. aqueum* leaf did not retard the growth of the rats.

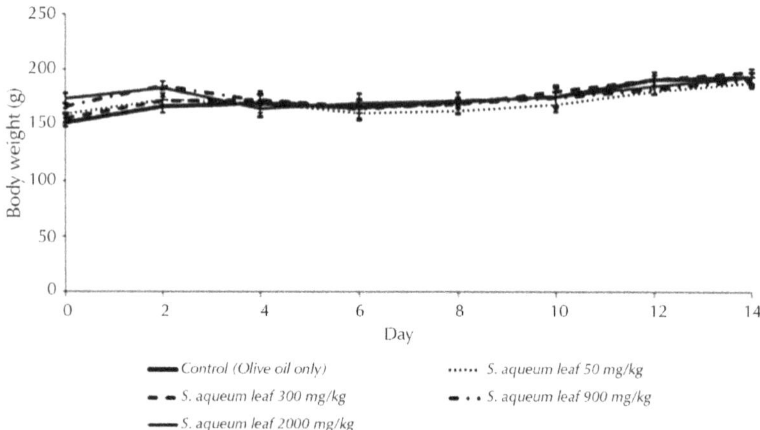

FIGURE 8 Body weight of rats in control and treated groups after administration of standardized ethanolic extract of *S. aqueum* leaf in subacute toxicity. Data indicated mean ± SEM, n=3. There are no significant ($p>0.05$) differences between the groups.

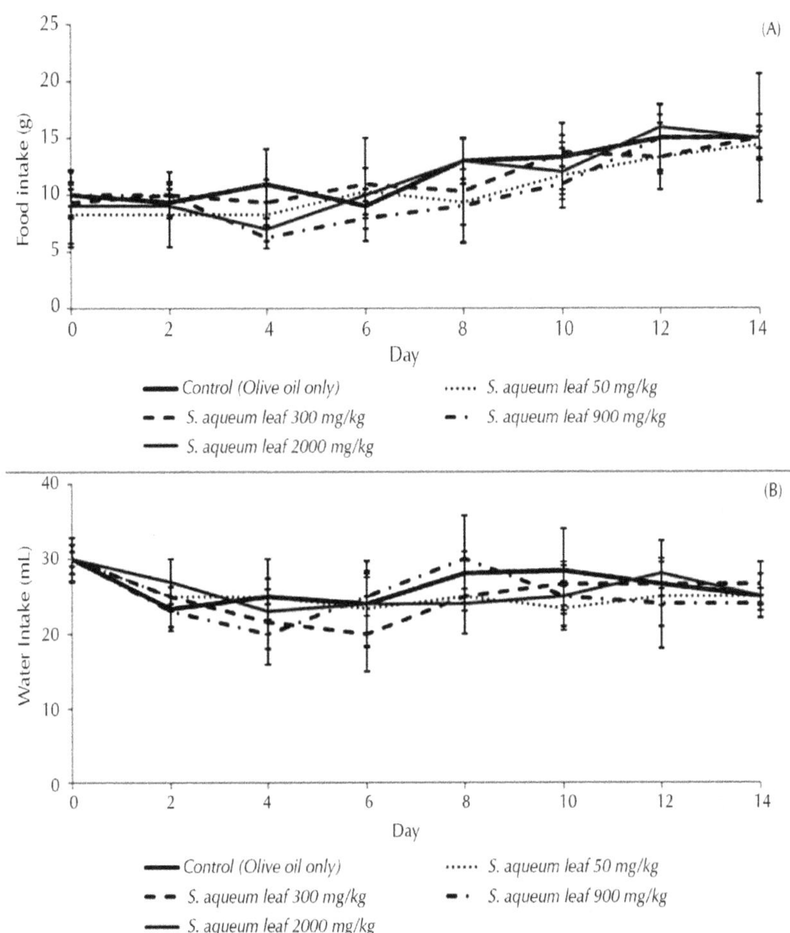

FIGURE 9 Consumption of (A) food and (B) water by rats in the control (olive oil as vehicle) and treated groups after administration of standardized ethanolic extract of *S. aqueum* leaf in subacute toxicity. Data indicated mean ± SEM, n =3. There are no significant (p>0.05) differences between the groups.

In addition, there were also no significant changes in the relative organ weight (Table 4) of rats treated with standardized ethanolic extract of *S. aqueum* leaf compared to the control. According to Demma et al. (2006), relative organ weight is more indicative of toxicity than absolute organ weight.

TABLE 4 Relative organ weight of rats in control and treated groups after administration of standardized ethanolic extract of *S. aqueum* leaf in subacute toxicity

		Relative Organ weight (%)			
		Heart	**Liver**	**Kidney**	**Pancreas**
Control	**Olive oil (vehicle)**	0.4 ± 0.1	4.1 ± 0.4	0.6 ± 0.1	0.7 ± 0.2
***S. aqueum* leaf**	**50 mg/kg**	0.4 ± 0.2	4.2 ± 0.4	0.5 ± 0.1	0.8 ± 0.2
	300 mg/kg	0.4 ± 0.1	3.9 ± 0.6	0.5 ± 0.2	0.6 ± 0.1
	900 mg/kg	0.5 ± 0.2	4.0 ± 0.5	0.7 ± 0.3	0.6 ± 0.3
	2000 mg/kg	0.5 ± 0.1	3.9 ± 0.2	0.6 ± 0.1	0.6 ± 0.1

Data shown as mean ± SEM, n = 3.

This was further supported by biochemical findings and histopathological observation conducted in all mentioned organs.The biochemistry data (Table 5) showed there were no significant differences in alanine transferase (ALT), alkaline phosphatase (ALP), creatinine, urea, and total protein levels of the rats treated with standardized ethanolic extract of *S. aqueum* leaf compared to the control.

TABLE 5 Biochemical tests performed on the sera taken from rats in control and treated groups after administration of standardized ethanolic extract of *S. aqueum* leaf in subacute toxicity

		Biochemical Tests				
		ALT	ALP	Creatinine	Urea	Total protein
		(U/L)	**(U/L)**	**(umol/L)**	**(mmol/L)**	**(g/L)**
Control	**Olive oil (vehicle)**	65 ± 5	281 ± 5	58 ± 6	7 ± 2	57 ± 6

TABLE 5 *(Continued)*

***S. aqueum* leaf**	**50 mg/kg**	65 ± 4	277 ± 4	57 ± 3	6 ± 1	54 ± 10
	300 mg/kg	62 ± 2	274 ± 4	56 ± 4	8 ± 2	55 ± 3
	900 mg/kg	64 ± 2	282 ± 6	58 ± 2	6 ± 2	57 ± 2
	2000 mg/kg	63 ± 2	280 ± 2	56 ± 2	7 ± 2	58 ± 2

Data shown as mean ± SEM, n = 3.

In addition, histopathological investigation of the organs (heart, liver, kidney, and pancrease) revealed no treatment-related microscopic changes (Figure 10).The rats from control and treated groups showed normal heart morphology (Figure 10(A)). The muscle fibers were healthy and there was no hypertrophy of the ventricular walls.Although the liver showed normal architecture in all the groups (Figure 10(B)), a mild non-specific inflammation was observed in the livers from rats in group 3 (900 mg/kg) and group 4 (2000 mg/kg).

In all the groups, the kidney showed adequate glomeruli and normal tubules (Figure 10(C)). However, the kidneys from the rats in group 3 (900 mg/kg) and group 4 (2000 mg/kg) showed some scattered glomerular atrophy and focal intestinal oedema (Figure 10(C)). The pancreas tissue showed normal morphology in all the groups, with maintenance of both endocrine and exocrine architecture (Figure 10(D)). In conclusion, no lesions or pathological changes attributable to administration of the standardized ethanolic extract of *S. aqueum* leaf were found in the organs of rats in the experimental groups. The findings suggest that the standardized ethanolic extract of *S. aqueum* leaf could be devoid of any toxic risk.

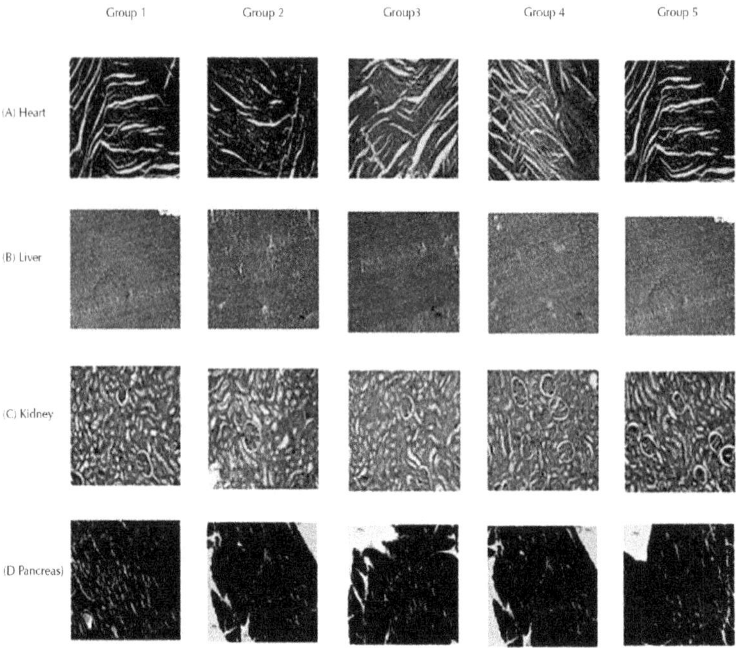

FIGURE 10 Photomicrographs from (A) the heart, showing normal architecture of the myocardium (H and E, 100x), (B) the liver, showing hepatocytes arranged around central veins with no evidence of necrosis or damage (H and E, 100x), with mild non-specific inflammation in the liver of groups 3 and 4, (C) the kidney, showing adequate glomeruli and normal tubules, with no evidence of glomerular damage or lumen casts, (H and E, 100x) with scattered glomerular atrophy and focal intestinal oedema in groups 3 and 4, and (D) pancreas, showing normal arrangement of acini and few islets (H and E, 100x).

4.3.10 ISOLATION AND IDENTIFICATION OF THE BIOACTIVE COMPOUNDS FROM S. AQUEUM LEAF

The ethanolic extracts of *S. aqueum* leaf (0.8 g) extracted from 5 g of plant material, was subjected into Gilson Preparative HPLC system as mentioned in methodology part. Six active compounds with α-glucosidase and α-amylase inhibitory activities were isolated from the ethanolic extracts at the retention times of 10.1, 13.8, 17.5, 48.7, 51.2, and 53.6 min, respectively (Figure 11(a)). The total yield of these six compounds from the crude extract of 0.8 g was only about 2.6% (20.5 mg from 0.8 g crude extract). The bioactive compounds were then analyzed on a Shidmazu Prominence UFLC-LCMS-IT-TOF (Manaharan et al., 2012). The bioactive compounds were identified as 4-hydroxybenzaldehyde (1, 0.2 mg), myricetin-3-O-rhamnoside (2, 1.3 mg), europetin-3-O-rhamnoside (3, 2.5 mg), phloretin (4, 3.2 mg), myrigalone-G(5, 5.4 mg) and myrigalone-B(6, 7.9 mg). The structures of the compounds are as shown in Figure 11(b), determined on the basis of MS and NMR data and comparison with those reported in literature. The presence of these six flavonoids in the *S. aqueum* leafextract may be contributing to its high antidiabetic activity.

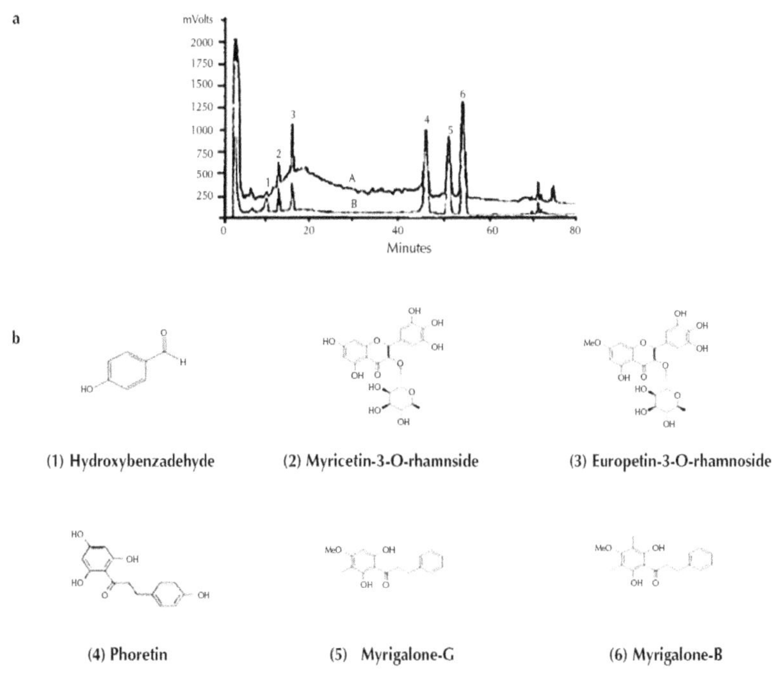

FIGURE 11 [a] Isolation of the six active compounds from *Syzygium aqueum* leaf extract using PREP-HPLC at retention times of 10.1, 13.8, 17.5, 48.7, 51.2, and 53.6 min, respectively. Solvent gradient consisted of 0–10% acetonitrile for 10 min, 10–85% acetonitrile for 70 min, and finally 100% acetonitrile for 5 min to recondition the column. Detection at wavelengths A: 210nm and B: 254 nm. [b] The chemical structures of the active compounds:(1)4-hydroxybenzaldehyde, (2) myricetin-3-O-rhamnoside, (3) europetin-3-O-rhamnoside, (4) phloretin, (5)myrigalone-G, and (6) myrigalone-B, respectively.

4.4 CONCLUSION

The ethanolic extract of *S. aqueum* leaf was shown to be effective antioxidant as well as an excellent inhibitor of the carbohydrate hydrolyzing enzymes, α-amylase and α-glucosidase and the key enzyme in the polyol pathway, aldol reductase, and prevent AGEs formation. We also identified for the first time the ability of six bioactive compounds; 4-hydroxybenzaldehyde, myricitrin, europetin-3-O-rhamnoside, phloretin, myrigalone-G, and myrigalone-B, from *S. aqueum* leaf to inhibit α-amylase and α-glucosidase at varying effectiveness. This investigations also revealed the extraordinary ability of *S. aqueum* leaf extract to reduce insulin resistance in 3T3-L1 adipocytes at a far more significant level than the antidiabetic drug TZD, by enhancing adipogenesis, promoting 2-NBDG uptake, and increasing adiponectin secretion. In addition, *S. aqueum* leaf extract was found to be not toxic to the 3T3-L1 cells. Acute and subacute toxicity studies of the standardized ethanolic *S.aqueum* leaf extract in animals, the LD_{50} was observed to be greater than 2000 mg/kg. Administration of the extract (50, 300,` 900, and 2000 mg/kg) to male SD rats for 14 days did not results in death or any toxicity effects in any of the experimental animals. There were no obvious changes in histological and biochemical and as well no significant differences in body weight and relative organ weight (heart, liver, kidney or pancreas) of the experimental groups compared to the control groups. This study also revealed the effectiveness of *S. aqueum* leaf ethanolic extract to reduce high blood glucose level in high fat diet and streptozotocin induced diabetes rat model.The results strongly suggest the antioxidant and antidiabetic potential of *S. aqueum* leaf extract. There are plenty of opportunities for nutraceutical and pharmaceutical industries to use *S. aqueum* leaf for the management of diabetes mellitus.

KEYWORDS

- **Antidiabetic**
- **Antioxidant**
- **Leaf extract**
- **Syzygium aqueum**

REFERENCES

1. American Diabetes Association. *Diabetes Care*, **31**(1), 562–567 (2008).
2. Alonso-Castro, A. J. and Salazar-Olivo, L. A. *J. Ethnopharm*, **118**(2), 252–256 (2008).
3. Angelika, S. and Petra, H. *Diabetes Res. Cli. Pract.*, **77**(1), 41–46 (2007).
4. Asare, G. A., Sittie, A., Bugyei, K., Gyan, B. A., Adjei, S., Addo, P., Wiredu, E. K., Nyarko, A. K., Otu-Nyarko, L. S., and Adjei, D. N. *J. Ethnopharm*,**134**, 938–943 (2011).
5. Baynes, J. W. *Diabetes*,**40**, 405–412 (1991).
6. Baynes, J. W. and Thorpe, S.R. *Diabetes*,**48**, 1–9 (1999).
7. Blanco, F. M. *Flora de Filipinas*., Gran edicion [Atlas 1] (1880),
8. Bouaboula, M., Hilairet, S., Marchand, J., Fajas, L., Fur, G. L., and Casellas, P. *Euro. J. Pharma*, **517**, 174–181 (2005).
9. Chang, C. W., Kim, S. C., Hwang, S. S., Choi, B. K., Ann, H. J., and Lee, M. Y. *Plant Sci.*, **63**(6), 1161–1168 (2002).
10. Chien, P. J.,Chien, Y. C., Lu, S. C., and Sheu, F. J. *Food and Drug Anal.*, **13**(2), 168–175 (2005).
11. Choi, S. S., Cha, B. Y., Lee, Y. S., Yonezawa, T., Teruya, T., Nagai, K.,et al. *Life Sci.*, **84**(25–26), 908–914 (2009).
12. Christensen, K. B., Minet, A., Svenstrup, H.,Grevsen, K., Zhang, H., Schrader, E., Rimbach, G., Wein, S., Wolffram, S., Kristiansen, K., and Christensen, L.P. *Phytotherapy Res.*, **23**, 1316–1325 (2009).
13. De Fronzo, R. A., Bonadonna, R. C., and Ferrannini, E. *Diabetes Care*,**15**(3), 318–368 (1992).
14. De Fronzo, R. A. *Annal Inter. Med.*,**131**(4), 281–303 (1999).
15. Demma, J., Gebre-Mariam, T., Asres, K., Evgetie, W., and Engindawork, E. *J. Ethnopharm.*, **111**, 451–457 (2006).
16. Diez, J. J. and Iglesias, P. Euro. *J. Endocrin.*,**148**(3), 293–300 (2003).
17. Feng, Y. Z., Liu, Y. M., Fratkins, J. Dm., and LeBlanc, M. H. *Brain Res. Bull.*,**66**, 120–127 (2005).
18. Fuente, J. A., Manzanaro, S., Martín, M. J., de Quesada, T. G., Reymundo, I., Luengo, S. M., et al. *J. Med. Chem.*, **46**(24), 5208–5221 (2003).
19. Gray, D. M. *New England J. Med.*, **29**, 1225–1230 (1995).
20. Gustavsson, J., Parpal, S., and Stralfors, P. *Mol. Med.*, **2**(3), 367–372 (1996).
21. Halliwell, B., and Gutteridge, J. M. C. *Free radicals in biology and medicine (3rd ed.)*, Oxford University Press, New York (1999).
22. Harizal, S. N., Mansor, S. M., Hasnan, J., Tharakan, J. K. J., and Abdullah, J. *J. Ethnopharm.*, **131**, 404–409 (2010).
23. Hassan, M., Yazidi, C. E., Landrier, J. F., Lairon, D., Margotat, A., and Amiot, M. *J. Biochem.Biophysic. Res. Comm.*, **361**, 208–213 (2007).
24. Hor, S. Y., Farsi, E., Lim, C. P., Ahmad, M., Asmawi, M. Z., and Yam, M. F.*J. Ethnopharm.*, (2011).
25. Ho, S. C., Wu, S. P., Lin, S. P., and Tang, Y. L. *Food Chem.*,**122**, 768–774 (2010).

26. Heo, S. J., Hwang, J. Y., Choi, J. I., Han, J. S., Kim, H. J., and Jeon, Y. J. *Euro. J. Pharm.*, **615**, 252–256 (2009).
27. Ichiki, H., Miura, T., Kubo, M., Ishihara, E., Komatsu, Y., Tanigawa, K., et al. *Biol. Pharmaceutical Bull.*, **21**(12), 1389–1390 (1998).
28. Joubert, E.,Winterton, P.,Britz, T. J, and Gelderblom, W. C. A. *J. Agri. FoodChem.*, **53**,10260–10267 (2005).
29. Jung, H. A., Yung, Y. J., Na, Y. Y., Jeong, D. M., Bae, H. J., Kim, D. W.,et al. *Food and Chem.Toxico*, **46**, 3818–3826 (2008).
30. Jung, H. A., Kim, Y. S., and Choi, J. S. *Food and Chem.Toxico*, **47**, 2790–2797 (2009).
31. Jung, E. Y., Lee, H. Y., Chang, U. J., Bae, S. H., Kwon, K. H., and Suh, H. J. *Food and Chem. Toxico*, **48**, 1677–1681 (2010).
32. Kador, P. F., Kinoshita, J. H., Tung, W. H., and Chylack Jr. L. T. *Inves.Ophthalm. Visual Sci.*, **19**, 980–982 (1980).
33. Kaneko, M., Bucciarelli, L., Hwang, Y. C., Lee, L., Yan, S.F., Schmidt, A. M., et al.*Ann. New York Acad. Sci.*, **1043**, 702–709 (2005).
34. Kao, W. F., Huang, D. Z., Tsai, W. J., Lin, K. P., and Deng, J. F. *Human and Exp. Toxico*, **11**(6), 480–487 (1992).
35. Kang, Y. and Kim, H. Y. *J. Ethnopharm.*, **92**, 103–105 (2004).
36. Kaur, L., Han, K. S., Bains, K., and Singh, H. *Food Chem.*, **129**, 1120–1125 (2011).
37. Kawanishi, Y., Noparatanawong, S., Kamohara, S., and Nakano, M. J. *American Diabetes Assoc.* , **103**(9), 36 (2003).
38. Kim, J. S., Hyun, T. k., and Kim, M. J. *Food Chem.*,**124**, 1647–1651 (2011).
39. Konan, N. A. and Bacchi, E. M. *J. Ethnopharm.*, **112**, 237–242 (2007).
40. Latiff, A. G., Omar, I. M. S., and Kadri, A. *J. Singapore Nat. Acad. Sci.*, **13**, 101–105 (1984).
41. Lee, D. S. and Lee, S. H. *FEBS Lett.*,**501**(1), 84–86 (2001).
42. Lee, M. J., Rao, Y. K., Chen, K., Lee, Y. C., andTzeng, Y. M. *J. Ethnopharm.*, **126**, 79–85 (2009).
43. Ling, L. T., Yap, S. A., Radhakrishnan, A. K., Subramaniam, T., Cheng, H. M., and Palanisamy, U. D. *Food Chem.*, **113**(4), 1154–1159 (2009).
44. Ling, L. T., Radhakrishnan, A. K., Subramaniam, T., Cheng, H. M., and Palanisamy, U. D. *Molecules*, **15**(4), 2139–2151 (2010).
45. Lio, K., Ohguchi, K., Inoue, H.,Maruyama, H., Araki, Y., Nozawa, Y., et al. *Phytomedicine* , **17**, 974–979 (2010).
46. Liu, J. P., Zhang, M., Wang, W. Y., and Grinsgard, S. *J. Ethnopharm.*, **115**(3), 173–183 (2004).
47. Lo, Y. C., Teng, C. M., Chen, C. F., Chen, C. C., and Hong, C. Y. *Biochem. Pharm.*, **47**(3), 549–553 (1994).
48. Manaharan, T., Ling, L. T., Appleton, D., Cheng, H. M., Masilamani, T., and Palanisamy, U.
49. D. *Food Chem.*, **129**(4), 1355–1361 (2011).
50. Marles, R. J. and Farnsworth, N. R. *Plants as sources of antidiabetic agents*. H. Wagner and N. R. Farnsworth (Eds.),*Economic and Medicinal Plant Research, vol. 6* (Chapter 4), Academic Press, London, pp. 149–187 (1994).

51. Matsuura, N., Aradate, T., Sasaki, C., Kojima, H., Ohara, M., Hasegawa, J., and Ubukata, M. *J. Health Sci.*, **48**, 520–526 (2002).
52. Maurizio, M., Conectta, B., Brunella, C., Stefonia, G., Valentina, N., and Elisabetta, S. *AnalyticaChimicaActa*, **617**, 192–195 (2008).
53. McCue, P. and Shetty, K. *Asia Pacific J. Cli. Nutr.*, **13**(1), 101–106 (2004).
54. Miliauskas, G., Venskutonis, P. R., and Van Beek, T. A. *Food Chem.*, **85**, 231–237 (2005).
55. Moghaddama, M. S., Anil Kumar, P., Bhanuprakash Reddy, G., and Gholea V. S.*J.Ethnopharm.*, **97**(2), 397–403 (2005).
56. Mohamed, A. K., Bierhaus, A., Schiekofer, S., Tritschler, H., Ziegler, R., Nawroth, P. P. *Biofactors Oxford England*, **10**(2–3), 157–167 (1999).
57. Mohamed, E. A. H., Lim, C. P., Ebrika, O. S., Asmawi, M. Z., Sadikun, A., and Yam, M. F.*J. Ethnopharm.*, **133**, 358–363 (2011).
58. Mukinda, J. T. and Syce, J. A.*J. Ethnopharm.*, **111**, 138–144 (2007).
59. Nishimura, C., Yamaoka, T., Mizutani, M., Yamashita, K., Akera, T., and Tanimoto, T. *ActaBiochem. Biophys.*,**1078**, 171–178 (1991).
60. Organisation of Economic Co-operation and Development (OECD). *The OECD guideline for testing of chemical*, 420 Acute Oral Toxicity. OECD, Paris, France, (2001a).
61. Organization of Economic Co-operation and Development (OECD). *The OECD guideline for testing of chemical*, 407 Repeated Dose Oral Toxicity-Rodent, 14–28 day study. OECD, Paris, France (2001b).
62. Palanisamy, U., Manaharan, T., Teng, L. L., Radhakrishnan, A. K. C., Subramaniam, T., and Masilamani, T. *Food Res. Int.*, **44**(7), 2278–2282 (2011).
63. Palanisamy, U. D., Ling, L. T., Manaharan, T., Sivapalan, V., Subramaniam, T.,Helme, M.H., and Masilamani, T. *Int. J. Cos. Sci.*, pp 1–7 (2011).
64. Park, S. Y., Lee, J. H., Kim, K. Y., Kim, E. K., Yun, S. J., Kim, C. D., et al. *Atherosclerosis*, **201**(2), 258–265 (2008).
65. Pinent, M., Blay, M. C., Salvado, M. J., Arola, L., and Ardevol, A. *Endocrin.*, **14**(11), 4985–4990 (2004).
66. Popovich, D. G., Li, L., and Zhang, W. *Food and Chem. Toxico*, **48**(6), 1619–1626 (2010).
67. Rathi, S., Grover, J. K., and Vats, V.*Phytotherapy Res.*, **16**, 236–243 (2002).
68. Roffey, B. W., Atwal, A. S., Johns, T., and Kubow, S. *J. Ethnopharm.*, **112**(1), 77–84 (2007).
69. Sanchez, G. M., Giuliani, L. R. E. A., Nunez-Sell′es, A. J., Davison, G. P., and Le′onfernandez, O. S. *Pharm. Res.*, **42**(6), 565–573 (2000).
70. Shobana, S., Sreerama, Y. N., and Malleshi, N. G. *Food Chem.*, **115**, 1268–1273 (2009).
71. Spranger, J., Kroke, A., Mohlig, M., Bergmann, M. M., Ristow, M., Boeing, H., et al. *Lancet*, **361**(9353), 226–228 (2003).
72. Tai, Y. T., But, P. P. H., Young, K., and Lau, C. P. *Lancet*, **341**(8830), 1254–1256 (1992).
73. Thomas, M. C., Baynes, J. W., Thorpe, S. R., and Cooper, M. E. *Curr. Drug Targets*,**6**(4), 453–474 (2005).
74. Tian, B. and Hua, Y. *Food Chem.*, **91**(3), 413–418 (2005).

75. Tongia, A., Tongia, S. K., and Dave, M. *Ind. J. Phys. Pharm.*, **48**, 241–244 (2004).
76. Tsao, T. S., Lodish, H. F., and Fruebis, J. *Euro. J. Pharm.*, **440**, 213–221 (2002).
77. Tsuduki, T., Kikuchi, I., Kimura, T., Nakagawa, K., Miyazawa. T. *Food Chemistry*, **139**(1–4), 16–23 (2013).
78. Tsuji-Naito, K., Saeki, H., and Hamano, M. *Food Chem.*,**116**(4), 854–859 (2009).
79. Vanherweghem, J. L., Depierreux, M., Tielemans, C., Abranowicz, D., Dratwa, M., Jadoul, M.,et al. *Lancet*, **341**, 387–391 (1993).
80. Wada, R. and Yagihashi, S. *Ann. New York Acad. Sci.*, **1043**, 598–604 (2005).
81. Wang, C. H., Cheng, X. M., Bligh, S. W. A., White, K. N., Branford-White, C. J., Wang, Z. T. *J. Pharmaceutical and Biomed. Anal.*, **449**(5), 1113–1117 (2007).
82. Wang, H., Du, Y. J., and Song, H. C. *Food Chem.*, **123**, 6–13 (2010).
83. Wang, D., Xu, K., Zhong, Y., Luo, X., Xiao, R., Hou, Y., et al. *J. Ethnopharm.*, **134**(1), 156–164 (2011).
84. World Health Organization, (2008). Prevalence data of diabetes worldwide. Available at http://www.who.int/mediacentre/factsheets/fs312/en/index.html 9 (accessed 16/7/09).
85. Wu, J. W., Hsieh, C. L., Wang, H. Y., and Chen, H. Y. *Food Chem.*, **113**, 78–84 (2009).
86. Wu, C.H., Hsieh, H.T., Lin, J.A., and Yen, G.C.*Food Chemistry*, **139**(1–4), 362–370 (2013).
87. Xiaoli,L., Zhao,M., Wang, J., Yang,B., and Jiang, Y.*J.Food Comp.Anal.*,**21**, 219–228 (2008).
88. Xu, A., Wang, H., Hoo, R. L. C., Sweeney, G., Vanhoutte, P. M., Wang, Y., et al. *Endocrin.*, **150**(2), 625–633 (2009).
89. Yao, X., Zhu, L., Chen, Y., Tian, J., and Wang, Y., *Food Chemistry*, **139** (1–4), 59–66 (2013).

CHAPTER 5

REVIEW ON NOVEL 2,4-THIAZOLIDINEDIONE DERIVATIVES AS POTENTIAL THERAPEUTIC AGENTS FOR TYPE II DIABETES

GANGADHARA ANGAJALA and RADHAKRISHNAN SUBASHINI

CONTENTS

ABSTRACT

The diabetes mellitus represents one of the most common endocrine disorders usually affecting nearly 6% people of the total world's population. India, the world's second most populous country now has more people with type-2 diabetes than any other nation. Thiazolidinedione's (TZDs) are an important classof antidiabetic drugs used for the treatment of type-2 diabetes mellitus. Novel 2,4-thiazolidinedione derivatives plays an important role in the design and discovery of active pharmacological agents. The compounds containing TZD nucleus shows promising activity in various categories such as antihyperglycemic, aldose reductase inhibitors, anti-arthritics, anti-inflammatory, and anticancer and so on. In this fast moving generation, more and more new drugs containing TZD nucleus have been reported by various scientist sall over the world. Biological importance of TZDs as an effective antihyperglycemic agents are available in literature in the form of short reviews, so there is a need to couple the latest information available in literature on the synthesis of novel 2,4-thiazolidinedione derivatives in order to better understand the current status of this nucleus for medicinal research and development.The synthesis of various novel 2,4-thiazolidinedione derivatives containing sulfonylurea's, flavonyl, and phthalazinone moieties are described along with their antihyperglycemic studies. The docking studies of the novel TZD were also performed in the active site of peroxisome proliferator-activated receptor gamma (PPARγ) receptor by using Molegro virtual docker.

5.1 INTRODUCTION

The diabetes mellitus is a clinical syndrome of multiple etiologies characterized by high blood sugar mainly due to deficiency or diminished action of insulin. The disease is usually chronic with metabolic disturbances of carbohydrate, protein, fat, and electrolytes. In rare cases over production of hormones which are antagonistic to insulin (e.g. glucagon, hormones of adrenaline, thyroid, and pituitary) also accounts for diabetes. The diabetes mainly divided into two major categories: Type-1 diabetes (insulin-dependent diabetes mellitus (IDDM)) usually develops at any age and rarely occurs when there is a family history of any form of diabetes. Type-2 diabetes (non-insulin dependent diabetes mellitus (NIDDM) usually develops in adulthood and is related to obesity, lack of physical activity, and unhealthy diets. According to the World Health Organization reports, it is estimated that more than 150 million people throughout the world suffered from diabetes of which 90% is type-2 and this figure usually doubles by the end of 2025. Despite the presence of known antidiabetic medicines in the pharmaceutical market, diabetes and its related complications still continue to be a major medical problem (Guo et al., 2006).

With the wide spread of fast-food outlets and more sedentary lifestyles, the prevalence of diabetes is rising alarmingly throughout the world. The major factors responsible for this change is urbanization, a rise in living standards and the spread of calorie-rich, fatty and fast foods cheaply available in cities to rich and poor alike. Another reason is the increased sedentariness that has resulted from the replacement of manual labor by service jobs and from the advent of video games, television and computers that keep people seated lethargically watching screens for hours every day.

The NIDDM is a complex, chronic metabolic disorder mainly associated with three basic pathophysiological abnormalities insulin resistance in target tissues, insulin resistance in skeletal muscle, liver, adipose tissue and excessive hepatic glucose output (Tuncbilek et al., 2003 and Bhat et al., 2004). The TZDs is a new class of orally active drugs that are particularly exciting because they decrease insulin resistance by enhancing the action of insulin at a level distal to the insulin receptor (Reginato et al., 1999 and Gaonkar et al., 2010). The molecular target of the TZDs is part of the nuclear receptor called peroxisome proliferator-activated receptorgamma (PPARγ) which controls the differentiation of adipocytes the metabolism of fatty acids and alters the expression of genes that are also regulated by insulin. The PPARγ mainly expressed in liver, activated macrophages, heart, skeletal muscle and colon but mostly abundant in adipocytes (Mourao et al., 2005 and Derosa et al., 2011).

The TZDs act as selective agonists to PPARγ, normally when activated by TZD derivative it binds to the 9-cis retinoic acid receptor to form a heterodimer. This subsequently binds to deoxyribonucleic acid (DNA) to regulate the genetic transcription and translation of various proteins involved in cellular differentiation, glucose and lipid metabolism. These, TZDs also shown to reduce plasmatic glucose, lipid and insulin levels also it can be used for treatment of diabetes mellitus type-2 (Da Costa et al., 2007 and Diatewa et al., 2009). The TZDs, which include troglitazone, pioglitazone and rosiglitazone are thought to sensitize target tissues to the action of insulin. Indeed, they are ineffective at lowering serum glucose levels in the absence of insulin (Hossain et al., 2007).Their mechanism of action is quite different from that of established antidiabetics such as sulfonylurea and biguanides. These compounds are synthetic, high affinity ligands of PPARγ and a member of the nuclear receptor super-family it controls the expression of genes involved in lipid and carbohydrate metabolism in the target tissues (Madhavan et al., 2011 and Herrera et al., 2011). The TZDs also gave an improvement of insulin resistance and insulin sensitivity parameter not reported with sulfonyl urea's (Sambasivarao et al., 2006). Furthermore, TZDs slowed the progression of coronary atherosclerosis in patients with diabetes and improved pressure values without increasing cardiovascular risk (Jawale et al, 2012).

The TZDs increases the expression of PPARγ in adipose tissue which results in increased fatty acid uptake and storage by increasing the transcription of fatty acid transport protein-1 and acyl-coenzyme-Asynthetase. Decreased circulating free fatty acid levels protect β cells, the liver and skeletal muscle from their toxic effects, thus improving insulin sensitivity. Such a phenomenon hasbeen termed the "fatty acid steal hypothesis" (Viral et al., 2013 and Maccari et al., 2007).

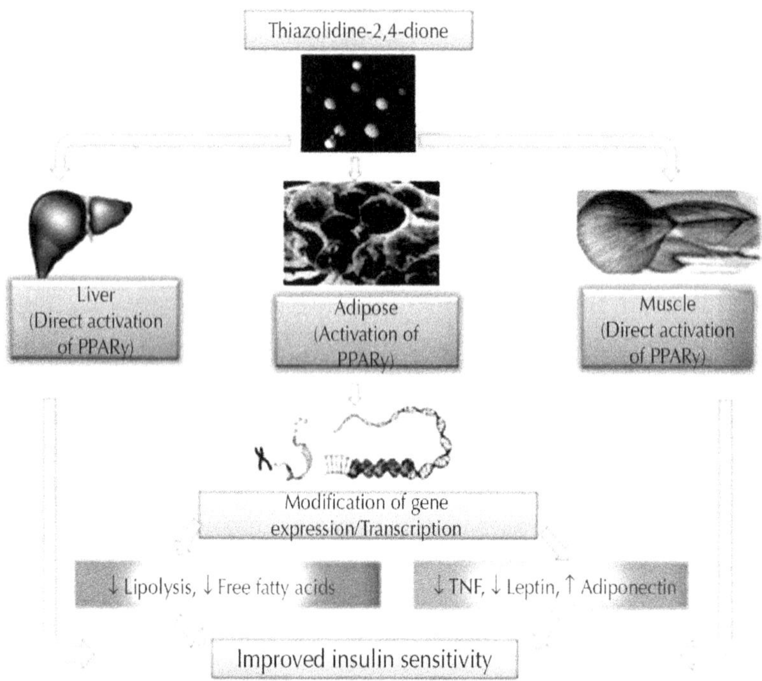

FIGURE 1 Mechanism of action of TZDs.

The TZD ring has been used as scaffold to develop a novel class of antidiabetic agents, encouraged by the literature report that toxicity of troglitazone is not due to the TZD ring (Figure 1).Thus there is a growing need for the effective therapies to achieve optimal glycemic control in the management of diabetes (Bozdag-Dundar et al., 2011 and Rakowitz et al., 2006).

Orally administered antihyperglycemic agents (OHAs) can be used either alone or in combination with other OHAs or insulin (Anna et al, 2003). Several TZDs derivatives are already released in the market with different brand names. Among them the most popular drugs include rosiglitazone (Avandia), pioglitazone (Actos) and troglitazone (Rezulin). All these drugs are proved to possess some side effects (Figure 2).

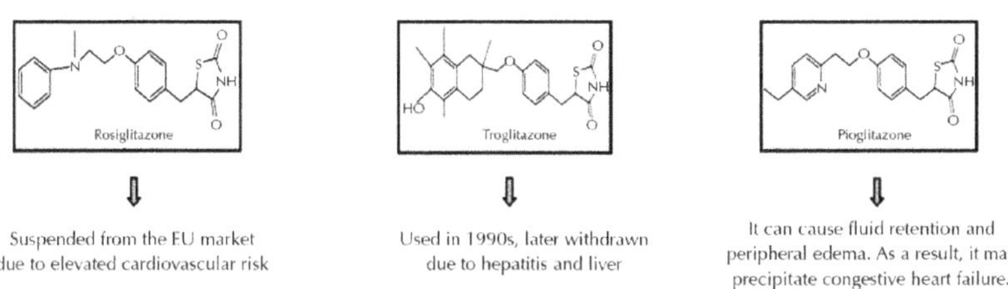

FIGURE 2 Structure of rosiglitazone, troglitazone, and pioglitazone, and its side effects.

Accordingly, there is a need for more effective, orally administered agents, particularly which normalize both the glucose and insulin levels (Rancic et al., 2012 and Youseff et al., 2010). It reveals that there is scanty information available on the molecules having both sulfonylurea and TZDs as their structural units. Considering the pharmacological importance of sulfonylurea's and TZDs and the side effects of the existing drugs, it was worthwhile to review the combination of drugs possessing two active moieties.

Several scientists expressed their opinion that the side effects of thiazolidine class of drugs were mainly due to the side chain of the heterocyclic moieties to which TZD has been attached. Here we are reporting the various synthetic methods in which the heterocyclic ring will be replaced with some Sulfonamides, arylidene, flavonyl, and phthalazinone. Sulfanilides are the basis of several groups of drugs which already proved to possess aldose reductase activity. Further combination of drugs also proved to enhance the antihyperglycemic effect, hence we are focusing to review various novel 2,4-thiazolidinedione derivatives possessing combination of both sulfanamides and TZD with the results of the docking studies, we hope that the final drug possess an enhanced antihyperglycemic activity with lesser side effects when compared to the existing drugs in the market.

5.2 EXPERIMENTAL WORK

Jawale et al., have reported synthesis and antihyperglycemic evaluation of new 2,4-thiazolidine diones having biodynamic aryl sulfonylurea moieties (Jawale et al., 2012) (Figure 3).

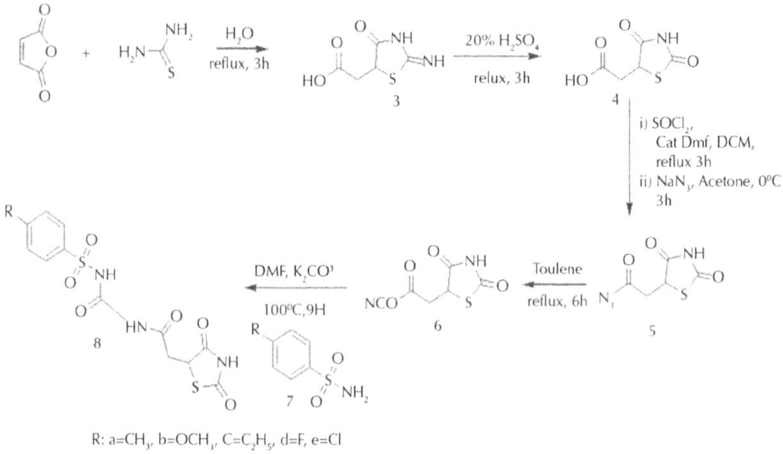

FIGURE 3 The formation of 1-(2,4-dioxothiazolidin-5-yl) methyl)-3-substitued benzene sulfonyl urea's.

The structure of the synthesized 3, 4, 5,and 6was confirmed on the basis of ^{1}H nuclear magnetic resonance (NMR) and ^{13}C NMR spectra. From the ^{1}H NMR spectra it has been delineated that sulfamyl protons of compounds 8(a-e) displayed their signals at δ 8.67–10.73 ppm confirms the presence of labile protons by deuterium oxide (D_2O) exchange.

Shakshi et al., have reported urea/thiourea catalyzed solvent free synthesis of 5-arylidenethiazolidine-2,4-diones (Shakshi et al., 2012) (Figure 4).

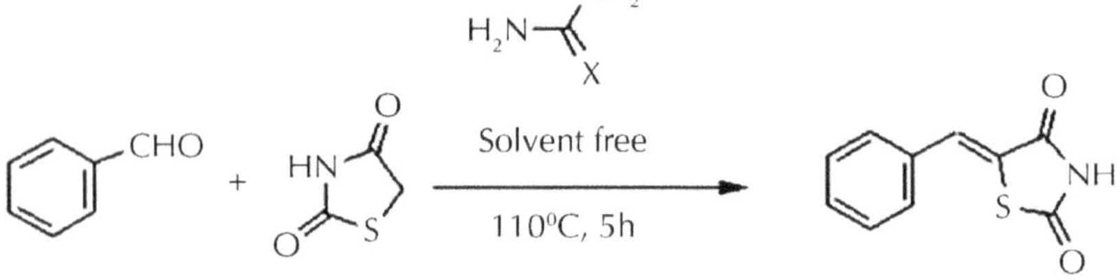

FIGURE 4 Theformation of (Z)-5-benzylidenethiazolidine-2, 4-dione.

Shashikant et al., have reported synthesis of 4-chloroacetyl-benzylidene-2,4-thiazolidinediones (Shashikant et al., 2012) (Figure 5).

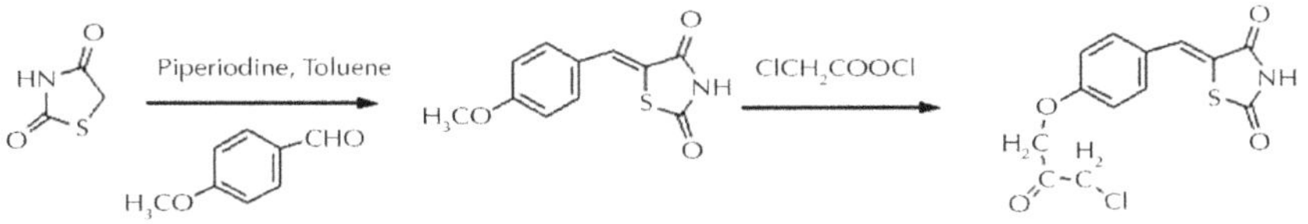

FIGURE 5 Theformation of (Z)-5-(4-(3-chloro-2-oxopropoxy) benzylidene) thiazolidine-2,4-dione.

Meral et al., have reported synthesis of some substituted flavonyl TZD derivatives (Meral et al., 2003) (Figure 6).

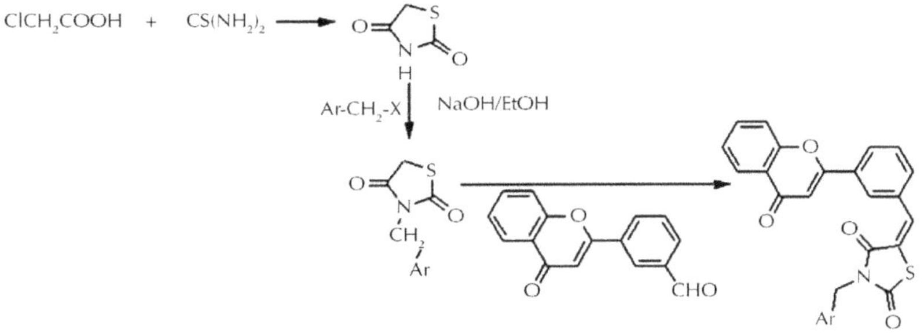

FIGURE 6 The formation of substituted flavonyl TZD derivatives.

Mourao et al., have reported synthesis of benzylideneTZDs (Mourao et al., 2005) (Figure7).

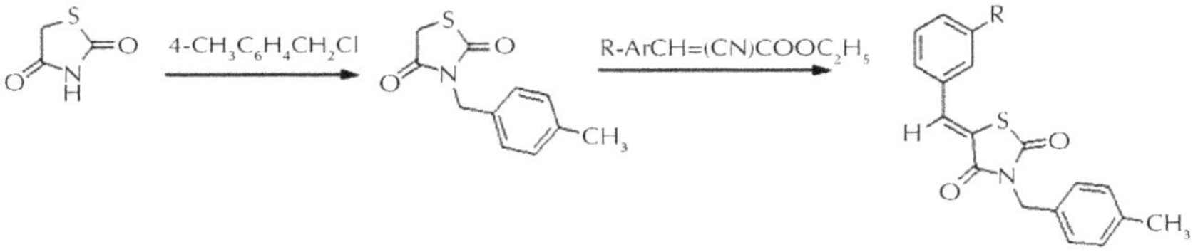

FIGURE 7 The formation of substituted benzylidene thiazolidine derivatives.

Madhavan et al., have reported synthesis of novel phthalazinone TZD derivatives. A process for the conversion of rosiglitazone to phthalazinones (Madhavan et al., 2001) (Figure 8).

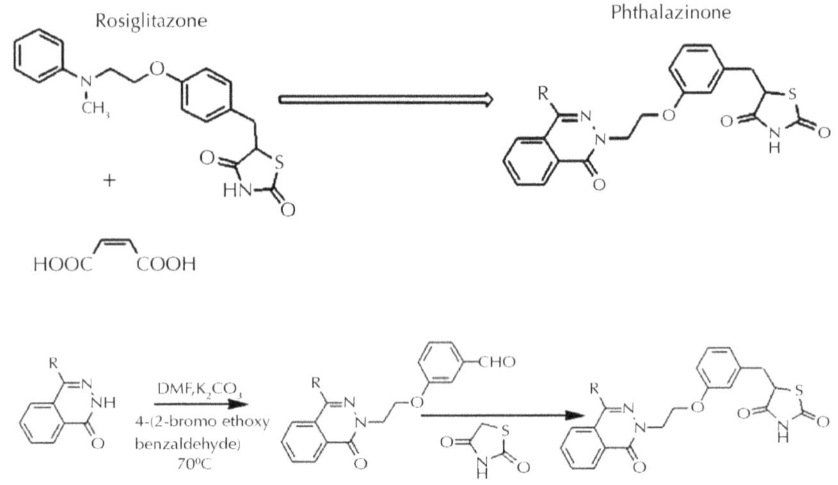

FIGURE 8 The formation of novel phthalazinone TZD derivatives.

5.3 ANTIHYPERGLYCEMIC ACTIVITY EVALUATION

5.3.1 SELECTION OF ANIMAL AND INDUCTION OF DIABETES

Male albino rats weighing 250–300 g were obtained from the animal house after approval from Institutional Animal Ethical Committee (1333/C/10/CPCSEA). The animals were maintained under standard condition of temperature (23 ± 2°C) and relative humidity (55 ± 10%) with 12 hr each of dark and light cycle. Rats were fed with standard pellet and tap water ad libitum. All experimental protocols were prepared and performed based on ethical committee guidelines.

5.3.2 CHEMICALS

Streptozotocin (STZ) used in this experiment was purchased from Himedia Bangalore, Glibenclamide from Sun Pharmaceuticals Limited, Baroda, India. All other chemicals used were of analytical grade.

5.3.3 INDUCTION OF DIABETES MELLITUS

Diabetes was induced in albino rats as per the method described by Kadnur and Goyal (2005) with slight modification. Briefly, after 18 h fasting rats were made diabetic by single administration of STZ (40mg/kg BW/ i.p) dissolved in 0.1M citrate buffer (pH 4.5), while the normal rats received citrate buffer as vehicle. After the injection they had free access to feed and 5% sucrose solution in order to overcome hypoglycemic shock. Blood glucose levels were estimated after 3 to 4 days of STZ injection in overnight fasted rats. Rats having blood glucose level more than 300 mg/dl were selected for further study.

5.3.4 EXPERIMENTAL DESIGN

Antidiabetic activity was studied in 42 rats (6 normal + 36 diabetic rats). They were grouped as follow:

- Group 1 received 1% Tween 80 in water after intraperitoneal injection of citrate buffer (0.1M).
- Group 2 received 1% Tween 80 in water after intraperitoneal injection of STZ (40 mg/kg body wt).
- Group 3 and 4 received different concentrations of the test sample (100, 200 and 300 mg/kg body wt) administered orally through intragastric tube after 48 h of STZ injection for 30 days.
- Group 5 received Glibenclamide (900 μg/kg body wt) administered orally through intragastric tube after 48 hr of STZ injection for 30 days.

The body weight and blood glucose level were monitored weekly once for 30 days. Blood samples were obtained by tail vein puncture of both normal and STZ induced diabetic rats and blood glucose level was measured using single touch glucometer. At the end of 31st day all the fasted rats were sacrificed by deep anesthesia. The blood samples were collected by cardiac puncture method and centrifuged at 4000 rpm for 20 min to remove serum from the clot and stored at 20 °C. Serum glucose and cholesterol level were estimated using commercially available reagent kits.

5.3.5 HISTOPATHOLOGICAL STUDY

Pancreas of control and compound treated animals were isolated for histopathological examination. Isolated pancreas after washing in phosphate buffered saline (PBS) solution stored in 10% Formalin. Paraffin sections of pancreas tissue were stained in haematoxylin and eosin for evaluation of β cells of islets in light microscope (David, 1991).

5.3.6 STATISTICAL ANALYSIS

The results are expressed as mean ± statistical difference (S.D). The S.D between the various derivatives of final compound and standard antidiabetic drug were determined using one-way analysis of variance (ANOVA). A difference in the mean P value < 0.01 was considered as significant.

5.3.7 HYPOGLYCEMIC EFFECT OF SYNTHESIZED COMPOUNDS

Treatment of the rats with STZ resulted in approximately 2.5-fold increase in blood glucose concentration in comparison to normal control rats. The effect of different concentration of test samples in lowering the blood glucose level of STZ induced diabetic rats were shown in Table 1. On administration of test sample and glibenclamide to the diabetic rats, blood glucose levels were reduced significantly (P< 0.01) from day one onwards, whereas the blood glucose remained consistently elevated in diabetic control rats throughout the period of study. Percentage reduction in blood glucose level was calculated (Figure 9) using the formula:

$$\% \text{ Reduction} = 1 - (n^{th} \text{ day treated}/0^{th} \text{ day treated})/(n^{th} \text{ day untreated}/0^{th} \text{ day untreated}) \times 100$$

where, n is the day of glucose measurement.

TABLE 1 Antihyperglycemic effect of different concentrations of the test samples reported by Jawale et al.

S.No	Dose (mg/kg body wt)	% Reduct-ioncom-pound a	% Reduct ion com-pound b	% Reduct ion com-pound c	% Reduct ion com-pound d	% Reduct ion com-pound e	% Reduct ion Glib-enclamide (Standard)
1	100	14.8±0.2	15.6±0.4	18.7±0.1	25.6±0.5	28.5±0.2	36.7±0.3
2	200	16.5±0.4	17.9±0.3	19.4±0.5	27.9±0.8	30.2±0.6	37.9±0.5
3	300	18.6±0.6	20.3±0.5	21.8±0.4	29.6±0.4	32.4±0.1	39.2±0.1

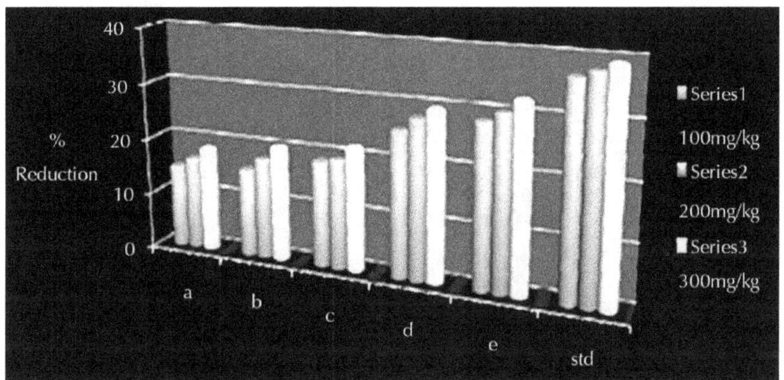

FIGURE 9 Percentage Reduction for final derivatives of *in vivo* active compounds at different concentrations on blood glucose level of STZ loaded rats.

5.4 DOCKING STUDIES

The docking analysis of compounds 8 (a–e) (Jawale et al)and glibenclamide were carried out by using Molegro Virtual Docker.v.4.0. The PPARγ receptor (ID-2Q8S) was taken from protein data bank. The derivatives of the final compounds were docked with the receptor and the interaction of ligands with the receptor was shown (Figure 10).

Docking view Secondary Structure view

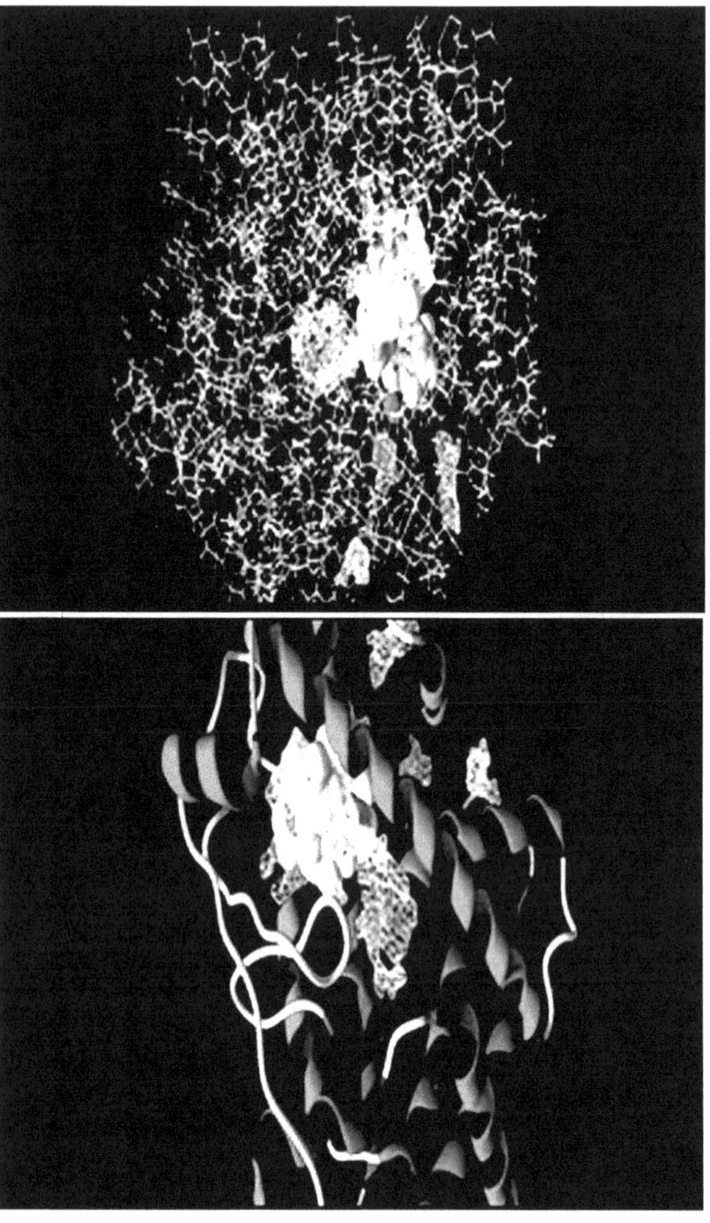

FIGURE 10 *(Continued)*

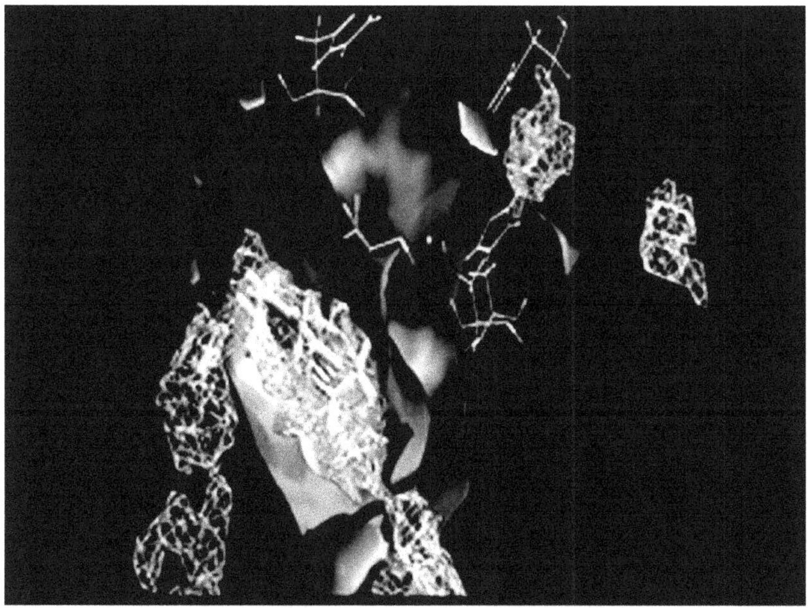

FIGURE 10 Electrostatic Interaction of 1-(2, 4-dioxothiazolidin-5-yl) methyl)-3-substitued benzene sulfonyl ureas (8a-e) with the PPAR-γ receptor.

5.5 DISCUSSION AND RESULTS

The most stable docking structures of various synthesized TZDs complexes with the PPARγ receptor are grouped under Figure 10 which clearly indicate that the ligands possessed strong binding interactions with the receptor. Further the presence of TZD moiety in the final synthesized derivatives enhances the antihyperglycemic activity. *In vivo* anti hyperglycemic activity evaluation showed, the average blood glucose profile of control and the experimental groups at various time intervals (Table 1). The results obtained from the variance analysis showed that most active compounds in this series are three out of the five studied synthetic compounds significantly ($p < 0.05$) inhibited the postprandial rise in the blood glucose level of STZ loaded rats. The compounds 8c, 8d, and 8e significantly inhibited the rise in postprandial hyperglycemia to the tune of 18.7% ($p < 0.01$), 25.6% ($p < 0.01$) and 28.5% ($p < 0.01$) respectively. The standard drug glibenclamide caused nearly 36.7% ($p< 0.001$) inhibition at 100 mg/kg body weight dose in sucrose loaded rats whereas on the other hand the compounds 8a and 8b exhibited very mild activity in terms of 14.8% and 15.6% respectively on normoglycemic rats.

5.6 CONCLUSION

In conclusion, it was reported that synthesis of various novel 2,4-thiazolidinedione derivatives in addition to this we also made an attempt to explain the versatile role of TZD nucleus for the treatment of type-2 diabetes. There is plethora information available on the biological activities of TZDs.The combination of two drugs into a single drug is getting more prominent in this fast moving generation. It was focused on antihyperglycemic activity of 1-(2,4-dioxothiazolidin-5-yl) methyl)-3-substitued benzene sulfonyl urea's 8(a–e) and also performed docking studies. The results clearly indicate that novel 2,4-thiazolidinedione derivatives along with sulfonyl urea's showed promising antidiabetic activity with minimum side effects.

KEYWORDS

- **Antihyperglycemic activity**
- **Diabetes mellitus**
- **Docking studies**
- **Sulfonylurea**
- **2,4-Thiazolidinedione**

ACKNOWLEDGMENT

The authors sincerely thankful to VIT University for providing all the research facilities for carrying out this review in paper form.

REFERENCES

1. Anna, G. *Life Sciences.*,**74**(5), 553–562 (2003).
2. Anna, G. *Experimental and Toxicologic Pathology.*, **56**(4–5), 321–326 (2005).
3. Bhat, B. A., Ponnala, S., Sahu, D. P., Tiwari, P., Tripathi, B. K., and Srivastava, A. K.*Bioorg. Med. Chem.*, **12**(22), 5857–5864 (2004).
4. Bozdag-Dundar, O., Evranos, B., Das-Evcimen, N., Sarıkaya, M., and Ertan, *R. Bioorg. Med. Chem.*, **16**(14), 6747–6751 (2008).
5. Bozdag-Dundar, O., Verspohl, E. J., Das-Evcimen, N., Kaup, R. M., Bauer, K., Sarıkaya, M., and Ertan, R. *Bioorg.Med. Chem.*, **16**(14), 6747–6751 (2008).
6. Da Costa Leite, L. F. C., Veras Mourao, R. H., de Lima, M. d. C. A., Galdino, S. L., Hernandes, M. Z., de Assis Rocha Neves, F., and da Rocha Pitta, I. *Eur. J. Med. Chem.*,**42**(10), 1263–1271 (2007).
7. David, S. K. *Handbook of histological and histochemical techniques, First ed.* C.S.B. Publishers., New Delhi, India, pp. 1–41 (1991).
8. Derosa, G. and Maffioli, P. *Diabetes Research and Clinical Practice.*,**91**(3), 265–270 (2011).
9. Diatewa, M., Samba, C. B., Assah, T. C. H., and Abena, A. A. *J.Ethnopharmacol.*, **92**(2–3), 229–232 (2004).
10. Gaonkar, S. L. and Shimizu, H. *Tetrahedron.*, **66**(18), 3314–3317 (2010).
11. Herrera, C., García-Barrantes, P. M., Binns, F., Vargas, M., Poveda, L., and Badilla, S. *J. Ethnopharmacol.*, **133**(2), 907–910 (2011).
12. Hossain, S. U. and Bhattacharya, S. *Bioorg. Med. Chem. Lett.*, **17**(5), 1149–1154 (2007).
13. Jawale, D. V., Pratap, U. R., Rahuja, N., Srivastava, A. K., and Mane, R. A. *Bioorg. Med. Chem. Lett.*, **22**(1), 436–439 (2012).
14. Kadnur, S.V. and Goyal, R. K. *Indian J Exp Biol.*, **43**(12),1161–1164 (2005).
15. Madhavan, G. R., Chakrabarti, R., Kumar, S. K. B., Misra, P., Mamidi, R. N. V. S., Balraju, V., and Rajagopalan, R.*Eur. J. Med. Chem.*,**36** (7–8), 627–637 (2001).
16. Maccari, R., Ottana, R., Ciurleo, R., Vigorita, M. G., Rakowitz, D., Steindl, T., and Langer, T. *Bioorg. Med. Chem. Lett.*, **17**(14), 3886–3893 (2007).
17. Mourao, R. H., Silva, T. G., Soares, A. L. M., Vieira, E. S., Santos, J. N., Lima, M. C. A., and Pitta,I.R. *Eur. J. Med. Chem.*,**40**(11), 1129–1133 (2005).
18. Rakowitz, D., Maccari, R., Ottana, R., and Vigorita, M. G. *Bioorg. Med. Chem.*, **14**(2), 567–574 (2006).
19. Rancic, M., Trišovic, N., Milcic, M., Uscumlic, G., and Marinkovic, A. Spectrochim. Acta, Part A, *Mol Biomol Spectrosc.*, **86**(0), 500–507 (2012).
20. Reginato, M. J. and Lazar, M. A.*Trends in Endocrinology & Metabolism.*, **10**(1), 9–13 (1999).
21. Sakshi, S. and Baldev,S. *Bioorg. Med. Chem. Lett.*, **22**, 5388–5391 (2012).
22. Sambasivarao, S. V., Soni, L. K., Gupta, A. K., Hanumantharao, P., and Kaskhedikar, S. G. *Bioorg. Med. Chem. Lett.*, **16**(3), 512–520 (2006).
23. Shashikant,P., Manisha,K., Jayashri,P., Santosh, D., Manjusha, S., Utkarsha, G., Punam,S., and Sushma,K. *Indian J. Chem.*, **51**(B), 1421–1425 (2012).

24. Sudipta, S., Debra, S. Z. C., Chern, Y.L., Winnie, W., Lee, S. N., Wai, K. C., Chun,W. Y., Eric, C.Y. C., and Han, K. H. *Eur. J. Pharmacol.*, **697**, 13–23 (2012).
25. Tuncbilek, M., Bozdag-Dundar, O., Ayhan-Kilcigil, G., Ceylan, M., Waheed, A., Verspohl, E. J.,and Ertan, R. *Il Farmaco.*, **58**(1), 79–83 (2003).
26. Youssef, A. M., Sydney White, M., Villanueva, E. B., El-Ashmawy, I. M., and Klegeris, A. *Bioorg. Med. Chem. Lett.*, **18**(5), 2019–2028 (2010).

CHAPTER 6

MOLECULAR MECHANISM OF S-OXIDATION OF ANTI-DIABETIC THIAZOLIDINEDIONE CLASS OF DRUGS: COMPUTATIONAL APPROACHES TO DRUG METABOLISM

NIKHIL TAXAK and PRASAD. V. BHARATAM

CONTENTS

ABSTRACT

The glitazones are the important class of anti-diabetic drugs, consisting of a thiazolidinedione (TZD) ring in their structure. The metabolic reactions of several important sulfide (-S-) containing drugs, such as glitazones and diclofenac involve *S*-oxidation as the first and essential step. However, the detailed mechanism of *S*-oxidation reaction of these drugs by cytochromes P450 (CPY) has not been explored at the molecular level. In this chapter, initially, a review of already reported computational studies, including quantum chemical studies, on *S*-oxidation is discussed. A database of sulfide and sulfoxide unit containing drugs was prepared. The molecular docking analysis was carried out to predict the probability of *S*-oxidation in these drugs. A comparative analysis has been carried out to establish a molecular docking protocol which can successfully predict the *S*-oxidation reaction. The molecular docking analysis was carried out on three major CYP isoforms using Glide software of Schrodinger package. The importance of oxygen atom on heme iron, (Cpd) I [iron (IV)-oxo] to mimic CYP450 in determining *S* as the site of metabolism (SOM) was critically analyzed. Thus, this chapter reviews the usefulnss of molecular docking and quantum chemical methods in providing significant details regarding SOM and mechanistic details for sulfide and sulfoxide unit containing drugs, which can be utilized as a protocol to predict SOM for any new lead, including anti-diabetic compounds, during the early phase of drug discovery.

6.1 INTRODUCTION

6.1.1 S-OXIDATION

Biotransformation involves the biochemical modification of xenobiotics (substances foreign to biological system of humans) including drug molecules to highly polar and easily excretable metabolites (Coleman, 2010). Flavoenzymes and CYPs are large families of monooxygenases, which perform these vital bioregulatory functions, such as detoxification of xenobiotics and biosynthesis of endogenous compounds (Montellano, 1995; Krueger and Williams, 2005; Cashman and Zhang, 2006). A variety of monooxygenase reactions are catalysed, such as hydroxylations, epoxidations, *N*- and *O*-dealkylation, and heteroatom (N, S) oxidation (Montellano, 1995; Lewis, 1996). The mechanisms of hydroxylation, epoxidation, and dealkylation by CYPs have been the attention of experimental and computational studies in the recent past. However, the molecular mechanism of *S*-oxidation has not been studied in detail. Sulfur oxidation is one of the important oxidative reaction mechanisms which plays a major role in phase I metabolism of drugs with sulfide unit (-*S*-) (Montellano, 1995; Brahmankar and Jaiswal, 2003). Sulfur containing drugs like troglitazone, pioglitazone, methimazole, cimetidine, artemiside, ranitidine, sulindac sulfide, and so on are reported to undergo change in metabolic state through sulfur oxidation process (Blake et al., 1995; Chung et al., 2000; Hamman et al., 2000; Nnane and Damani, 2003).

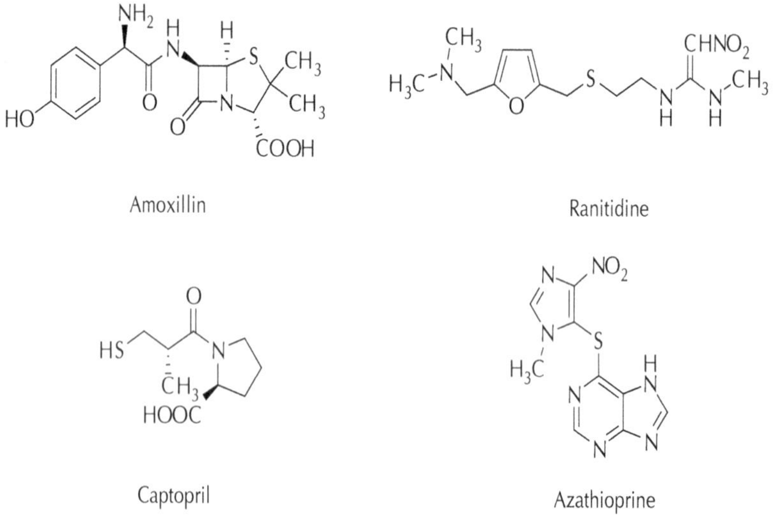

Amoxillin

Ranitidine

Captopril

Azathioprine

FIGURE 1 Structures of some sulfide-based drugs.

Many therapeutic drugs possess a sulfide pharmacophore. The sulfides are typically excellent sulfide-containing substrates for flavin-containing monooxygenase (FMO) and are readily converted to the sulfoxide (Nnane and Damani, 2003). The sulfide-containing drugs (see Figure 1), for which FMO is active in *S*-oxygenation to sulfoxides, include captopril, ranitidine, azathioprine, thioridazine, amoxicillin, *S*-methyl-N,N-diethyldithiocarbamate (metabolite of disulfiram), clindamycin, albendazole, and fenbendazole (Taxak et al., 2011). Sulfur has two unpaired electrons and can be oxidized twice to give sequentially a sulfoxide and a sulfone. First stage *in vivo* oxidation is generally known to be reversible and the second stage oxidation is known to be irreversible. The chemistry, thermodynamical control, enzyme specificity and so on associated with *S*-oxidation needs to be understood. Thorough understanding of the sulfur oxidation process at molecular level is an essential first step in the prediction of complex pathway of metabolite generation and its action. Thus, the well-known example of glitazones were considered for the study owing to the reasons mentioned later.

6.1.2 METABOLISM IN TZD AND TOXICITY

The glitazones (see Figure 2) are insulin sensitizers useful for the treatment of type-II diabetes mellitus (Saltiel and Olefsky, 1996; Mudaliar and Henry, 2001; Lehrke and Lazar, 2005; Montagnani and Gonnelli, 2013). They are agonists for the peroxisome proliferator activated receptor gamma (PPARγ), a member of the nuclear hormone receptor superfamily involved in lipid homeostasis (Saltiel and Olefsky, 1996; Mudaliar and Henry, 2001; Lehrke and Lazar, 2005). They bind strongly to PPARγ in adipocytes to promote adipogenesis and fatty acid uptake (in peripheral but not visceral fat). The rosiglitazone (RGZ) and pioglitazone (PGZ) constitute the TZD class of drugs, employed in the treatment of type-II diabetes mellitus, however, one of the member of glitazones, troglitazone has already been withdrawn from market owing to its hepatotoxicity (Gale, 2001).

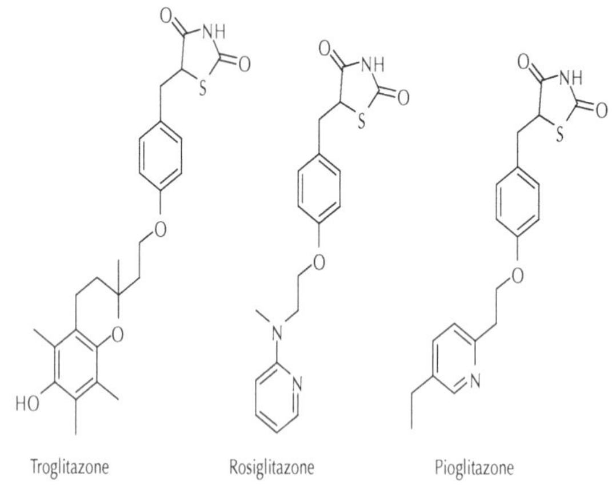

Troglitazone Rosiglitazone Pioglitazone

FIGURE 2 Structures of glitazone class of drugs.

In some countries, RGZ has also been withdrawn due to cardiovascular complications, and PGZ has been withdrawn due to bladder cancer. The clinical use of TZDs is limited, owing to several adverse effects, such as body-weight gain, congestive heart failure, bladder cancer, and so on (Cariou et al., 2012). There are certain hypothetical mechanisms proposed, where it has been demonstrated that the TZD ring in troglitazone and PGZ could undergo oxidative cleavage leading to reactive isocyanate (ISC) intermediate responsible for toxicity (see Figure 3) (Kiyota et al., 1997; Kassahun et al, 2001; Prabhu et al., 2003; He et al., 2004; Liu et al., 2004; Reddy et al., 2005; Baughman et al., 2005; Uchiyama et al., 2010). However, the mechanistic details of formation of metabolites (*S*-oxide) have not been explored at the molecular level.

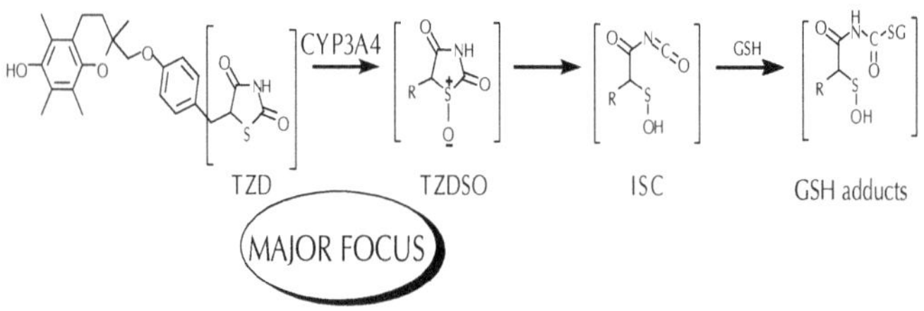

CYP3A4 GSH

TZD TZDSO ISC GSH adducts

MAJOR FOCUS

FIGURE 3 The process of TZD ring oxidation and formation of isocyanate reactive intermediate and GSH adducts leading to toxicological consequences.

Many recent works propose mechanisms with respect to oxidation of TZDs and their metabolic pathways from various *in vitro* studies. Kassahun et al. suggested that the reactive oxidative metabolites lead to the hepatotoxicity of the withdrawn drug troglitazone (2001). Reddy et al. suggested that the involvement of quinine-methide metabolites in the withdrawal of troglitazone, whereas initial *S*-oxidation leading to TZD ring scission played a minor role (2005). It has also been observed that the TZD ring bearing glitazones form *S*-oxidation based ring opened products *in vivo* (Liu et al., 2004; Baughman et al., 2005). Liu et al. carried out metabolic studies on 2, 4-thiazolidinedione containing PPAR α/γ agonist MK-0767, by elucidating the *in vitro* biotransformation pathways (see Figure 4) (2004).

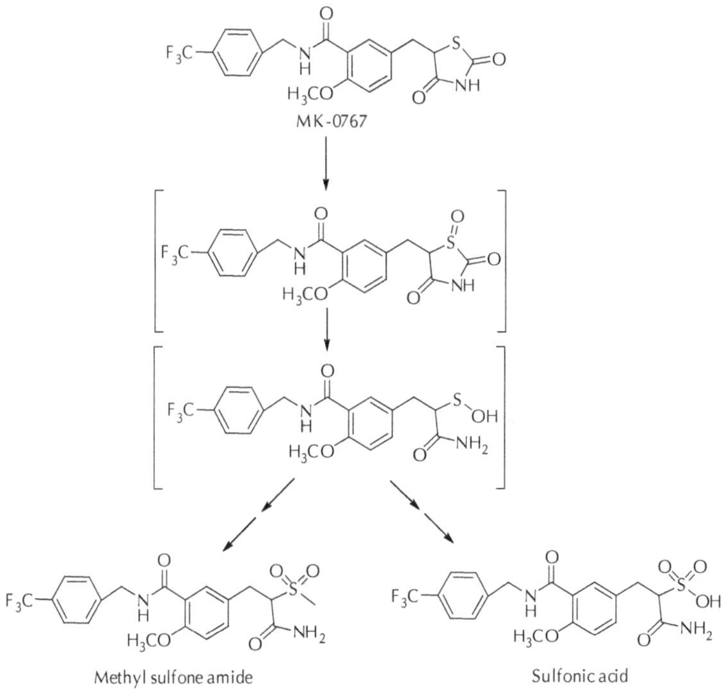

FIGURE 4 The TZD ring opened metabolites *via* *S*-oxidation of MK-0767.

The CYP3A4-mediated metabolic activation of PGZ was studied in detail by Baughman et al. highlighting the role of ring-opened reactive intermediates in toxicity of PGZ (2005). Uchiyama et al. reported the ring-opened metabolites generated by oxidation of TZD ring in PGZ and RGZ (2010). Hulin et al. proposed that the *S*-oxidation in glitazones is responsible for the rapid racemization in these antidiabetic agents (1996). The group investigated the effect of single and double *S*-oxidation in TZDs computationally, according to which reversible *S*-oxidation is responsible for the observed rapid racemization (see Figure 5) (Bharatam and Khanna, 2004). Saha et al. reported the bioisosteric replacement of the TZD ring with pyrrolidinedione heterocyclic system to improve their safety profiles (2012).

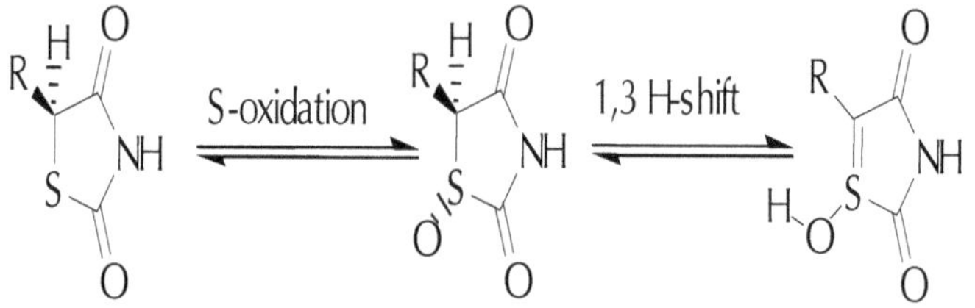

FIGURE 5 Tautomerism in TZD after *S*-oxidation.

The literature indicates that TZD derivatives have come under a scanner owing to their toxicological implications, thus, it becomes necessary to establish molecular level details of the CYP-catalyzed biochemical reactions occurring on TZD ring.

The quantum chemical calculations using *ab initio* molecular orbital (MO) and density functional methods have been reported to be useful in describing the detailed mechanistic aspects of *S*-oxidation and TZD ring opening. The group reported *ab initio* MO and density functional theory (DFT) calculations using Gaussian 03 package (Taxak et al., 2011, Taxak et al., 2012). The B3LYP/6-31+G (d, p) basis set was utilized for all the geometry optimizations, related to *S*-oxidation of TZD ring. The effect of solvent molecules was also analyzed, using explicit water molecules in the transition state calculations at the same levels of geometry optimization. The process of oxygen transfer to the sulfur atom of TZD ring was elucidated with different oxidants such as H_2O_2, HOONO, and C4a-hydroperoxy-flavin (to mimic flavoprotein monooxygenases (FMOs)).

The mechanism of oxygen transfer involves the nucleophilic attack of sulfur atom on the electrophilic oxygen atom of hydrogen peroxide. This results in the formation of TZD sulfoxide (TZDSO) and water as the side product (Taxak et al., 2011).

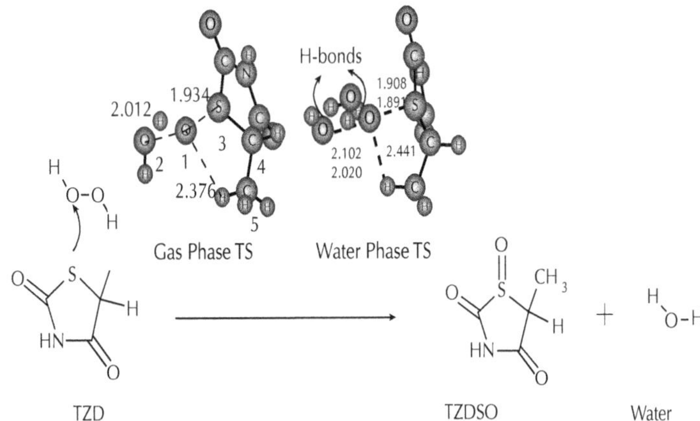

Nuclephilic attack of S atom on electrophilic oxygen atom of HOOH with a barrier of 32.49 and 28.55 kcal/mol in gas phase and water phase respectively.

FIGURE 6 The transition state geometries for the process of S oxidation of methylthiazolidinedione with HOOH in gas and aqueous (explicit water) phase. All the distances are in Å unit.

The 3D structures of the transition states on the S-oxidation path in gas phase and involving explicit water molecules is shown in Figure 6. In the gas phase, it can be observed that the S-O distance in transition state is 1.93 Å, and the O_1-O_2 distance is elongated to 2.01 Å. This indicates the proximity of S to O_1, along with the elimination of water molecule. This is confirmed by the O-O-H angle (40.28°) and suitable distance for hydrogen transfer (1.39 Å). Also, an additional C_5-H-O_1 hydrogen bond interaction (O_1-H-C (chiral) 2.37 Å) was observed. The energy barrier was observed to be 32.49 kcal/mol, which reduced to 28.55 kcal/mol on addition of one explicit water molecule. The hydrogen bond network between HOOH and explicit water molecule in the transition state complexes is clearly visible from the structures. Thus, the barrier for the *S*-oxidation is lowered after the inclusion of water molecule, due to the stabilization of transition state geometries (Taxak et al., 2011).

Recently, Taxak et al. reported the novel protonated intermediate, TZDSOH$^+$ (Figure 7), an elusive missing link on the metabolic path of glitazones, which plays a critical role in their toxicity (2012). It was reported that the proton transfer in TZDSO occurs *via* hydronium ion catalysis. The nucleophilic attack on TZDSOH$^+$ and ISC reactive intermediates were assessed, where the nucleophilic adducts of TZDSOH$^+$ were observed to be highly stable. This indicated that observed glutathione (GSH) adducts in mass spectral studies originate from TZDSOH$^+$ without involving ISC intermediate (Taxak et al., 2012).

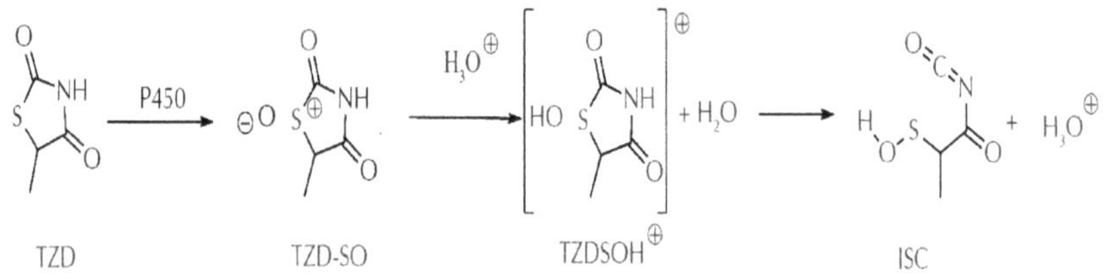

FIGURE 7 The CYP450 mediated *S*-oxidation of TZD ring and protonation of TZD ring to TZDSOH$^+$ (novel intermediate) on the metabolic pathway of glitazones.

Thus, these studies on the biochemical pathway of TZD ring metabolism would be useful in designing novel alternative anti-diabetic compounds with lesser toxicity. Raza et al. have synthesised several thiazolidin-4-one and thiazinan-4-one derivatives analogous to RGZ for their antidiabetic effects (Raza et al., 2013). The molecular docking studies have also been reported to be helpful in understanding the binding interactions of several drugs in the active site of CYPs. Hence, molecular docking methodology was adopted in this study for sulfide and sulfoxide unit containing drugs.

In thischapter, we report the detailed *S*-oxidation mechanism using molecular docking methods. Since, the biotransformation of TZDs is carried out by CYP450, it becomes essential to establish the critical role played by these enzymes using molecular docking methodology. The role of high-valent iron (IV)-oxo Cpd I, the active species of CYP450 has also been elucidated.

6.2 METHODOLOGY

6.2.1 MOLECULAR DOCKING

The molecular docking is a powerful and highly potential technique in molecular modeling (Cohen et al., 1990). This technique is helpful in understanding the interaction between the substrate and the receptor by estimating the best conformational fit between them (Lengauer and Rarey, 1996). The docking is a computational methodology to study the changes in the conformations of drug and to estimate the free energy change (ΔG^o) associated with this process. In this method, several likely docking models are constructed interactively and the energy minimization studies are carried out on each one of them. Keeping track of 3D complementarity of the molecular shape and sub-molecular properties between a drug and the active site of the receptor is very important in carrying out docking studies. Several scoring parameters such as interaction energy, strain energy, and so on can be calculated to estimate the strength of the interaction. On the basis of relative scaling parameters, the relative importance of the drugs can be estimated.

Grid-based ligand docking with energetics (Glide) approximates a complete systematic search of the conformational, orientation, and positional space of the docked ligand. It utilizes the sampling algorithms and descriptor matching, and is a highly coherent approach where the algorithm and scoring functions are optimized simultaneously. It is high-speed flexible docking software from Schrödinger, which utilizes van der Waals and electrostatic grids of the receptors and hierarchical filters for the conformational selection of the ligand. It possesses the specific advantages for docking of flexible ligands as discussed below and carries out exhaustive search. The general principle involves the representation of the shape and properties of the protein receptor on a grid. This grid is defined in the form of a rectangular box and it confines the ligand within the receptor. The best binding mode is identified through Monte Carlo sampling and the binding poses for ligands are ranked by using accurate scoring function. This software predicts the binding affinities faster with higher accuracy and thus, gives a higher probability of success in drug discovery programs.

6.2.2 COMPARISON WITH OTHER DOCKING SOFTWARE: GENETIC OPTIMIZATION FOR LIGAND DOCKING (GOLD) AND FLEXX

A large variety of docking softwares are available, where mostly differ with respect to their implementation. The treatment of ligand during docking differs in these softwares. Glide removes the terminal rotamer groups from the ligands while, FlexX adopts an incremental build-up strategy (Friesner et al., 2004; Friesner et al., 2006). The FlexX divides the non-cyclic bonds of the ligands, and uses the resulting base fragments as the starting points for the docking procedure. Thereafter, the correct rotameric state of each group is added, which is chosen by evaluating a specific scoring function for the fragment. On the other hand, gold GOLD treats the whole individual ligand as the entire entity, instead of fragmenting it. Molecular docking software also differs in the implementation of the search strategy. Glide uses incremental build-up approach, whereas, GOLD uses the genetic algorithm approach in exploring the conformational flexibility of ligands. Kontoyianni et al. have reported a higher success rate of Glide and GOLD, while evaluating the ability of several docking tools (2004). Friesner et al. discussed that Glide software can handle up to 35 rotatable bonds for non-covalently bound ligands (with ten to twenty rotatable bonds) and for other ligands (2004). Bissantz et al. and Cross et al. reported the higher efficiency of Glide in screening of virtual libraries (2000, 2009). There are differences in the preparation of the protein sites, where GOLD and FlexX retain the original PDB coordinates for non-hydrogen atoms. Halgren et al. discussed that GOLD and FlexX donot use the hard 12–6 Lennard-Jones vdW potential and thus, are lesser sensitive to the details of protein preparation, which is not the case with Glide (2004). Thus, several studies report the use of molecular docking software with their respective advantages and limitations.

6.2.3 GENERAL PARAMETERS CHOSEN FOR DOCKING USING GLIDE

The first step in a docking experiment involves the generation of the receptor grid. Van der Waals and electrostatic potentials are evaluated using the Optimized Potential for Liquid Simulations (OPLS)-2005 force field (Perola et al., 2004). Van der Waals interaction energies are calculated using the hard 6–12 Lennard–Jones potential, and the Coulomb formula is used for electrostatics with the net ionic charge on formally charged groups reduced approximately by 50% (Friesner et al., 2004; Friesner et al., 2006). The Glide involves the computation of fields (representing properties and shape of receptors) prior to docking. The binding site is defined by a rectangular box, which confines the ligand within the receptor site. Exhaustive search of torsional minima is carried out to generate the set of initial ligand conformations, which are thereafter, clustered in a combinatorial fashion. The search involves an initial rough positioning and scoring phase, which gradually narrows the search space and aids in the reduction of the number of poses to a few hundred. The selected poses are subsequently minimized and this procedure results in the generation of 5–10 lowest-energy poses. These poses are subjected to Monte Carlo Sampling to examine the torsional minima. The minimized poses are thereafter rescored using GlideScore.

The best pose is examined using Emodel which combines gscore and internal energy strain. GlideScore contains van der Waals and Coulomb energy terms, rewards for hydrophobic interactions and for polar but non-hydrogen-bonding groups in a hydrophobic environment, a hydrogen bonding term handling neutral-neutral, neutral-charged and charged-charged hydrogen bonds differently, a metal binding term and penalties for freezing rotatable bonds and inadequate solvation of functional groups not involved in close contacts (Friesner et al., 2004; Friesner et al., 2006). Parameters chosen for GLIDE jobs comprise of two sets; first one belongs to the parameters used for grid generation, while second refers to parameters used for docking.

6.2.4 LIGANDS

A database of ligands was prepared on the basis of presence of sulfide or sulfoxide unit, and their important pharmacological activity. The ligands were selected on the basis of following criteria: (a) Should have distinct pharmacological activity and are drug molecules, (b) Contain sulfide or sulfoxide unit. The ligands were built and minimized using Powell method embedded in Sybyl 7.1 (Sybyl, version 7.1, 2005). The minimized 3D structures were subjected to LigPrep module of Schrodinger software package version 9.2 and the output single ".sdf" file was used for the docking in Glide software (Schrödinger, Inc., 2006; Friesner et al, 2004).

6.2.5 PROTEINS

The selected CYP3A4 (pdb id: 2V0M) and 2C9 (pdb id: 1R9O) crystal structures were prepared using protein preparation wizard of Schrodinger package 2009. The in-house homology model of CYP2C19 was also utilized in the study (Patel et al., 2012). The heme iron was modeled as Fe^{+2}. For molecular docking with oxygen atom on heme iron (mimic Cpd I), the oxygen atom was placed at a distance of 1.9 Å from heme iron (see Figure 8).

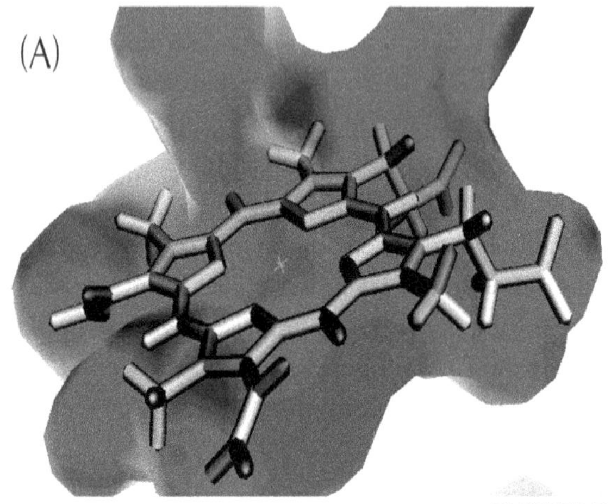

FIGURE 8 *(Continued)*

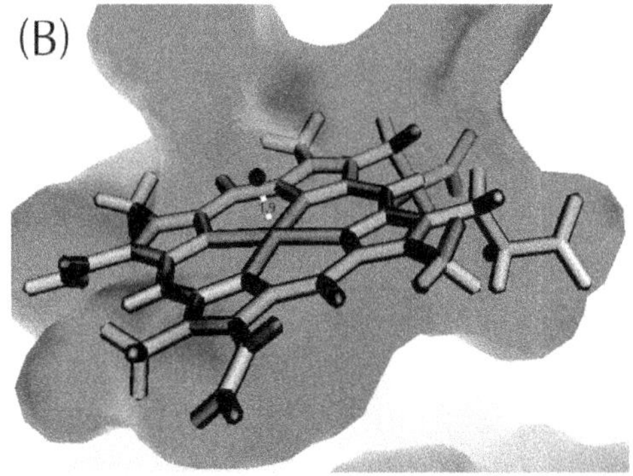

FIGURE 8 (A) Structure of heme-porphyrin without O atom, and (B) Structure of heme-porphyrin with O atom (shown as black) on heme iron (Fe), placed at a distance of 1.90 Å.

The parameters chosen included the use of OPLS 2001 as the force field, with a scaling factor: 0.80 (with partial charge cut-off of 0.25). A grid box of size 20 Å (with 10 Å internal box) with the coordinates X: 0.284, Y: 1.622, Z: 0.621 (with O); and X: 1.896, Y: 1.327, Z: 0.192 (without O) was chosen. The standard precision was utilized for docking study. The scoring functions utilized were gscore and Emodel. The number of poses saved per ligand was set as 20.

The metric of success in case of docking was set to the criteria of being the SOM within a certain distance from heme iron (6 Å, unless specified otherwise) in a docking pose (de Graaf et al., 2006). Top three docking poses were scanned (unless specified otherwise) for the evaluation of success rates in the docking analysis.

6.3 DISCUSSION AND RESULTS

6.3.1 MOLECULAR DOCKING ANALYSIS OF MAJOR SULFIDE-UNIT CONTAINING DRUGS INTO THE ACTIVE SITE OF CYP450

The drug metabolism is the one of the major determinant, apart from physicochemical properties, that characterizes a successful drug candidate from several novel compounds. The combinations of several quantitative and qualitative methods have evolved to determine the rate of metabolism and the SOM. It has been observed that the close interaction between the metabolism scientists and medicinal chemists are crucially important for this process. The identification of metabolites is crucial for drug safety and efficacy studies, as the metabolic alterations alter several properties of the molecules. Significant technological advances in mass spectrometry (MS) and utilization of molecular modeling approaches to metabolite identification have been observed in the last decade (Pahler and Brink, 2012).

The molecular docking methods offer a variety of tools to identify a suitable pose between a substrate and enzyme for metabolism (Leach, 2001; Morris and Lim-Wilby, 2008). This implies that the site of metabolism of a drug can be successfully predicted using molecular docking analyses. Although molecular docking analyses theoretically optimize favourable interactions between ligand and enzyme to estimate the binding mode and SOM predictions, these methods heavily rely on a well-defined active site. Therefore, the availability of a validated crystal structure or homology model of the P450 enzyme is a prerequisite for reliable SOM prediction in substrates. The currently available docking algorithms are probabilistic rather than deterministic, hence every docking exercise is not expected to provide the exact pose, but provides an acceptable pose. Currently, popular molecular docking software do not account for the induced fit effects. Hence, it is required to develop protocols based on molecular docking for SOM prediction.

A database of sulfide and sulfoxide unit containing drugs was prepared based on their metabolism by respective CYP isoforms: 3A4, 2C9 and 2C19 (see Table 1). These drugs have various sites of metabolism, and not necessarily the sulfide or sulfoxide unit. The molecular docking analysis was carried out using Glide software to determine whether *S* is shown to be the site of metabolism in these drugs. The distance for site of metabolism was taken to be within 6Å. Unconstraint molecular docking was carried out in two sets of three CYP isoforms. The two sets comprise of CYP450 having Fe without oxygen and other having Fe with oxygen (mimic Cpd I). The top ranked and top three rank poses were analyzed on the basis of Glide g score.

TABLE 1 Database of drug molecules with sulfide or sulfoxide unit, along with their SOM and metabolizing CYP isoforms

Drug	Site of Metabolism	Success/ Failure (for major CYP isoform)	CYP isoform
Clopidogrel	O, S-oxidation (not reported)	Y	3A5, 3A4, 2B6
Esomeprazole	S, O, ring	N	2C19,3A4,1A2
Fulvestrant	S	N	3A4
Lansoprazole	S	Y	2C19, 2C9
Metixene	S, N	Y	2D6, 3A4
Montelukast	S, C	Y	3A4, 2C8, 2C9
Pantoprazole	O, S-oxidation (not reported)	Y	2C19
Quazepam	C,N, S-oxidation (not reported)	Y	3A4, 2C9, 2C19
Quetiapine	S	Y	3A4(mainly), 2D6(minor)
Rabeprazole	S	Y	2C19, 3A4
Ranitidine	S,N	Y	2C19
Retapamulin	N, S-oxidation (not reported)	N	3A4
Ritonavir	isopropyl carbon, S-oxidation (not reported)	Y	3A4, 2C9, 2D6
Sulindac	S	N	FMO2, CYP2D6, CYP3A4, and CYP4A11
Tiagabine	S-oxidation (not reported)	N	3A
Ticlodipine	C, ring, S-oxidation (not reported)	Y	2C19, 3A4, 2B6
Troglitazone	S (but conjugation)	N	2C19, 3A4

TABLE 1 *(Continued)*

Zileuton	N, S-oxidation (not reported)	Y	1A2, 2C9 and 3A4
ziprasidone	S-oxidation (not reported)	Y	3A4

6.3.2 SUMMARY OF MOLECULAR DOCKING RESULTS

The molecular docking results for all the drugs molecules in all CYP isoforms are summarized in Table 2. Molecular docking results are based on the distances between iron of heme and the *S* atom on the substrates (within 6Å) in the first ranked pose as well as top three ranked docking poses. It is observed from the docking results that the substrates in CYP3A4 with O atom enjoy a higher success rate in predicting *S* atom to be the site of metabolism.

Comparison of CYP Isoforms: The CYP isoforms having O atom above heme iron were found to give better results as compared to those without oxygen atom. Among the CYP isoforms, all the six substrates of CYP2C9 were successfully docked (100%), and *S* was observed to be the site of metabolism.

TABLE 2 Molecular docking results for all substrates in their respective CYP isoforms

Protein	Oxygen atom on Fe	Scoring function	Number of Substrates	S atom Within <6 Å distance from Fe		
				I rank pose	Top III	% success
CYP3A4	No	gscore	16	5	9	56
CYP2C19	No	gscore	7	1	2	28
CYP2C9	No	gscore	6	3	5	83
CYP3A4	Yes	gscore	16	7	8	50
CYP2C19	Yes	gscore	7	2	4	57

TABLE 2 *(Continued)*

CYP2C9	Yes	gscore	6	6	6	100
CYP3A4	No	Emodel	16	3	6	37
CYP2C19	No	Emodel	7	2	2	28
CYP2C9	No	Emodel	6	5	5	83
CYP3A4	Yes	Emodel	16	7	9	56
CYP2C19	Yes	Emodel	7	2	2	28
CYP2C9	Yes	Emodel	6	5	6	100

The CYP2C19 showed least successful results in molecular docking. The major CYP isoform CYP3A4 showed a success rate of 56% for its substrates. Table 3 shows the Glide energies (binding energies) along with gscore for the top three poses for *S*-oxidation reaction in few ligands. Table 3 also shows the delta energy change for three poses of respective ligands, indicating the most favorable conformation of the respective ligand.

TABLE 3 Glide energies, gscore and delta energy change for the top three poses of few docked substrates

Substrate	CYP 3A4 with O atom on heme iron				CYP 3A4 without O atom on heme iron			
	Pose number	gscore	Glide energy	Δ Energy change	Pose number	gscore	Glide energy	Δ Energy change
Clopidogrel	1	–7.16	–30.99	6.13	1	–6.06	–19.69	1.26
	2	–6.85	–37.12	0.00	2	–5.89	–20.95	0.00
	3	–6.34	–34.55	2.57	3	–5.50	–20.68	0.27
S-omeprazole	1	–6.64	–39.20	4.72	1	–5.90	–29.78	2.59
	2	–6.60	–43.92	0.00	2	–5.63	–23.15	9.22
	3	–6.57	–41.94	1.98	3	–5.11	–32.37	0.00

TABLE 3 *(Continued)*

Rabe-prazole	1	−6.33	−44.02	0.76	1	−5.58	−29.36	0.63
	2	−6.10	−44.78	0.00	2	−5.42	−25.31	4.68
	3	−6.09	−43.15	1.63	3	−5.14	−29.99	0.00
Ritona-vir	1	−9.52	−71.39	0.00	1	−8.02	−43.72	1.64
	2	−9.00	−63.23	8.16	2	−7.70	-45.36	0.00
	3	−8.13	−61.62	9.77	3	−7.04	−44.58	0.78
Trogli-tazone	1	−6.37	−44.07	0.57	1	−6.64	−38.59	0.00
	2	−6.32	−44.64	0.00	2	−6.35	−35.01	3.58
	3	−6.22	−40.24	4.40	3	−6.02	−31.13	7.46
Zileuton	1	−6.57	−31.39	0.65	1	−6.22	−27.07	0.66
	2	−6.33	−31.50	0.54	2	−6.06	−27.73	0.00
	3	−6.28	−32.04	0.00	3	−5.85	−24.38	3.35

It was observed that most of the ligands acquire the most stable conformation in pose number 2 during molecular docking analysis in CYP3A4 isoform (with and without oxygen atom on heme iron). Troglitazone, anti-diabetic drug acquired most stable conformation in pose number 1 during docking without oxygen atom on heme iron, whereas the most stable conformation was observed in pose number 2 during molecular docking with oxygen atom on heme iron.

6.3.3 COMPARISON OF SCORING FUNCTION

Glide uses Emodel and gscore scoring function with their exhaustive search algorithm. The comparison of scoring functions show that the Glide gscore predicted S atom as site of metabolism in for 3A4, 2C9, and 2C19 better than the Glide Emodel. Figures 9 and 10 illustrate the molecular docking analysis of Troglitazone (anti-diabetic drug) and Zileuton in predicting the binding pose for the process of *S*-oxidation, with and without O atom on heme iron.

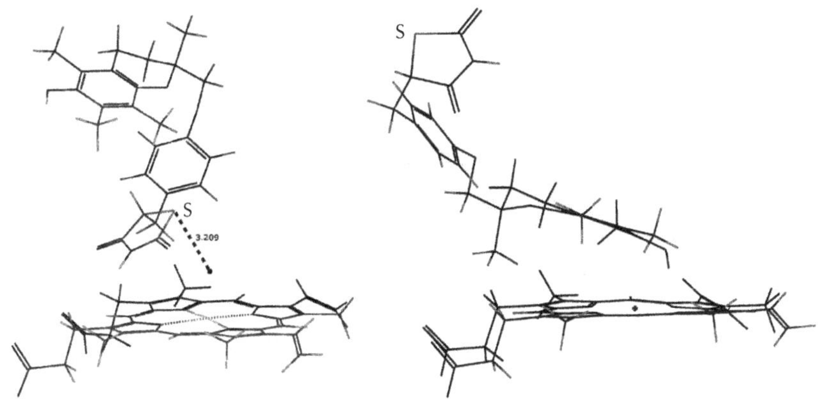

FIGURE 9 (A) Docking pose of troglitazone successful in CYP3A4 with O atom on heme iron, and (B) unsuccessful docking pose of troglitazone in CYP3A4 without O atom on heme iron.

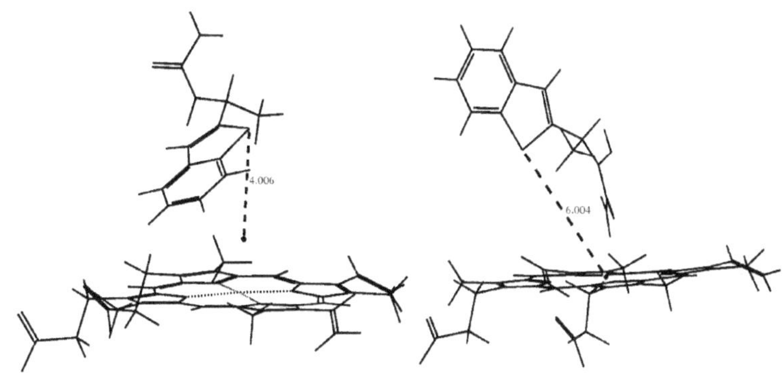

FIGURE 10 (A) Successful first rank docking pose of Zileuton in CYP3A4 with O atom on heme iron, and (B) unsuccessful docking pose of Zileuton in CYP3A4 without O atom on heme iron.

The analysis predicted *S* as the site of metabolism with a higher success rate, while docking with CYP having oxygen atom on heme iron, as compared to CYP without oxygen atom on Fe atom. This type of molecular docking analysis can form the basis for determining molecular mechanism of *S*-oxidation by quantum chemical methods.

Overall, this molecular docking study ascertains the protocol for SOM predication for a new molecule, determining its metabolites and would be helpful in elucidating the metabolic pathway. We discussed the docking analysis of sulfide or sulfoxide unit containing drugs, considering anti-diabetic glitazones and developed a protocol which can be applied to any new molecule. This study also highlighted the contribution of oxygen atom on heme iron leading to sulfoxidation. This is also discussed the toxic metabolites such as TZD ring-opened metabolites in case of glitazones, which can be avoided by searching for alternative heterocyclic rings as a selective and safer choice in future anti-diabetic drug design.

6.4 CONCLUSION

The site of metabolism prediction for a new molecule or chemical entity whether it is synthesized or virtually proposed, are important in the early phase of drug discovery to guide efforts of a medicinal chemist in designing leads with reduced liability to undergo metabolism. Here, molecular docking methodology (Glide) has been proposed to predict SOM for sulfide-unit containing drugs, such as anti-diabetic glitazones. It was observed that unconstrained molecular docking using Glide software was helpful in predicting SOM for ligands metabolized by specific CYP isoforms. The scoring and ranking of substrates should be carried out using gscore and Emodel scoring functions. Glide docking tool proved handy in our study for sulfide and sulfoxide unit containing compounds by identifying the metabolic sites. This is a general study for predicting the metabolic profile for sulfide and sulfoxide unit containing compounds. Hence, a more specific study for SOM prediction for anti-diabetic agents can be carried out using the same protocol as established in this study. This would be useful in guiding medicinal chemists to synthesize anti-diabetic compounds with better metabolic properties and helpful in determining their metabolites (active or toxic).

Three major CYP isoforms; CYP3A4, 2C9, and 2C19 were utilized in the study. It was observed that docking carried out in CYP isoforms with O atom on Fe increased the success rate, and thereby highlighting the importance of oxygen atom and implicating the role of Cpd I in oxidation reactions. This oxygen atom attached to heme iron is transferred from CYP to the incoming substrate for the process of *S*-oxidation. The molecular docking analysis predicted *S* as the metabolic site in 12 out of 19 substrates (success rate of 63%). Hence, molecular docking can be employed in predicting and analyzing SOM for a new molecule (with potential activities and specifically for anti-diabetic compounds), and guiding the medicinal chemists during the early stages of drug discovery.

KEYWORDS

- **Anti-diabetic**
- **Computational chemistry**
- **Drug metabolism**
- **Molecular mechanism**
- **S-oxidation**
- **Thiazolidinedione**

REFERENCES

1. Bissantz, C., Folkers, G., and, Rognan, D. Protein-based Virtual Screening of Chemical Databases. 1. Evaluation of Different Docking/Scoring Combinations. *J. Med. Chem.*, **43**, 4759–4767 (2000)
2. Baughman, T. M., Graham, R. A., Wells-Knecht, K., Silver, I. S., Tyler, L. O., Wells-Knecht, M., and Zhao, Z. Metabolic activation of pioglitazone identified from rat and human liver microsomes and freshly isolated hepatocytes. *Drug Metab. Dispos.*, **33**, 733–738 (2005).
3. Bharatam, P. V. and Khanna, S. Rapid racemization in thiazolidinediones: A quantum chemical study. *J. Phys. Chem. A.*, **108**, 3784 (2004).
4. Blake, B. L., Rose, R. L., Mailman, R. B., Levi, P. E., and Hodgson, E. Metabolism of thioridazine by microsomal monooxygenases: relative roles of P450 and flavin-containing monooxygenase. *Xenobiotica*, **25**, 377–393 (1995).
5. Brahmankar, D. M. and Jaiswal, S. B. *Biopharmaceutics and Clinical Pharmacokinetics- A Treatise*, Vallabh Prakashan, Delhi (2003).

6. Cariou, B., Charbonne, B., and Staels, B. Thiazolidinediones and PPARγ agonists: time for a reassessment. *Trends Endocrin. Metab.*, **23**, 205–215 (2012).
7. Cashman, J. R. and Zhang, J. Human flavin-containing monooxygenases. *Ann. Rev. Pharmacol. Toxicol.*, **46**, 65–100 (2006).
8. Chung, W. G., Park, C. S., Roh, H. K., Lee, W. K., and Cha, Y. N. Oxidation of ranitidine by isozymes of flavin-containing monooxygenase and cytochrome P450. *Jpn. J. Pharmacol.*, **84**, 213–220 (2000).
9. Cohen, N. C., Blaney, J. M., Humblet, C., Gund, P., and Barry, D. C. Molecular modeling software and methods for medicinal chemistry. *J. Med. Chem.*, **33**, 883–894 (1990).
10. Coleman, M. Drug Biotransformational Systems–Origins and Aims. *In Human Drug Metabolism: An Introduction*, John Wiley and Sons, UK, pp 13–18 (2010).
11. Cross, J. B., Thompson, D. C., Rai, B. K., Baber, J. C., Fan, K. Y., Hu, Y., and Humblet, C.
12. Comparison of Several Molecular Docking Programs: Pose Prediction and Virtual Screening Accuracy. *J. Chem. Inf. Model.*, **49**, 1455–1474 (2009).
13. de Graaf, C., Oostenbrink, C., Keizers, P. H. J., van der Wijst, T., Jongejan, A., and Vermeulen, N. P. E. Catalytic site prediction and virtual screening of cytochrome P450 2D6 substrates by consideration of water and rescoring in automated docking. *J. Med. Chem.*, **49**, 2417–2430 (2006).
14. de Montellano, P. O. *Cytochromes P450: Structure, Mechanism and Biochemistry*, Plenum, New York, (1995).
15. Foresman, J. B. and Frisch, A. E. *Exploring Chemistry with Electronic Structure Methods*, Gaussian, Inc., Pittsburgh, PA (1995).
16. Friesner, R. A., Banks, J. L., Murphy, R. B., Halgren, T. A., Klicic, J. J., Daniel, T. M., Repasky, M. P., Knoll, E. H., Shelley, M., Perry, J. K., Shaw, D. E., Francis, P., and Shenkin, P. S. Glide: A New Approach for Rapid, Accurate Docking and Scoring. 1. Method and Assessment of Docking Accuracy. *J. Med. Chem.*, **47**, 1739–1749 (2004).
17. Friesner, R. A., Murphy, R. B., Repasky, M. P., Frye, L. L., Greenwood, J. R., Halgren, T. A., Sanschagrin, P. C., and Mainz. D. T. Extra Precision Glide: Docking and Scoring Incorporating a Model of Hydrophobic Enclosure for Protein-Ligand Complexes. *J. Med. Chem.*, **49**, 6177–6196 (2006).
18. Gale, E. A. M. Lessons from the glitazones: a story of drug development. *The Lancet*, **357**, 1870–1875 (2001).
19. Halgren, T. A., Murphy, R. B., Friesner, R. A., Beard, H. S., Frye, L. L., Pollard, W. T., and Banks, J. L.. Glide: A New Approach for Rapid, Accurate Docking and Scoring. 2. Enrichment Factors in Database Screening. *J. Med. Chem.*, **47**, 1750–1759 (2004).
20. Hamman, M. A., Haehner-Daniels. B. D., Wrighton, S. A., Rettie. A. E., and Hall, S. D. Stereoselective sulfoxidation of sulindac sulfide by flavin-containing monooxygenases. Comparison of human liver and kidney microsomes and mammalian enzymes. *Biochem. Pharmacol.*, **60**, 7–17 (2000).
21. He, K., Talaat, R. E., Pool, W. F., Reily, M. D., Reed, J. E., Bridges, A. J., and Woolf, T. F. Metabolic Activation of Troglitazone: Identification of a Reactive Metabolite and Mechanisms Involved. *Drug Metab. Dispos.*, **32**, 639–646 (2004).

22. Hulin, B., Newton, S. L., Lewis, D. M., Genereux, P. E., Gibbs, M. E., and Clark, D. A. Hypoglycemic Activity of a Series of α-Alkylthio and α-Alkoxy Carboxylic Acids Related to Ciglitazone. *J. Med. Chem.*, **36**, 3897–3907 (1996).
23. Kassahun, K., Pearson, P. G., Tang, W., McIntosh, I., Leung, K., Elmore, C., Dean D., Wang, R., Doss, G., and Baillie, T. A. Studies on the metabolism of troglitazone to reactive intermediates in vitro and in vivo. Evidence for novel biotransformation pathways involving quinone methide formation and thiazolidinedione ring scission. *Chem. Res. Toxicol.*, **14**, 62–70 (2001).
24. Kiyota, Y., Kondo, T., Maeshiba, Y., Hashimoto, A., Yamashita, K., Yoshimura, Y., Motohashi, M., and Tanayama, S. Studies on the Metabolism of the New Antidiabetic Agent Pioglitazone - Identification of Metabolites in Rats and Dogs. *Arzneimittel-Forschung*, **47**, 22–28 (1997).
25. Kontoyianni, M., McClellan, L. M., and Sokol, G. S. Evaluation of Docking Performance:
26. Comparative Data on Docking Algorithms. *J. Med. Chem.*, **47**, 558–565 (2004).
27. Krueger, S. K. and Williams, D. E. Mammalian flavin-containing monooxygenases: structure/function, genetic polymorphisms and role in drug metabolism. *Pharmacol. & Ther.*, **106**, 357–387 (2005).
28. Leach, A. R. *Molecular Modelling: Principles and Applications*, Addison-Wesley Longman Ltd. (2001).
29. Lehrke, M. and Lazar, M. A. The many faces of PPARgamma. *Cell*, **123**, 993–999 (2005).
30. Lengauer, T. and Rarey, M. Computational Methods for Biomolecular Docking. *Curr. Opin. Struct. Biol.*, **6**, 402–406 (1996).
31. Liu, D. Q., Karanam, B. V., Doss, G. A., Sidler, R. R., Vincent, S. H., and Hop, C. E. C. In vitro metabolism of MK-0767 [(+/-)-5-[(2,4-dioxothiazolidin-5-yl)methyl]-2-methoxy-N-[[(4-trifluoromethyl)-phenyl] methyl]benzamide], a peroxisome proliferator-activated receptor alpha/gamma agonist. II. Identification of metabolites by liquid chromatography-tandem mass spectrometry. *Drug Metab. Disp.*, **32**, 1023–1031 (2004).
31. Lewis, D. F. *Cytochromes P450: Structure, Function and Mechanism*, Taylor and Francis, London, (1996).
32. Montagnani, A. and Gonnelli, S. Antidiabetic therapy effects on bone metabolism and fracture risk In Diabetes. *Obesity and Metabolism*, DOI: 10.1111/dom.12077 (2013).
33. Morris, G. M. and Lim-Wilby, M. Molecular Docking Methods. *Mol. Biol.*, **443**, 365–382 (2008).
34. Mudaliar, S. and Henry, R. R. New Oral Therapies for Type 2 Diabetes Mellitus: The Glitazones or Insulin Sensitizers. *Annu. Rev. Med.*, **52**, 239–257 (2001).
35. Nnane, I. P. and Damani, L. A. Involvement of cytochrome P450 and the flavin-containing monooxygenase(s) in the sulphoxidation of simple sulphides in human liver microsomes. *Life Sciences*, **73**, 359–369 (2003).
36. Pähler, A. and Brink, A. Software aided approaches to structure-based metabolite identification in drug discovery and development. *Drug Discovery Today, Technologies* (In Press) (2012).

37. Patel, D. S., Ramesh, M., and Bharatam, P. V. CytochromeP450 isoenzyme specificity in the metabolism of anti-malarial biguanides: molecular docking and molecular dynamics analyses. *Med. Chem. Res.*, **21**, 4274–4289 (2012).
38. Perola, E., Walters, W. P., and Charifson, P. S. A Detailed Comparison of Current Docking and Scoring Methods on Systems of Pharmaceutical Relevance. *PROTEINS: Structure, Function, and Bioinformatics*, **56**,235–249 (2004).
39. Prabhu, S., Fackett, A., Lloyd, S., McClellan, H. A., Terrell, C. M., Silber, P. M., and Li, A. P. Identification of glutathione conjugates of troglitazone in human hepatocytes. *Chem. Biol. Interact.*, **142**, 83–97 (2002).
40. Razaa, S., Srivastava, S. P., Srivastava, D. S., Srivastava, A. K., Haq, W., and Katti, S. B. Thiazolidin-4-one and Thiazinan-4-one Derivatives Analogous to Rosiglitazone as Potential Antihyperglycaemic and Antidyslipidemic Agents. *Eur. J. Med. Chem.*, http://dx.doi.org/10.1016/j.ejmech.2013.01.054 (2013).
41. Reddy, V. B. G., Karanam, B. V., Gruber, W. L., Wallace, M. A., Vincent, S. H., Franklin, R. B., and Baillie, T. A. Mechanistic studies on the metabolic scission of thiazolidinedione derivatives to acyclic thiols. *Chem. Res. Toxicol.*, **18**, 880–888 (2005).
42. Saha, S., Chan, D. S. Z., Lee, C. Y., Wong, W., New, L. S., Chui, W. K., Yap, C. W., Chan, E. C. Y., and Ho, H. K. Pyrrolidinediones reduce the toxicity of thiazolidinediones and modify their anti-diabetic and anti-cancer properties. *Eur. J. Pharmacol.*, **697**, 13–23 (2012).
43. Saltiel, A. R. and Olefsky, J. M. Thiazolidinediones in the Treatment of Insulin Resistance and Type II Diabetes. *Diabetes*, **45**, 1661–1669 (1996).
43. Schrödinger, Inc., New York, NY (2006).
44. Scott, A. P.; Radom, L. Harmonic Vibrational Frequencies: An Evaluation of Hartree–Fock, Møller–Plesset, Quadratic Configuration Interaction, Density Functional Theory, and Semiempirical Scale Factors. *J. Phys. Chem.*, **100**, 16502–16513 (1996).
45. *Sybyl, version 7.1*, Tripos International, St. Louis, MO (2005).
46. Taxak, N., Dixit, V., and Bharatam, P. V. Density Functional Study on the Cytochrome-Mediated S-Oxidation: Identification of Crucial Reactive Intermediate on the Metabolic Path of Thiazolidinediones. *J. Phys. Chem. A*, **116**, 10441–10450 (2012).
47. Taxak, N., Parmar, V., Patel, D. S., Kotasthane, A., and Bharatam, P. V. S-Oxidation of Thiazolidinedione with Hydrogen Peroxide, Peroxynitrous Acid, and C4a-Hydroperoxyflavin: A Theoretical Study. *J. Phys. Chem. A*, **115**, 891–898 (2011).
48. Uchiyama, M., Fischer, T., Mueller, J., Oguchi, M., Yamamura, N., Koda, H., Iwabuchi, H., and Izumi, T. Identification of Novel Metabolic Pathways of Pioglitazone in Hepatocytes: N-Glucuronidation of Thiazolidinedione Ring and Sequential Ring-Opening Pathway. *Drug Metab. Dispos.*, **38**, 946–956 (2010).

CHAPTER 7

ROLE OF WOUND DRESSINGS IN THE MANAGEMENT OF CHRONIC AND ACUTE DIABETIC WOUNDS

ROBIN AUGUSTINE, NANDAKUMAR KALARIKKAL, and SABU THOMAS

CONTENTS

ABSTRACT

People with diabetes are at increased risk for complications of wound healing for several reasons. A greater understanding of the molecular mechanism of diabetes and advances in biomaterial research has led to significant advancements in the management of diabetic wounds. These advances have saved thousands of patients from lower extremity amputation. Most of these amputations could easily be prevented with good foot care and wound treatment. Thus it is crucial for health care professionals working across the acute community interface to manage diabetic wounds effectively. The future of diabetic wound healing lies in the development of more effective smart wound dressings. Development of these kinds of therapies will require multidisciplinary translational research teams. This chapter outlines how current advances in molecular biology, polymer technology, and biomaterials can be incorporated into a multidisciplinary translational research approach for formulating novel smart wound dressings for diabetic wound treatment. It also provides an overview of recent advances in biomaterial research for the management of diabetic wounds and the different kind of wound dressings available in the market aimed on diabetic wounds.

7.1 INTRODUCTION

The diabetes forms a multisystem disorder that retards the wound healing process and makes it more complicated. The complications due to diabetes lead to physiological changes in tissues and cells which may delay healing and complications. It has been estimated that every 30 sec, someone loses a lower limb as a result of diabetes (Boulton et al, 2005). For a diabetic patient, even a small foot sore can become an ulcer that, if not rightly treated, can lead to amputation. The chance of amputation for people with diabetes is many times higher than for those who do not has it. People with diabetes are at increased risk for complications of wound healing due to several abnormalities associated with it. The diabetes decreases blood flow, so injuries are slower to heal than in people who do not have it. People with clogged arteries in their legs are more likely to get wounds, have wound infections, and have problems with wound healing. The diabetes patients often have narrowed arteries make it harder for blood to get to the wound which may retard healing, and increase the chance of get infected. Further many people with diabetes also have neuropathy–reduced sensation in their hands or feet as a result, minor trauma to the skin of the foot is often neglected and becomes infected (Sweitzer et al, 2006). Generally people with diabetes will have a weakened immune system. If the natural defenses are malfunctioning, even a minor wound may become susceptible to bacterial colonization. Due to these factors, it is important for health care teams working across the acute community interface to manage diabetic wounds effectively.

The diabetic wound care has become an integral part of diabetes treatment and a thorough understanding of diabetic wound care and advances in wound care technology has led to significant advancements in the management of diabetic wounds. These advances have spared thousands of patients the trauma of lower extremity amputation.The Figure 1 summarizes the factors that contribute to the onset of chronic diabetic wounds.

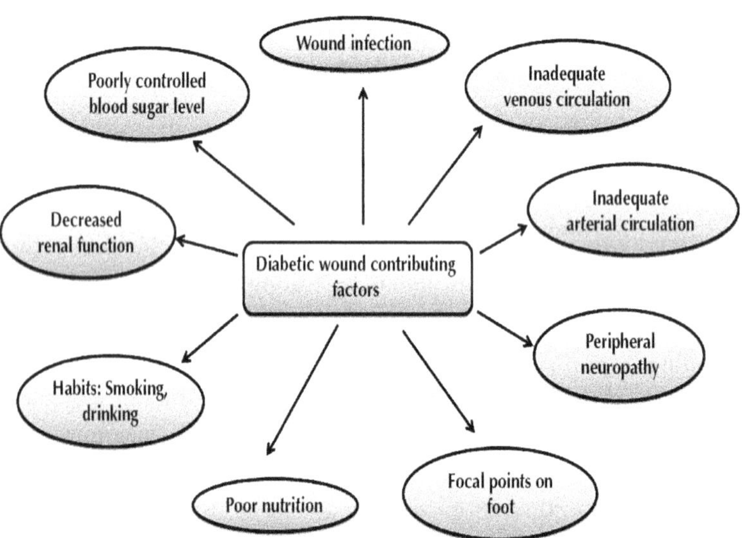

FIGURE 1 Risk factors that contribute to chronic diabetic wounds.

It has been known for many years that wounds in diabetic patients can take longer to heal than similar wounds in non-diabetics (Mulder, 1998). Wound healing in diabetes is a complex process, characterized by a chronic inflammation phase. In diabetic wound healing, the distribution of macrophage phenotypes being altered in the diabetic patient compared to normal wound repair (Helen et al, 2006). The major effects of diabetes on the wound healing process are the impairment of cellular proliferation for most cell types (Sank, 1994; Hehenberger, 1998; Lerman, 2003), increased apoptosis of endothelial cells (Lorenzi et al, 1985; Baumgartner, 1995; Darby, 1997), impairment of blood vessel regrowth (Loots, 1998; Singer and Clark, 1999), inadequate flow through blood vessels (Singer and Clark, 1999; Greenhalgh, 2003), and decreased collagen deposition at the wound site (Black, 2003). Furthermore, it is likely that growth factor expression is altered (Shukla, 1998; Wetzler, 2000; Robson, 2001; Greenhalgh, 2003), and nitric oxide secretion (Bulgrin, 1995; Zykova, 2000) and macrophage removal to the lymph nodes may also be impaired (Bellingan, 1996).

The diminished peripheral blood flow, impaired angiogenesis, and vasculogenesis are characteristic of poorly healing wounds in diabetic patients, particularly in lower extremities (Brem and Tomic, 2007; Gallagher et al, 2007). Low partial pressure of oxygen reduces the activity of enzymes producing reactive oxygen species (ROS) (Gordillo and Sen, 2003). As a consequence, the differentiation of myofibroblasts (MFB), the cells responsible for wound contraction, is impaired. The expression of α-smooth muscle actin, the main component of MFB cytoskeleton, decreases with reduced supply of oxygen, as shown in the cells transferred from 21% to 2% oxygen atmosphere. The MFB lose their ability to contract matrix *in vitro* and possibly the wound *in vivo* (Modarressi et al, 2010). On the other hand, when human dermal fibroblasts are exposed to 2% oxygen, they produce more transforming growth factor (TGF-β1) that mediates the increase in mRNA levels of procollagen I (Falanga et al, 1993). Low oxygen tension is also a stimulus for the proliferation of human adult and neonatal dermal fibroblasts (Falanga and Kirsner, 1993).

Feet and ankles are the regions most susceptible to diabetic wound complications. Since, these areas are dynamic than in other parts of the body and are prone to swelling, which can inhibit healing. But it is quite a difficult task for people with diabetes to avoid foot wounds due to the presence of more calluses, dry skin, and nerve damage. These are the major risk factors of diabetic foot ulcers which can lead to infections. Along with loss of sensation in the feet, many people with diabetes also have vision problems. So, they may be unable to feel or visually detect small wound until it becomes serious.

An experiment on diabetic rats showed that the amount of α-smooth muscle actin, took longer time to form in diabetic wounds, suggesting that wound contraction may be delayed in the diabetic animals. Further, the procollagen I expression in the diabetic wounds was very poor than healthy animals. The rate of apoptosis in diabetic wounds was higher than the normal wounds (Ian et al, 1997).

7.2 CLASSIFICATION OF DIABETIC WOUNDS

There two well accepted systems for the classification of diabetic wounds: The Wagner system and the Texas system.

7.2.1 WAGNER SYSTEM

The diabetic foot ulcers may be classified using the Wagner classification system. Wagner system is based primarily on wound depth and comprises of six wound grades. Grade 0 foot ulcers have intact skin with bony malformations or dry keratinized skin that increases the potential for ulceration, grade 1 involves ulceration of the dermis, grade 2 has ulceration involving tendons and joints, grade 3 extends to the bone and causes osteomyelitis, grade 4 shows localized gangrene, and grade 5 has gangrene involving a major portion of the foot (Wagner et al, 1987).

Failure of the Wagner classification to specifically deal with infection and ischemia within each grade has been realized and hybrid systems have been formulated to explain these important attributes of foot ulcers. A modified system which only amends modifiers for ischemia (A) and infection (B) to the well-known Wagner system is presented in the table

1, realizing that grades 3 through 5 usually have some degree of infection underlying within these lesions.

TABLE 1 Wagner hybrid system of wound classification

Grade	Lesion
0	**No open lesions: may have deformity or cellulites**
A	Ischemic
B	Infected
1	**Superficial Ulcer**
A	Ischemic
B	Infected
2	**Deep ulcer to tendon, or joint capsule**
A	Ischemic
B	Infected
3	**Deep Ulcer with abscess, osteomyelitis**
A	Ischemic
B	Infected
4	**Localized gangrene- forefoot or heel**
A	Ischemic
B	Infected
5	**Gangrene of entire foot**
A	Ischemic
B	Infected

7.2.2 TEXAS SYSTEM

Armstrong et al., proposed a new system for the classification of diabetic wounds that have been validated to predict outcome of wound (1998). They have considered infection, peripheral vascular disease, and wounds of increasing depth, and that the cumulative effect of these comorbidities to a greater likelihood of amputation. The system of classification is given in Table 2.

TABLE 2 Texas system of diabetic wound classification

Grade/depth					
		Grade			
	Depth	**0**	**I**	**II**	**III**
Stage/Comorbidities:	**A**	Pre- or post-ulcerative lesion completely epithelialized	Superficial would not involving tendon, capsule or bone	Would penetrating to tendon or capsule	Would penetrating to bone or joint
	B	Pre- or post-ulcerative lesion completely epithelialized with infection	Superficial would not involving tendon, capsule or bone with infection	Would penetrating to tendon or capsule with infection	Would penetrating to bone or joint with infection
"Is the wound infected, ischemic, or both?"	**C**	Pre- or post-ulcerative lesion completely epithelialized with ischemia	Superficial would not involving tendon, capsule or bone with ischemia	Would penetrating to tendon or capsule with ischemia	Would penetrating to bone or joint with ischemia

TABLE 2 *(Continued)*

D	Pre- or post-ulcerative lesion completely epithelial-ized with infection and ischemia	Superficial would not involving tendon, capsule or bone with infection and isch-emia	Would penetrating to tendon or capsule with infec-tion and ischemia	Would penetrating to bone or joint with infection and isch-emia

7.3 WOUND DRESSINGS

The wound healing is a native process of regenerating dermal and epidermal tissues. When an individual is wounded, a set of complex biochemical actions take place in a closely orchestrated cascade to repair the damage. These events can be classified into inflammatory, proliferative, and remodeling phases and epithelialization. The treatment of the wounds has evolved from the ancient times. Initially, application of dressing material was aimed at inhibition of bleeding, protection of the wound from environmental irritants as well as water and electrolyte disturbances. The skin plays an important role in homeostasis and the prevention of invasion by microorganisms. The skin generally needs to be covered with a dressing immediately after it was damaged. The wound management has seen many changes over the past few decades. A large variety of wound dressings have been applied to wounds since ancient times, for effective healing of a wound, a suitable material had to be used to cover the wound in order to prevent any infection. Historically, honey pastes, plant fibers, and animal fats were used as wound dressing materials (Majno, 1975; Thomas, 1990; Doshi and Reneker, 19954; Formhals, 1934).

Wound dressings are extensively used in the treatment of ulcers in people with diabetes. There are many types of dressings that can be used, which also vary substantially in cost. Nowadays, with new biopolymers and fabrication techniques, a wound dressing material is expected to have extraordinary properties which enhance the healing process of a wound.

With the right choices of biopolymers used for these fibrous materials, they could enhance the healing of wounds significantly compared with the conventional fibrous dressing materials, such as gauze. These bandages could be made such that they contain bioactive ingredients, such as antimicrobial, antibacterial, and anti-inflammatory agents, which could be released to the wounds enhancing their healing. In an active wound dressing (AWD), the main purpose is to control the biochemical states of a wound in order to aid its healing process. For a fantabulous design of a functional wound dressing material, characteristics of the wound type, wound healing time, physical, mechanical, and chemical properties of the bandage must be taken into consideration. Ultimately, the main purpose is to achieve the highest rate of healing and the best aesthetic repair of the wound (Thomas S, 1990).

Today's moist wound healing principles are based on pioneering work by Winter (1962) and later by Hinman and Maibach (1963). A wound dressing material should function to protect the wound, absorb extra body fluids from the wound area, destroy the pathogenic microorganism, improve the appearance and sometimes accelerate the healing process. The wound healing is a dynamic process and the performance requirements of a dressing can change as healing progresses. However, it is widely accepted that a warm, moist environment encourages rapid healing and most modern wound care products are designed to provide these conditions. The wound dressing material should provide a physical barrier to a wound, but be permeable to moisture and oxygen. Extensive literature supports the benefits of moist wound healing (Seaman, 2002; Mulder et al, 1998; Choucair and Phillips, 1996; Turner, 1997; Carver and Leigh, 1992; Higgins and Ashry, 1995: Doughty, 1992: Haimowitz and Margolis, 1997). Fluid balance in burn injury is very important since heavy loss of water from the body by exudation and evaporation may lead to a fall in body temperature and increase in the metabolic rate. Besides this, dressing should have certain other properties like ease of application and removal, and proper adherence so that there will not be any area of non-adherence left to create fluid-filled pockets for the proliferation of bacteria.

Numerous wound dressing materials are available and are also being investigated (Harsh et al, 1991). Hydrogels combine the features of moist wound healing with good fluid absorbance and are transparency to allow the monitoring of healing. *In situ* forming hydrogels that fabricated in to the shape of wound defect will have advantages over the use of shaped hydrogel scaffolds it would enable conformability of the dressing on wounds without wrinkling or fluting. Most commercially available dressing in the form of membranes and sheets are problematic as far as the conformability is concerned and the *in situ* formed dressings will therefore be superior to preformed dressings.

7.3.1 SELECTION OF A WOUND DRESSING MATERIAL

The wound requires a protective barrier to promote the healing. Passive dressings such as gauze and tulle can act to cover the wound from external environment. Gauze can stick to the wound and disrupt the wound bed when removed, thus are suitable for minor wounds. Tulle is greasy gauze suitable for minimal to moderate exudates. Interactive dressings contain polymeric films, foams and hydrogels which are permeable to water and atmospheric oxygen. Such dressings are advantageous for heavily exuding wounds and good barriers against invasion of bacteria to the wound and the pathogenesis (Andreia and Artur, 2011). Bioactive dressings produced from a variety of biopolymers like collagen, hyaluronic acid, chitosan (CS), alginate (AL), and elastin have the ability to alter or confront the physiological condition of the wound and promote the healing (Falabella 2006; Queen et al. 2004). These dressings usually contain active ingredients such as antimicrobials and wound healing agents (Queen et al. 2004). Considering the above features, wound dressing materials are designed to manage critical conditions such as infection in the local wound environment beyond mere exudate management.

Choosing the right treatment option is the essential step in the management of all kinds of chronic wounds (Katarzyna et al., 2013). The selection of a most appropriate wound dressing material for the treatment of a wound can be complicated and clarity concerning dressing form and function is in great deal a hurdle to overcome (Carville, 1999). Before selecting a suitable wound dressing, it is crucial to identify the intention or principal aim of the suggested treatment. It is essential to evaluate the whole patient, diagnose causative disease pathology and assess the patient's opinion before choosing the dressing (Schultz et al, 2003). Apart from the availability and use of novel dressings, wound management requires an understanding of the process of tissue repair and the knowledge of the characteristics of the dressings available (Carolina and Geoff, 2006).

The dressing selection should have the main objectives of promoting and maintaining a favorable environment to facilitate healing (Eaglstein, 1997). Most of the published clinical data support the use of dressings that promote micro environmental factors, such as optimal oxygen tension, pH, and humidity, which stimulate more rapid wound healing, in particular those that support a moist wound environment. In addition, the choice of dressing will be influenced by clinical factors, such as the type of wound, position, presence of debris or infection, level of exudate, and patient comfort. Effective wound management requires the understanding of the type of wound and healing process. The physical, mechanical, and chemical properties of the dressing must also be taken into consideration. The new biomaterials to be applied as wound dressings should create a moist environment around the wound, effective oxygen circulation, cellular guidance, and low bacterial load.

Wound treatment decisions must be patient centered. Local wound care starts with a thorough assessment of the wound and a comprehensive collection of data about the patient's overall status. Wound assessment is the cumulative process of observation of the actual wound, as well as observing the patient, data collection, and evaluation. Consideration of the etiology of the wound is essential for proper care. Wound care products must be individualized for the particular wound. For example, a venous stasis ulcer might require a highly absorptive dressing, as well as the necessary compression therapy. Furthermore, checking for ankle-brachial index and/or toe pressures using Doppler technology is part of the total care of a patient with a peripheral vascular ulcer or history of diabetic neuropathies (Okan et al, 2007).

For many patients, weekly reassessment will provide the indices of a successful treatment and guide decisions that suggest product changes. As the wound characteristics change, the choice of the wound dressings should also change. Indeed, several different types of products may be needed as the wound progresses through the stages of healing. After a thorough wound assessment is completed, choosing dressings and treatments becomes a clinical decision that includes the patient's overall expected outcome. Treatment goals may aim to achieve a clean wound, heal the wound, maintain a clean wound bed, prevent wound deterioration, contain odor or exudates, reduce pain, or to place the patient in another setting to continue care. Clinicians should match the wound assessment characteristics with the dressing characteristics or function. The goal of care then becomes using the right product on the right wound at the right time. For example, a granular, non-draining moist or wet wound needs to maintain a moisture balance contributing to healing. The primary dressing choice would be a product that maintains a moist environment but does not cause maceration or desiccation of the wound bed. The goal of dressing selection for a necrotic draining diabetic wound is to loosen or soften the eschar for surgical debridement or to assist in autolytically debriding the wound, absorbing the excess exudate, and preventing trauma to surrounding tissue. A wound that is dry and necrotic and non-healable would not benefit from moist wound healing. Treatment would focus on maintenance care, keeping the wound protected and assessing for any signs of infection. Further it is important to remember that one of the primary goals of care is the prevention of wound-related infection. Infection is a common complication of all open wounds including diabetic wounds. Open wounds are colonized with bacteria, which means that low numbers of bacteria are always present on the wound surface (Doughty, 2010). Antimicrobial or antiseptic dressing can be used to manage wounds that are critically colonized with bacteria, which provide sustained release of various agents, such as silver or cadexomer iodine (Rodeheaver, 2007).

According to National Pressure Ulcer Advisory Panel and European Pressure Ulcer Advisory Panel, it is necessary to reassess the wound status when completing dressing changes so that most suitable treatment can be implemented (2009). Selection of wound dressing should also include an evaluation of the patient's outcome of care. Acute care patients with length of stays of 4–5 days commonly will not attain healing as their outcome, but will achieve a moist, clean wound bed that supports the healing environment. Home care and long-term-care circumstances may have a goal of healing or maintaining the current status of the wound based on the overall health status of the patient. Wound outcomes need to be patient focused and naturalistic to the length of time for which a patient gets care (Sharon and Elizabeth, 2012).

One example of an increased understanding of the cellular biology of wound healing and technology is the use of growth factors in wound care. All growth factors are proteins that are secreted by cells and have the ability to stimulate cell division, a positive action during the wound healing process (Davidson, 2010). Growth factors are now available-derived from either a patient's own human platelets or in a drug form dispensed in a tube to apply to wounds. Research continues as to what combination, what quantity, and when growth factors will best enhance wound healing.

Tissue engineering is a fascinating technology which provides new options for wound management by the use of skin equivalents or substitutes for healing chronic wounds. The use of gene therapy in wound healing by regulating the expression of key molecules like growth factors is the future perspective yet to be seen.

Current decisions on choice of wound dressing if any, mostly based on dressing costs and selecting the most useful management properties offered by each dressing type, for example, the management of wound exudate (Dumville et al, 2011).

7.3.2 SPECIALIZED WOUND DRESSINGS

Desirable characteristics for wound dressings must incorporate the principles of wound healing and the nature of wound. The conventional wound dressing materials are not suitable for acute and chronic wounds as far as rapid healing of a wound is concerned. For this purpose functionalized biological and biochemical bandages were developed. One of the main advantages of using such specialized wound dressing materials is the modified chemical environment confronting the physiological conditions in accordance with the nature of the wound and facilitates more rapid healing (Liane et al., 2013). In addition, frequent changing of the wound dressing also can be avoided. These materials produced more promising clinical results as compared to the conventional wound dressing materials. The bioactive wound dressing materials are produced from a variety of biopolymers such as pectin, collagen, hyaluronan, CS, AL, elastin, and so on. Nowadays, biopolymers containing active ingredients, such as antimicrobials and antibiotics, are extensively used in wound dressing materials against contaminations and infections. Incorporation of potential wound healing and anti-inflammatory agents in such dressing materials are also under active research.

Nowadays the research and development focus more on interactive materials that can facilitate the healing process by addressing specific issues in non-healing wounds rather than simply using natural materials to just cover and conceal the wound. These novel dressings much link with the proteolytic wound environment and the bacteria load to promote the healing process. Recently, the wound dressing research is revolving about the substitution of synthetic polymers by natural proteinaceous materials such as silk fibroin, keratin, and elastin to deliver bioactive agents to the wounds in a controlled fashion. The improved properties of these dressings, like the release of antibiotics and growth factors, are advantageous for situations like diabetic foot ulcers.

For diabetic wounds, especially for diabetic foot ulcers, many such specialized wound dressing materials like hydrocolloids and hydrogels with improved wound healing have been tried (Daichi et al., 2010)

7.4 CHARACTERISTICS OF A WOUND DRESSING MATERIAL FOR DIABETIC WOUNDS

As in the case of general wound dressings, the diabetic wound also should be covered with materials that alleviate symptoms, provide wound protection, encourage healing, reduce wound dehydration and offer proper aeration. A schematic representation of essential properties of a diabetic wound dressing material is given in Figure 2. Wound dressings have been fabricated to preserve such an environment while also controlling the growth of microorganisms, allowing gaseous exchange, and thermally insulating the wound, which allows painless removal. A good wound dressing must also fit virtual issues such as permitting the observation of the wound and rendering mechanical support and conformability. Further the dressings must also be cost effective (Jones, 1998).

While treating diabetic wounds utmost importance must be given to the level of moisture in the wound. Non-adhesive dressings are simple, inexpensive, and well tolerated. Foam and AL dressings are highly absorbent and effective for heavily exuding diabetic wounds. Hydrogels encourage autolysis and may be advantageous in managing chronic diabetic ulcers containing necrotic tissue. Dressings incorporated with antimicrobials like silver and povidone-iodine can assist in handling wound infection. Occlusive dressings should be avoided for infected wounds. Heavily exuding diabetic ulcers need frequent change to reduce maceration of surrounding skin (Hilton et al., 2004).

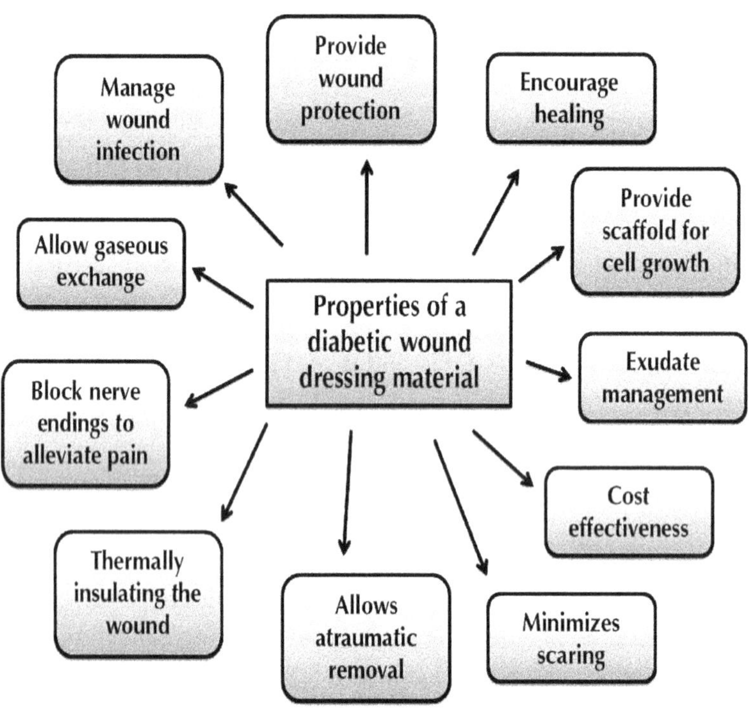

FIGURE 2 Essential properties of a wound dressing material used for diabetic wounds.

7.5 TYPES OF WOUND DRESSINGS SUITABLE FOR DIABETIC WOUNDS

There are different schools on the ideal dressing in diabetes. The principles of moist wound healing are generally followed. This is good practice for uncomplicated acute surgical wounds. However, chronic diabetic wounds must be monitored for infection every 1–2 days, so dressings designed for optimum use over longer periods are not ideal. Adhesive borders on modern dressings provide improved contact with the wound bed. However, care must be taken to avoid damaging surrounding skin on removal. Infected wounds produce increased exudate, so dressings' exudate-handing capability should be considered, ALs are often useful. All ALs have similar properties, but differences in manufacture affect the absorptive capabilities of various products. Those with needled fibers are dense and liable to form a fibrous mat in the presence of thick exudates. This obstructs drainage and can undermine neighboring tissue. Use of ALs is best restricted to wounds exuding large amounts of thin exudate.

Antimicrobials are being introduced into numerous wound dressings with evidence of effectiveness being studied (Ovington, 2010). Silver preparations or cadexomer iodine dressings may be used to reduce bacteria in colonized or infected wounds (Schultz et al., 2003). However, dressings are not a replacement for systemic therapy for infection. Bulky dressings are likely to increase intra-shoe pressures.

The wound care and the management improved a lot during the past few decades and technology was still advancing in the field of wound care. Even though many current technologies are improving and expanding, and many new methods are still being developed and researched, wet-to-dry gauze remains a popular dressing with healthcare providers. (Ovington, 2010). Skin substitutes have shown promise as a "smart" dressing, which can deliver specific growth factors to the wound. This method of gene theory is the newest and latest research that is being tested. In addition, wound pain has emerged as a needed focal point in wound care management. Pain at dressing removal is a frequent complaint heard from patients who have their wounds dressed with gauze dressings that have dried into their wound. Dressings that do not cause skin damage upon removal are now available.

There a large number of wound dressing materials in the market claimed to have application potential in diabetic wounds. They are briefly discussed as follows.

7.5.1 NON-ADHERENT OR LOW-ADHERENCE DRESSING

Various types of non-adherent or saline-soaked gauze dressings are often regarded as standard treatment for diabetic ulcers. These dressings are designed to be atraumatic and to provide a moist environment for wound healing. These wound dressings are advantageous in the sense that they are simple and relatively inexpensive but are not designed to specifically managing infection. They can be safely used in combination with antibiotic treatments. Non-adherent silicone-based dressings have been developed to minimize damage to the wound bed and surrounding tissue. They can be especially useful in fragile or friable skin like diabetic wounds where regular change of dressing is necessary. Silicone is also inert (Thomas, 2003), which makes it suitable for patients with an increased risk of sensitivity, such as those with diabetic foot ulcers.

Adaptic Touch® (Systagenix) silicone dressing is a non-adherent, flexible, open- mesh primary wound contact layer comprised of cellulose acetate coated with a soft tack silicone. It is designed to stay in place unassisted during dressing application and to be atraumatic with regard to both the wound and surrounding skin during dressing change. The atraumatic nature of the dressing will help to reduce pain during dressing changes.

A new generation of non-adherent primary wound dressing called the lipidocolloid dressings has been developed to combine desirable properties of hydrocolloids with those of petrolatum gauze. The first example of this new class of dressing is Urgotul®. Urgotul® is suggested for the treatment of superficial acute or chronic exuding diabetic wounds at the granulation and re-epithelialization stages of the wound healing. It should usually be changed once in every 2–3 days, but can be left in place for longer (6 days) on low or lightly exuding wounds. As a result of the low adherence to the wound, painless, and atraumatic removal are to be expected (Moody, 1992; Hollinworth, 1995; Williams, 1996). In practice, this has been found to be the case (Benbow, 2002)

Urgotul® is composed of a 100% polyester crosswise open weave impregnated with hydrocolloid polymers dispersed within a petrolatum impregnated mesh. Its macroscopic aspect is that of a non-greasy light and soft gauze which adapts itself easily to wound shape. Urgotul® will not fray, so no microfibers will be released into the wound. In contact with exudate, hydrocolloid polymers are hydrated and constitute with the petrolatum part of the dressing, a lipidocolloid interface which is designed to reduce adhesion to the wound surface. Urgotul® has an appreciable fluid absorptive capacity. The lipidocolloid interface is very cohesive, preventing release of petrolatum on to the wound surface and facilitating dressing removal. In addition, the open weave of the polyester is non-deformable and maintains the 500 μm size when impregnated, thus reducing the growth of granulation tissue growing through and the consequent risk of trauma on removal (Meaume et al., 2002).

7.5.2 HYDROCOLLOIDS

Hydrocolloids are special class of wound dressings that are widely used in clinical practice to manage diabetic wounds. Generally term hydrocolloid depicts the family of wound management products fabricated from colloidal or gel forming materials combined with other materials such as adhesives and elastomers (Joshua et al., 2008). Hydrocolloid dressings are semipermeable to vapor, occlusive to wound exudate, and absorbent. They are normally introduced as an absorbent layer on a film or foam. Hydrocolloids are also indicated for granulating and epithelializing diabetic wounds. They bear colloidal materials, such as carboxymethylcellulose (CMC), gelatin, and pectin (Joshua et al., 2008). When the dressing comes into touch with wound exudate it absorbs fluid and terns into gel which creates a moist environment that can promote healing process (Heenan, 1998). Hydrocolloid materials are designed in such a way that to be occlusive, trapping exudate within the dressing and hydrating the wound. This makes them the second most popular choice of dressing (behind non-adherent) for all diabetic foot ulcers in a study of British diabetic specialist nurses and chiropodists (Fisken and Digby, 1997). Hydrocolloid dressings are designed to be left on the wound for prolonged periods, this is useful in managing clean diabetic ulcers but not when regular wound inspection is required. Thus, these dressings are probably more useful in preventing, rather than treating, infection within a wound (Hilton et al, 2004).

Knowles et al. (1993) attempted a retrospective study on the use of Granuflex hydrocolloid dressing (ConvaTec, Deeside) and other dressings in the treatment of diabetic foot ulcers. Their findings suggest that healing and infection rates were similar in the Granuflex group when compared with the other groups. They concluded that Granuflex is equally effective and safe to use as other dressings commonly used on diabetic foot ulcers. Gill (1999) reviewed the literature on the use of hydrocolloids on the diabetic foot and suggested that the concerns regarding the use of hydrocolloids on diabetic foot ulcers has mainly focused on subjective reports of adverse effects, which a great deal developed due to the inappropriate use of these dressings.

Examples of hydrocolloid dressings include Granuflex™ and Aquacel ™ (Conva Tec, Hounslow, UK), Comfeel™ (Coloplast, Peterborough, UK), and Tegasorb™ (3M Healthcare, Loughborough, UK) (Joshua et al., 2008).

7.5.3 HYDROGELS

Hydrogels are swellable, insoluble and hydrophilic materials made from synthetic polymers such as poly(methacrylates) and polyvinylpyrrolidine. Some dressings such as Nu-gel™ (Johnson and Johnson, Ascot, UK) and Purilon™ (Coloplast) are hydrogel/AL combinations. Hydrogels are similar to hydrocolloid dressings in that they are designed to facilitate autolysis of necrotic tissue, but they differ in that they donate moisture to extensively dry wounds. Examples include Aquaform (Maersk Medical) and Intrasite Gel (Smith and Nephew). Hydrogels can be applied either as an amorphous gel or as elastic, solid sheet or film depending upon the amount of exudate present in wounds. To prepare the sheets, the polymeric components are cross-linked so that they physically entrap water. The sheet form of hydrogel dressings can absorb and retain significant quantity of exudate from exuding diabetic ulcers. When applied to the wound as a gel, hydrogel dressings usually require a secondary covering such as gauze and need to be changed frequently (Debra, 1998). The sheet form, do not need a secondary dressing since these are designed as a semi-permeable polymer film backing, with or without adhesive borders which controls the transmission of water vapour through the dressing. In addition the sheets can be cut to fit around the wound due to their flexible nature. The gels are used as primary dressings whereas the hydrogel films may be used as primary or secondary dressings.

Hydrogel dressings can lead to maceration when applied to wounds that are moderately to heavily exuding. Thus, these should be used carefully on patients with limb ischemia, because dry gangrene could potentially rapidly progress to wet gangrene, with serious outcomes. Even though there exist a hesitation to apply hydrogels to infected wounds; *in vitro* studies have shown that hydrogels will not enhance bacterial growth (McCulloch, 1993). Morgan (2002) suggested that, hydrogels are suitable to apply on all the stages of wound healing excluding heavily exuding or infected wounds (Morgan, 2002).

A novel layered hydrogel composing of AL, CS, and poly(γ-glutamic acid) (PGA) has been reported by Yen-Hsien Lee et al. They have examined the effect of the hydrogels on wound healing in type 1 diabetic rat model induced by streptozotoxin (STZ). After grafting to full-thickness wounds, layered AL-CS-PGA has shown higher rate of wound healing than conventional AL hydrogels. The histological examination indicated AL-CS-PGA treated wounds showed increased collagen regeneration and epithelialization (Yen et al., 2012).

7.5.4 FOAMS

Foam dressings comprise of porous polyurethane foam or polyurethane foam film, sometimes with adhesive borders. Foam-based wound dressings are another popular choice for diabetic foot management. These dressings possess the ability to absorb large quantity of exudate, provide thermal insulation to the wound, and are comfortable. There have been a few published data on their use in diabetic foot ulceration and none on their use in infection (Hilton, 2004). However, their absorbency and comfort would theoretically make them a suitable choice. A new foam dressing

(Avance) impregnated with bactericidal silver has recently been introduced. Foam dressings maintain a moist environment around the wound, provide thermal insulation and are convenient to wear. They are highly absorbent, absorbency being controlled by foam properties such as texture, thickness and pore size. The open pore structure also gives a high moisture vapour transmission rate (MVTR). Examples include Allevyn (Smith and Nephew) and Cavicare (Smith and Nephew).

According to a review carried out Dumville et al. there is no research evidence to suggest that foam wound dressings are more effective in healing foot ulcers in people with diabetes than other types of dressing. Pooled data from two studies comparing foam and AL dressing found no statistically significant difference in ulcer healing. Similarly there is no evidence to suggest, diabetic foot ulcers healed when foam dressings compared with hydrocolloid (matrix) dressings. But while considering other advantages like conformability, exudate uptake capacity etc. (Dumville et al., 2011).

7.5.5 ALGINATES

A wide variety of different AL based wound care products are currently available in the market. They are conformable into cavity wounds to provide hemostasis, highly absorbent and are atraumatic and cause little pain at dressing change. The AL dressings occur either in the form of freeze-dried foams (porous sheets) or as flexible fibers. The use of ALs as dressings roots primarily from their ability to form gels upon contact with wound exudates which attribute to the high exudate uptake capacity. The high absorption occurs via strong hydrophilic gel formation, which limits wound secretions and minimizes bacterial contamination (Heenan, 1998). The ALs rich in mannuronate, such as Sorbsan™ (Maersk, Suffolk, UK) form soft flexible gels upon hydration whereas those rich in guluronic acid, like Kaltostat™ (Conva Tec), form firmer gels upon absorbing wound exudate. Some contain calcium AL fibre such as Sorbsan™ and Tegagen™ (3M Healthcare). Comfeel Plus™ is a hydrocolloid/AL combination dressing.

It is important to ensure that AL dressing is removed from the cavity wound since if it is retained may leads to infection. Calcium AL dressing inhibited growth of *Staphylococcus aureus in vitro*, with a bacteriostatic property on *Pseudomonas*, *Streptococcus pyogenes*, or *Bacteroides fragilis* (Cazzaniga et al., 1992). The ALs are safe to use on infected foot ulcers, if the dressings are regularly changed. The AL dressings may have a pharmacological function due to the action of the calcium ions present in the dressing which is known to enhance wound healing. Schmidt and Turner reported that calcium AL has a role in the wound healing process and may help in the production of mouse fibroblast (Schmidt and Turner, 1986. This process was further confirmed *in vitro* by Doyle et al. (1996). They have shown that calcium AL increased proliferation of fibroblasts but not their motility. This suggests that the effects of the dressing may have been mediated by calcium ions released from the AL and therefore calcium AL may improve some cellular aspects of wound healing but not others.

7.6 BIOACTIVE WOUND DRESSINGS

The active ingredients used in wound management have revolutionized alongside the pharmaceutical agents and dressings used to deliver them. Traditional dressings commonly used to deliver drugs include plain gauze and paraffin impregnated gauze (tulle gras). The modern dressings used to deliver active agents to wounds include hydrocolloids, hydrogels, ALs, polyurethane foam/films, and silicone gels. Some of the commonly used active compounds and the dressings (and novel polymer systems) used to deliver them to wound sites are described below.

7.6.1 ANTIMICROBIAL DRESSINGS

Following surgery, patients with diabetes are at higher risk of wound infections as their immune response may be compromised (Mulder et al., 1998). Even though, detecting infection is usually based on clinician's assessment using the signs of inflammation, the response to infection may be less pronounced due to the distinct pathophysiology of diabetes. Thus, it is crucial to use antibacterial dressings in diabetic patients. These are act as covers that deliver antibacterial agents such as silver or polyhexamethylene biguanide (PHMB). Antimicrobial dressings are available as film dressings, non-adherent barriers, absorptive products, island dressings, sponges, impregnated woven gauzes, nylon fabric, or a combination of these materials where an antimicrobial agent get incorporated. These are prescribed for people with diabetes to reduce the risk of infection in partial and full-thickness wounds. A large range of antimicrobial dressings are available with various indications and it is laborious to describe all of them. A common few type of such materials are discussed as follows.

7.6.2 IODINE PREPARATIONS

Although it has been speculated that iodine delays healing and is cytotoxic, they are commonly-used in low concentration as slow release iodophors to improve healing rates and are effective as highly potent antimicrobials with a broad spectrum of activity, including antibiotic-resistant strains like Methicillin-resistant *Staphylococcus aureus* (MRSA) (Gordon, 1993). Cadexomer-iodine and povidone-iodine are the two major iodine preparations. Povidone-iodine has been used as a skin antiseptic for years, but its antimicrobial effect on wounds is under debate (Lammers et al., 1990). A randomized controlled trial of cadexomer-iodine versus saline-soaked gauze on clean foot ulcers showed no significant difference in healing between the groups (Apelqvist and Ragnarson, 1996). Despite the lack of evidence, many clinicians consider iodine preparations to be appropriate dressings for infected diabetic foot ulcers (Hilton et al., 2004).

7.6.3 SILVER-IMPREGNATED DRESSINGS

Silver has been used as a topical antimicrobial agent for acute and chronic wounds for the past few decades. The medical uses of silver include its incorporation into wound dressings, and its use as an antibacterial coating in biomaterials. Wound dressings containing silver sulfadiazine or silver nanomaterials are used to treat external infections. It has been traditionally delivered as silver nitrate or as silver sulfadiazine such as Flamazine ointment. The antimicrobial effects of silver are complex, including direct inhibition of bacterial cell respiration, inactivation of intracellular enzymes, and alterations to the cell membrane (Russell and Hugo, 1994). Silver-impregnated dressings may be suitable for use for infected diabetic foot ulcers. Examples include Acticoat and Actisorb 220. There have been no randomized controlled clinical trials of these dressings in diabetic foot ulceration. However, reports of accelerated wound reepithelialization (Olson et al, 2000) and beneficial antibacterial action in the treatment of burns (Tredget et al., 1998) are encouraging.

Recently, silver nanoparticles incorporated wound dressings have got considerable attention in wound bioburden reduction and in anti-inflammation, as they can release Ag^{+} ions at a greater rate than bulk silver, by virtue of their large surface area. If released from dressings, they also have the potential to cross biological compartments (Wilkinson et al., 2011).

7.6.4 HONEY DRESSING ON AN INFECTED DIABETIC FOOT ULCER

Honey is known to inhibit broad spectrum of bacteria ranging from Acinetobacter species to Yersinia ruckeri (Blair, 2009). It has been demonstrated in vitro that the gel of L-Mesitran Tulle is capable to successfully destroy MRSA, Extended-spectrum Beta-Lactamases (ESBL) and other antibiotic resistant bacteria (Stephen et al., 2011). This study reflected these in vitro findings in vivo with two patients infected with P. aeruginosa. In the wounds featured in this case report, debridement took place quickly, one of the key features of honey-based products (White, 2005; Molan, 2006). The stimulation of angiogenesis by honey-based products (Rossiter, 2010) is clearly demonstrated by the rapid epithelialization described in this evaluation. Emergence of resistant strains and the financial burden of modern dressings have revived honey as cost-effective dressing particularly in developing countries. Its suitability for all stages of wound healing suggests its clinical effectiveness in diabetic foot wound infections.

A study conducted on thirty infected diabetic foot wounds using honey dressing, complete healing was achieved in 43.3% of ulcers. Decrease in size and healthy granulation was observed in another 43.3% of patients. Bacterial load of all ulcers was significantly reduced after the first week of honey dressing. This study proves that commercial clover honey is a clinical and cost-effective dressing for diabetic wounds in developing countries (Moghazy, 2010).

7.6.5 GROWTH FACTOR IMPREGNATED WOUND DRESSINGS

Various strategies have been employed to encourage the healing process in acute wounds. These strategies usually involve administering a therapeutic stimulus that is reasoned to trigger a healing response (eg, growth factors, cell lines, and tissue substitutes) (Menke et al., 2007; Steed, 2003; Chen et al., 1997).

The wound healing ability of growth factors are mediated through the stimulation of angiogenesis and cellular proliferation, which leads to both the production and the degradation of the extracellular matrix and also plays a role in cell inflammation and fibroblast activity (Komarcevic, 2000). Growth factors therefore affect the inflammatory, proliferation and migratory phases of wound healing (Dijke, 1989). A variety of growth factors have been reported which participate in the process of wound healing including, epidermal growth factor (EGF), platelet derived growth factor (PDGF), fibroblast growth factor (FGF), TGF-β1, insulin-like growth factor (IGF-1), human growth hormone, and granulocyte-macrophage colony-stimulating factor (GM-CSF) (Greenhalgh, 1996). Most of these growth factors are recombinant proteins and the selection of appropriate dressing is crucial for effective release and action at the wound site. Introducing the growth factor at the right time and under the right circumstance appears to be pivotal. Vascular endothelial growth factor (VEGF) might have a capital role in conditions where vascularization is limited, as in the diabetic wound.

7.7 COLLAGEN BASED WOUND DRESSINGS IN DIABETIC WOUND MANAGEMENT

Collagen, which is produced by fibroblasts, is the most abundant protein in the human body which is involved in all three phases of the wound healing cascade. It stimulates cellular migration and contributes to new tissue development. Collagen deposition and remodelling contribute to the increased tensile strength of the wound, which is approximately 20% of normal by three weeks after injury, gradually reaching a maximum of 70% of that of normal skin (Desmouliere et al., 1995). Although epithelial structures can heal by regeneration, connective tissues cannot and depend on the process of repair mostly by the formation of collagenous scar tissue (Berry et al., 1998), predominantly of type I, which serves to restore tissue continuity, strength and function. Because of their chemotactic properties on wound fibroblasts, collagen dressings encourage the deposition and organization of newly formed collagen, creating an environment that fosters healing. Collagen-based biomaterials stimulate and recruit specific cells, such as macrophages and fibroblasts, along the healing cascade to enhance and influence wound healing. These biomaterials can provide moisture or absorption, depending on the delivery system. Collagen dressings are easy to apply and remove and are conformable. Collagen dressings are usually formulated with bovine, avian, or porcine collagen. Oxidized regenerated cellulose, a plant based material, has been combined with collagen to produce a dressing capable of binding to and protecting growth factors by binding and inactivating matrix metalloproteinases in the wound environment. The increased understanding of the biochemical processes involved in chronic wound healing allows the design of wound care products aimed at correcting imbalances in the wound microenvironment. Traditional advanced wound care products tend to address the wound's macro environment, including moist wound environment control, fluid management, and controlled transpiration of wound fluids. The newer class of biomaterials and woundhealing agents such as collagen and growth factors are targets specific defects in the chronic wound environment. *In vitro* laboratory data point to the possibility that these agents benefit the wound healing process at a biochemical level. Considerable evidence has indicated that collagen-based dressings may be capable of stimulating healing by manipulating wound biochemistry (Cynthia and Richard Simman, 2010).

A large variety of collagen dressings have been developed to encourage wound repair, especially of non-infected, chronic, and indolent skin ulcers. Along with the critical collagen functions, several other factors pertaining to poor wound healing, directly affect collagen metabolism. Diabetes forms such an extrinsic factor, in which hyperglycemia reduces normal collagen synthesis and induces non-enzymatic glycosylation of collagen and keratin, leading to formation of abnormal rigid collagen and promote tissue breakdown (Black et al., 2003).

7.7.1 ALKALINE-TREATED COLLAGEN AND ATELOCOLLAGEN GELS

Daichi et al. developed an intelligent wound dressing comprising components that encourage wound healing. Apart from conventional dressings, this is a gel-type dressing that bears basic factors needed by cells in a complex of alkaline-treated collagen and atelocollagen. One method of collagen solubilization utilizes proteases, enzymes that break the cross-links between collagen molecules, as indicated in the following figure. Collagen obtained through solubilization is called Atelocollagen. The *in vivo* study on genetically diabetic mice had shown that the collagen-gel induced the formation of granulation tissue, with wound contraction caused by migration of epidermal cells from the surrounding tissue. By day 14, wound area had decreased to 37% for the untreated side as compared to 22% on the collagen-gel side, indicating that collagen gel was associated with significantly greater wound contraction. Moreover, there were a lot of blood vessels on the collagen-gel side. Collagen-gel dressing is most effective for dry, open wounds, that is, those with minimal effusion, and it may also be effective for depressed open wounds. Collagen-gel dressing is supposed to be very useful in treating wounds such as skin defects and skin ulcers (Daichi et al., 2010).

7.7.2 CHITOSAN-CROSS LINKED COLLAGEN SPONGE

Wei Wang et al. reported a better wound-dressing to enhance diabetic wound healing using CS-cross linked collagen sponge containing recombinant human acidic FGF. Collagen cross linked with CS showed several advantages required for wound dressing, including the uniform and porous ultrastructure, less water-imbibition, small interval porosity, and high resistance to collagenase digestion and slow release of FGF from the dressing. Diabetic rats showed less body-weight gain as compared to non-diabetic rats. It suggests that FGF impregnated CS-cross linked collagen sponge is an ideal wound-dressing to improve the recovery of healing-impaired wound such as diabetic skin wound, which provides a great potential use in clinics for diabetic patients in the future (Wei Wang, et al., 2008).

7.7.3 COLLAGEN AS ACELLULAR DERMAL SKIN SUBSTITUTE

In the field of bioengineered skin substitute, collagen is proving effective for skin constructs (such as Dermagraft® and Apligraf®). Nevertheless, the compelling experimental data around the value and potential influence of collagen in the healing of stalled traumatic and surgical wounds, or 'hard-to-heal' chronic ulcers of all types, including diabetic, venous leg and pressure ulcers, clearly remains attractive for many scientific groups and manufacturers.

This product deserves special interest as it has been the subject of prolonged and in-depth research and marketing. It is a matrix dressing containing regenerated cellulose and collagen which has been shown experimentally to modulate proteases, metalloproteinases and elastase in open wounds (Cullen et al., 2002; Hart et al., 2002) by 'protecting' platelet-derived growth factor (PDGF) and other growth factors in the wound. There is also clinical trial evidence that Promogran may be able to handle exudate and accelerate healing in venous and diabetic ulcers (Vin et al., 2002; Veves et al., 2002), but the clinical significance of this is open to doubt (Cullen et al, 2002b). There is a plethora of case reports and small patient series, which are supportive, but these have a high risk of publication bias.

7.7.4 PROTEASE ABSORBENT COLLAGEN DRESSING

Impaired wound healing and non-healing ulceration in diabetes might be due to high levels of matrix metalloproteases (MMPs) which contribute to wound chronicity. The local treatment with a protease inhibitor has a beneficial effect on wound healing. Thus, the topical use of protease inhibitors might influence wound healing and promote transition from a chronic to an acute wound. Application of protease inhibitory modulating matrix (the OCR/collagen Promogran matrix, Ethicon) which is incorporated in wound dressings. Even though there was not much difference between mRNA levels of MMPs as well as of IL-1β and TNF-α in both treated and untreated. In addition, MMP levels in wound tissue (analyzed by ELISA) were also not significantly different between both groups. However, IL-1β was increased on 8th day in the treatment group ($P = .01$) only. Interestingly, a significant reduction of the MMP-9/TIMP-2 ratio in the group is being treated with the ORC/collagen. These wounds exhibited a more rapid healing rate when treated with the ORC/collagen matrix (Ralf et al., 2006).

7.8 SMART WOUND DRESSINGS FOR DIABETIC WOUNDS

The future of diabetic wound healing lies in the exploitation of more effective artificial "smart" matrix skin substitutes. A smart biomaterial is just like a smart boy or girl who is able to manage the things very well in accordance with the circumstances. Thus, it should be able to behave in accordance with the circumstances and manage the critical situations without the effort of an external influence.

Similarly a smart wound dressing should be able to manage the following strategies:

- Able to absorb excess exudate whenever it is formed on the wound bed
- Able to give optimum aeration and moisture to promote healing
- Able to deliver wound healing agents in a controlled manner
- Able to deliver antimicrobial agent at the time of infection

These smart matrices can release a number of growth factors, cytokines, and bioactive peptide fragments in a temporally and spatially specific, event-driven manner. The controlled and focal release of these agents should enhance optimal tissue regeneration and repair of full-thickness wounds. Development of these kinds of therapies will require multidisciplinary translational research teams (Sweitzer et al., 2006). Further, it also should have all optimal features of a standard wound dressing material like ability to maintain a moist environment at the wound/dressing interface, remove excess exudate, have thermal insulation properties, allow gaseous exchange, be impermeable to bacteria, in and out of the wound environment, be free of particles and toxic wound contaminants, permit trauma, and facilitate pain-free removal (Dealey, 1993).

7.8.1 SMART EXUDATE MANAGEMENT

A new wound dressing material marketed under the trade name, TheraGauze™, which is designed to either release or absorb moisture based on conditions at the wound's surface. This product represents a new class of smart dressings which are capable of dynamically adapting to existing conditions at the wound surface and to different needs across the wound surface. TheraGauze™ consists of a proprietary inert polymer which is integrated into a non-woven polyester/rayon substrate. During the manufacturing process, release of alcohol in a specially controlled environment creates a vertically oriented matrix of hundreds of thousands of microscopic channels that decrease in a fractal pattern and are bordered by millions of vertically oriented polymer chains. A randomized clinical trial designed to compare treatment of foot ulcers in patients with diabetes to compare with that of saline wet to dry dressings and the preliminary results are extremely positive in favor of the use of TheraGauze™ to heal wounds (Adam Landsman, 2013).

7.8.2 SMART ANTIMICROBIAL DRESSING

A considerable effort has been made to make the wound dressings with the ability to fight against the pathogenic bacteria entering in the wound bed by incorporating antibacterial agents. This may be antibiotics and chemicals like silver nitrate or iodine. Jenkins and his colleagues from the Department of Chemistry at the University of Bath have shown that pathogenic bacteria can be used as the agents of their own destruction by releasing toxins that rupture nanocapsules containing an antimicrobial agent. It has been already demonstrated that this simple vesicle system can be used as a 'nano-Trojan horse' for controlling bacterial growth and infection. These nanocapsules can be integrated into wound dressings, which will automatically detect pathogenic bacteria and respond to this by releasing an antibiotic into the wound, and changing color to alert medical staff. The work attempts to engineer a 'smart' wound dressing material that only releases an encapsulated antimicrobial agent in the presence of pathogenic bacteria, without responding to harmless bacteria. A schematic representation of this material is given in Figure 3. The use of certain specific toxins or enzymes produced by the pathogenic bacteria, the property that makes some bacteria pathogenic by presenting them with capsules which bacterial toxins attack. Inside the capsules is an antimicrobial or a dye which will destroy the bacteria or act as cues for the detection of infection (Jin et al., 2010).

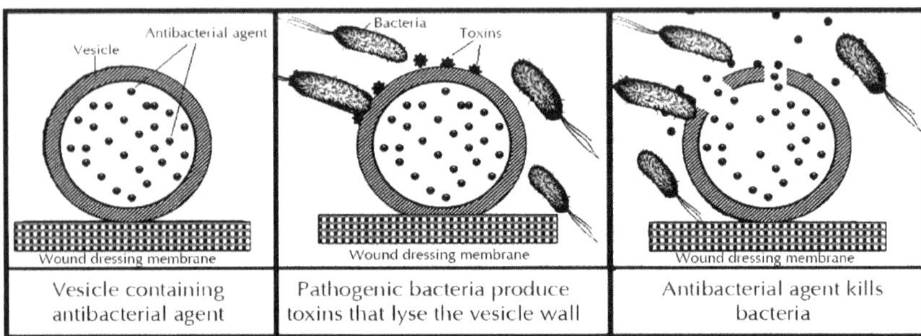

FIGURE 3 Schematic diagram of responsive antimicrobial system (Giant Unilamellar Vesicle (GUV)) with encapsulated antimicrobial. Toxins secreted by pathogenic bacteria lyse the vesicle and release the antimicrobial agent, eventually destroys the pathogenic bacteria (Adapted from Jin et al., 2010.).

The researchers have demonstrated the effectiveness of their system for two pathogenic species of bacteria, *P. aeruginosa* and *S. aureus*. A non-pathogenic strain of *E. coli*, which does not secrete toxins or membrane lysing agents, was used as a control system.

In another study by Victoria et al., a microgel based smart wound dressings for the controlled delivery of antimicrobial drugs by utilizing pH as a stimulus has been proposed. In commercially available hydrogel/gauze wound dressings, the gel swells to adsorb wound exudates and provide an efficient non adhesive particle barrier. Colloidal gel particles termed as microgels, as a result of their very high surface area to volume ratio compared to bulk gels, they have a much faster response to external stimuli such as temperature or pH. In response to either an increase or decrease in solvent quality these porous networks shrink and swell reversibly. When swollen the interstitial regions within the polymer matrix are available for further chemistry; such as the incorporation of small molecules. The reversible shrinking and swelling as a function of external stimuli provides a novel drug release system. As the environmental conditions of a wound change over its lifetime, tending to increase in pH if there is an infection combining these discrete polymeric particles with a substrate such as cotton, results in a smart wound dressing (Victoria et al, 2006).

7.8.3 SMART WOUND DRESSING TO CONTROL MOISTURE AND REDUCE PAIN

Controlling moisture content is a critical challenge in wound healing. Dry and desiccated wounds rapidly lead to necrosis and diminished angiogenesis. Conversely, wounds which are too moist will show localized maceration, which leads to separation of dermal layers and increases the risk of skin slough and infection. The problem most commonly encountered when trying to control fluid content is that every wound requires a different amount of moisture control. Ideally, a dressing that continually adapts to existing conditions would be able to provide optimal moisture content to enhance healing.

A smart wound dressing marketed under the trade name TheraGauze™ which utilizes the Skin Moisture Rebalancing Technology (SMRT) polymer to regulate moisture so precisely, it finds its application potential in diabetic wound care. TheraGauze™ consists of an inert polymer which is integrated into a non-woven polyester/rayon substrate. During the manufacturing process, release of alcohol in a specially controlled environment creates a vertically oriented matrix of hundreds of thousands of microscopic channels that decrease in a fractal pattern and are bordered by millions of vertically oriented polymer chains. A materials analysis of this dressing has characterized the, TheraGauze™ polymer as "biomimetic", a man-made substance that simulates a natural process exudate management. This structure enables TheraGauze™ to dynamically absorb or release fluid differentially across the wound surface. Although, the polymer itself is very good at regulating moisture over small areas, there needs to be a more coordinated mechanism to add or remove fluid from the area, once the contact areas have filled (or emptied). This is where the "canals" separating the polymer chains come in. This network works like a capillary bed, dividing up into finer and finer extensions, in order to move fluid into the dressing. This coordinated movement of fluid allows the surface moisture content to be maintained perfectly, while managing the ingress and egress of larger volumes of fluid just off the wound surface.

In its current formulation, the SMRT TheraGauze™ polymer is also hydrated with propylene glycol (PG).

A randomized, multicenter study conducted by Landsman et al, examined outcomes from treatment of diabetic foot ulcers with TheraGauze and TheraGauze in conjunction with becaplermin (brand name Regranex), a recombinant "PDGE-BB" available as a topical gel used for diabetic foot ulcers. They have also compared these outcomes with data from the literature that used saline-moistened gauze and becaplermin. Wounds in which moisture content was regulated with TheraGauze showed more rapid change in wound area and a higher percentage of wounds closure at 12 and 20 weeks regardless of whether becaplermin was used (Landsman, 2010).

A boot-like dressing, the Kerraboot® dressing maintains a moist, humid environment, which is optimal for wound healing (http://www.rnao.org, 2005). Exudate, or discharge, that remains on a wound can delay healing. The Kerraboot allows exudate to drain away from the wound and into the absorbent pad, where it forms a soft, conformable gel at the base of the boot. Kerraboot also reduces wound odour. Some wounds may require daily boot changes, while others may be changed less frequently, depending on the amount of exudate. Kerraboot may reduce nursing staff time for wound care and enable patients to change their own dressings at home. Dressing changes are also less painful, as the wounds are not covered by contact dressings (Harvey et al., 2005). A randomized controlled trial compared 14 adult participants who received Kerraboot with 16 participants who received a hydrocellular foam dressing (Allevyn®) for the treatment of diabetic foot ulcers confirmed rate of wound healing is almost the same (Edmonds et al., 2006).

7.9 NEGATIVE PRESSURE WOUND THERAPY (NPWT)

The NPWT is one of the oldest forms of medicinal therapy using a vacuum dressing to promote healing in acute or chronic wounds. The NPWT has been a proven technology for non-healing wounds. Clinical studies have proven its effectiveness for a variety of acute and chronic wounds (Graeme and Jagdeep, 2012). The therapy involves the controlled application of sub-atmospheric pressure to the local wound environment, using a sealed wound dressing connected to a vacuum pump. For the past decade there has been a substantial increase in the use of NPWT and today it offer clinicians with an important choice for the proper management of acute wounds and chronic. Presently, negative pressure wound NPWT is extensively used for the treatment of several types of wounds. Patients with diabetes frequently develop foot ulcers due to atherosclerosis that blocks blood flow to the extremities and peripheral neuropathy that prevents the sensation of discomfort due to the mechanical stress on or injury to the feet. These complications of diabetes increase the chance of induction of ulcers on pressure-bearing regions of the feet. There are five mechanisms by which the application of negative pressure to a wound may aid in the healing process:

- Stimulation of granulation tissue formation,
- Continuous removal of exudate,
- Continuous wound cleansing after adequate primary surgical debridement,

- Wound retraction and
- Reduction of interstitial edema.

There are a few clinical evidences to support the application of these kinds of dressings in foot wounds in patients with diabetes. Armstrong et al. investigated to find out whether NPWT improves the proportion and rate of wound healing after partial foot amputation in patients with diabetes. The assigned 162 patients into 16 weeks, 18 centres, randomized clinical trial in the USA. More patients healed in the NPWT group than in the control group. The rate of wound healing, based on the time to complete closure, was faster in the NPWT group than in controls. The rate of granulation tissue formation, based on the time to 76–100% formation in the wound bed, was faster in the NPWT group than in controls (Armstrong et al., 2005).

Gustavo et al. carried out randomized controlled trial in diabetic patients with a foot amputation wound to treatment with NPWT or standard wound dressing to evaluate the efficacy of NPWT compared with standard wound dressing to heal diabetic foot amputation wounds. The NPWT was prepared with a polyurethane ether foam dressing, a Nelaton catheter, a transparent adhesive drape and continuous negative pressure of 100 mm Hg. The wound was treated every 48–72 hr and evaluated weekly. The average time to reach 90% of granulation was lower in NPWT group than the control group. They have shown that, NPWT reduces the granulation time of diabetic foot amputation wounds by 40%, compared with the standard wound dressing (Gustavo et al., 2009).

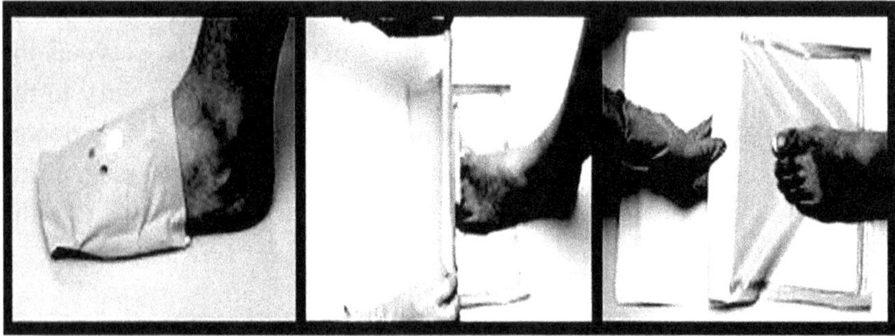

FIGURE 4 Application of Kalypto Forefoot wound dressing (http://www.diamondrx.com).

7.10 FOOT WOUND DRESSINGS (DIABETIC FOOT WOUNDS, TOE WOUNDS)

The Kalypto Forefoot wound dressing is ideal for hard to treat wounds on the foot. The Kalypto foot wound dressing is designed for the forefoot (toe area). It creates an envelope type wound dressing which the front of the foot is placed. The dressing can be concealed in a large sock, or wrapped with an ace-bandage type material. Kalypto negative pressure wound dressing is easy to use and patients prefer it. From the patient's perspective, they are not required to carry a heavy wound pump with them. The Kalypto wound vacuum eliminates that issue as there is no collection canister. (http://www.diamondrx.com/foot-wound-dressing accessed on 11-01-2013)

7.11 CONCLUSION

Diabetes retards the wound healing process and makes it more complicated. Like other wounds diabetic wound also should be covered with materials that alleviate symptoms, provide wound protection, encourage healing, reduce wound dehydration and offer proper aeration. Apart from these there should be a special consideration about the devastations associated with diabetic wounds. The AL, collagen or other conventional wound dressings also have multifunctional role in diabetic wound management. Controlling moisture content is a critical challenge in wound healing. Thus smart wound dressings that can manage excess wound exudates successfully are the preferred candidates for chronic diabetic wounds. Hydrocolloids, hydrogels, foams, and ALs are extensively used in wound dressings due to their excellent exudate management capacity. To reduce the load of pathogens in the diabetic wound bed, smart antimicrobial dressings are also in the translational research. Negative pressure wound therapy has been a proven technology for non-healing diabetic wounds. Tissue engineering is a fascinating technology which provides new options for wound management by the use of skin substitutes for healing chronic wounds. The use of gene therapy in wound healing by regulating the expression of key molecules like growth factors is the future perspective yet to be exploited. Even though there are many factors that determine the choice of a wound dressing for a diabetic wound, current decisions on choice of wound dressing is mostly based on dressing costs and selecting the most useful management properties offered like management of wound exudates. Finally, a rationalized evidence-based approach should be implemented to wound care and dressing selection to effectively manage chronic and acute diabetic wounds.

KEYWORDS

- **Active wound dressing (AWD)**
- **Diabetes**
- **Texas System**
- **Wagner System**
- **Wound healing**

REFERENCES

1. Adam, Landsman. A New "Smart" Wound Dressing to Control Moisture Content and Reduce Pain. Technical report, http://www.solublesystems.com/files/PDF/Ther-aGauze_Whitepaper.pdf, accessed on 21/01/2013.
2. Andreia, V. and Artur, C. P. *Appl Microbiol Biotechnol*, **90**, 445–460 (2011).
3. Apelqvist, J. *Acta Derm Venereol*, **76**, 231–235 (1996).
4. Armstrong, D. G. and Lavery, L. A. Diabetic Foot Study Consortium. *Lancet.*, **12**, **366**(9498), 1704–1710 (2005).
5. Armstrong, D. G., Lavery, L. A., and Harkless, L. B. *Diabetes Care.*, **21**, 855–859 (1998).
6. Baumgartner-Parzer, S. M. *Diabetes.*, **44**(11), 1323–1327 (1995).
7. Bellingan, G. J. *J. Immunol.*, **157**(6), 2577–2585 (1996).
8. Black, E. *Arch. Surg.*, **138**(1), 34–40 (2003).
9. Blair, S. *Antibacterial activity of honey*. In: Rose Cooper, Peter Molan and Richard White (Eds). Honey in Modern Wound Management Wounds UK, London (2009).
10. Boulton, A. J., Vileikyte, L., Ragnarson-Tennvall, G., and Apelqvist, J. *Lancet.*, **366**, 1719–1724 (2005).
11. Brem, H. and Tomic-Canic M. *J. Clin. Invest.*, **117**, 1219–1222 (2007).
12. Bulgrin, J. P. *Wounds.*, **7**, 48–57 (1995).

13. Carolina, W. and Geoff, S. *J. Pharma Practice Research*, **36**(4) (2006).
14. Carver, N. and Leigh, I. M. *Int. J. Dermatol.*, **31**, 10–18 (1992).
15. Carville, K. General principles of wound management. In: *The care of wounds*: a guide for nurses. Oxford: Black well Science,pp. 49–67 (1999).
16. Cazzaniga, A. L., Masrshall, D. A., and Mertz, P. M. Proceedings of the 5th annual Symposium on Advanced Wound Care (New Orleans). *The effect of calcium alginate dressing on the multiplication of bacterial pathogens in vitro*, p. 139 (1992).
17. Chen, S. M., Ward, S. I., Olutoye, O. O., Diegelmann, R. F., Kelman, C. I. *Wound Repair Regen.*, **5**, 23–32 (1997).
18. Choucair, M. and Phillips, T. *Wounds.*, **8**(5), 165–172 (1996). *Cirugía Española (English Edition)*, **86**(3), 171–177 (2009).
19. Cynthia, A. F. and Richard, S. *The Journal of the American College of Certified Wound Specialists*, **2**(3), 50–54 (September 2010).
20. Daichi, C., Tetsushi, T., Hiroyuki, K., Hisako, H., Hisako, F., Hideyuki, S., Hideto, S., Yoshiyuki, M., Ichiro, S., Mitsuyoshi, I., and Tsuyoshi, T. *Sian J Oral Maxillofac Surg.*, **22** (2), 61–67 (2010).
21. Darby, I. A. *Int. J. Biochem. Cell Biol.*, **29**(1), 191–200 (1997).
22. Davidson, J. Growth factors and extracellular matrix in wound repair. In J. McCulloch and L. Kloth (eds). *Wound Healing Evidence-Based Management*. 4th ed.: F. A. Davis (Ed.), pp. Philadelphia, PA 35–43 (2010).
23. Debra, J. B. and Cheri, O. *Wound healing: Technological innovations and market overview*. 2:1–185 (1998).
24. Dijke, P. and Iwata, K. K. *Biotechnology*, **7**, 793–798 (1989).
25. Doshi, J. and Reneker, D. H. *J. Electrostatic.*, **35**, 151 (1995).
26. Doughty, D. B. Principles of wound healing and wound management. In R. A. Bryant (ed). *Acute and Chronic Wounds: Nursing Management*. St. Louis, MO: Mosby, 31–68 (1992).
27. Doughty, D. B. Saxe Healthcare Communication 2010, **4**(3), 1, 5–7.
28. Doyle, J. W., Roth, T., and Smith M. *J Biomed Mater Res*, **32**, 561–568.
29. Dumville, J. C., Deshpande, S., O'Meara, S., and Speak, K. *Cochrane Database Syst. Rev.*, 9. Art. No.: CD009111. DOI: 10.1002/14651858.CD009111.pub2 (2011).
30. Eaglstein, W. H. and Falanga, V. *Surg. Clin. N. Am.*, **77**, 689–700 (1997).
31. Edmonds, M., Foster, A., Jemmott, T., Kerr, D., Malik, R., Knowles, A., Jude, E., Chadwick, P., Rahaman, L, and Murray, N. *Wounds UK*, **2**(1), 25–30 (2006).
32. Falabella, A. F. *Dermatol Ther.*, **19**, 317–325 (2006).
33. Falanga, V. and Kirsner, R. S. *J. Cell Physiol.*, **154**, 506–510 (1993).
34. Falanga, V., Martin, T. A., Takagi, H., Kirsner R. S., Helfman, T., Pardes, J., Ochoa, M. S. *J. Cell Physiol.*, **157**, 408–412 (1993).
35. Fisken, R. A., Digby, M. *J. Br. Podiatr. Med.*, **52**, 20–22 (1997).
36. Formhals A. US patent, 1975504 (1934).
37. Gallagher, K. A., Liu, Z. J., Xiao, M., Chen, H., Goldstein, L. J., Buerk, D. G., Nedeau, A., Thom, S. R., and Velazquez, O. C. *J. Clin. Invest.*, **117**, 1249–1259 (2007).
38. Gill, D. *J Wound Care*, **8**(4), 204–206 (1999).
39. Gordillo, G. M. and Sen, C. K. *Am. J. Surg.*, **186**, 259–263 (2003).
40. Gordon, J. *Postgrad Med J*, **69**(Suppl 3), 106–16 (1993).

41. Graeme, E. G. and Jagdeep, N. *J. Plastic, Reconstructive & Aesthetic Surgery*, **65**(8), 989–1001 (2012).
42. Greenhalgh, D. G. *Clin. Plast. Surg.*, **30**(1), 37–45 (2003).
43. Greenhalgh, D. G. *J Trauma. Inj Infect Crit Care*, **41**, 159–167 (1996).
44. Gustavo, S., Manuel, E., Mauricio, M., Edgardo, S., José, I. F., Oliva, C., Sanhueza, A., Manuel, V., and Carlos, M. *Cir Esp.*, **86**(3), 171–177 (2009).
45. Haimowitz, J. E. and Margolis, D. J. Moist wound healing. In D. Krasner and D. Kane (eds). Chronic Wound Care, In A Clinical Source Book for Healthcare Professionals, Second Edition, Health Management Publications, Inc., Wayne PA, pp. 49–56 (1997).
46. Harvey, D. *Br J Community Nurse*, **11**(6), S28–S30 (2006).
47. Heenan, A. *World Wide Wounds.*, **1**, 1–7 (1998).
48. Hehenberger, K. *Wound Repair Regen.*, **6**(2), 135–141 (1998).
49. Waugh, H. V. and Sherratt, J. A. *B. Math. Biol.*, **68**, 197–207 (2006).
50. Higgins, K. R. and Ashry, H. R. *Clin. Podiatr. Med. Surg.*, **12**, 31–40 (1995).
51. Hilton, J. R., Williams, D. T., Beuker, B., Miller, D. R. and Harding, K. G. *Clin. Infect. Dis.*, **39**, S100–S103 (2004).
52. Hinman, C. D and Maibach, H. *Nature*, **200**, 377–378 (1963).
53. Ian, A. D., Teresa, B., Tim, D. H., and Donald, G. M. *Int. J. Biochem. Cell Biol.*, **29**(1), 191–200 (1997).
54. Jin, Z., Andrew, L. L., Geraldine, M., and Toby, A. J. A. *J. AM. CHEM. SOC.*, **132**, 6566–6570 (2010).
55. Jones, V. *Diabetic Foot.*, **1**, 48–52 (1998).
56. Joshua, S. B., Kerr, H. M., Howard, N. E. S., and Gillian, M. E. *J Pharm Sci*, **97**(8), 2892–2923 (2008).
57. Katarzyna, S. T., Magdalena, C., Anna, K., and Jan, S. *J Am Acad Dermatol*, **68**(4), e117–e126 (2013).
58. Komarcevic A. *Med Pregl*, **53**, 363–368 (2000).
59. Lammers, R. L., Foume, M., and Callahan, M. L. *Ann Emerg Med*, **19**, 709–714 (1990).
60. Landsman, A, Agnew, P., Parish, L., Joseph, R., and Galiano, R. D. *J Am Podiatr Med Assoc*, **100**(3), 155–160 (2010).
61. Lerman, O. *Am J Pathol*, **162**(1), 303–312 (2003).
62. Liane, I. F. M., Ana M. A. D., Eugénia, C., and Hermínio, C. deSousa. *Acta Biomater*, http:/ /dx.doi.org /10.1016/ j.actbio.2013.0 3.033 (2013).
63. Loots, M. A. *J Invest Dermatol*, **111**(5), 850–857 (1998).
64. Lorenzi, M., Cagliero, E., and Toledo, S. *Diabetes*, **34**(7), 621–627 (1985).
65. Majno, G. *The Healing Hand: Man and Wound in the Ancient World.* Harvard University Press, Cambridge (1975).
66. McCulloch D. Proceedings of 2nd European Conference on Advances in Wound Management. London: MacMillan; 1993. *An investigation into the effects of Intrasite Gel on the in-vitro proliferation of aerobic and anaerobic bacteria* [poster]; p. 207.
67. Meaume, S., Senet, P., Dumas, R., Carsin, H., Pannier, M., and Bohbot, S. *British Journal of Nursing*, **11**(16), (2002).
68. Menke, N. B., Ward, K. R., Witten, T. M., Bonchev, D. G., and Diegelmann, R. F. *Clin Dermatol*, **25**, 19–25 (2007).

69. Modarressi, A., Pietramaggiori, G., Godbout, C., Vigato, E., Pittet, B., and Hinz, B. *J Invest. Dermatol*, **130**, 2818–2827 (2010).
70. Moghazy A. M., Shams, M. E., Adly, O. A., Abbas, A. H., El-Badawy, M. A., El-sakka, D. M., Hassan, S. A., Abdelmohsen, W. S., Ali, O. S., and Mohamed B. A. *Diabetes Research and Clinical Practice*, **89**(3), 276–281 (2010).
71. Molan, P. *Int J Low Extrem Wounds*, **5**(1), 40–54 (2006).
72. Morgan, D. A. *Hosp Pharmacist*, **9**, 261–266 (2002).
73. Mulder, G. D. Clinician's Pocket Guide to Chronic Wound Repair. In *Wound Care Communications, Network*, 4th edn. Springhouse Corp., Springhouse, PA,. pp. 58–67 (1998).
74. National Pressure Ulcer Advisory Panel and European Pressure Ulcer Advisory Panel. Prevention and Treatment of pressure ulcers: *Clinical practice guideline*. Washington, DC: National Pressure Ulcer Advisory Panel; (2009)
75. Okan, D., Woo, K., Ayello, E. A., and Sibbald, R. G. *Adv. Skin Wound Care*, **20**, 39–53 (2007).
76. Olson, M. E., Wright, J. B., Lam, K., and Burrell, R. E. *Eur J Surg*, **166**, 486–489 (2000).
77. Ovington, L. Dressings and skin substitutes. In J. McCulloch, L. Kloth (Eds.) *Wound Healing Evidence-Based Management*. 4th ed. Philadelphia, PA: FA Davis; 180–93 (2010).
78. Queen, D., Orsted, H., Sanada, H., and Sussman, G. *Int Wound J.*, **1**, 59–77 (2004).
79. Ralf, L., Carola, Z., Markus, M., Kirsten, R., and Hendrik, L. *J. Diabetes and its Complications*, **20**(5), 329–335 (2006).
80. Robson, M. C., Steed, D. L., and Franz, M. G. *Curr Probl Surg*, **38**(2), 65–140 (2001).
81. Rodeheaver, G. Wound cleansing, wound irrigation, wound disinfection. In D. Krasner, G. Rodeheaver, R. G. Sibbald, (Eds.) *Chronic Wound Care: A Clinical Source Book for Health Care Professionals*. 4th ed. Malvern, PA: HMP Communication; (2007).
82. Russell, A. D, and Hugo, W. B. *Prog. Med Chem*, **31**, 351–370 (1994).
83. Sank, A. *J. Surg Res*, **57**(6), 647–653 (1994).
89. Schmidt, R. J., and Turner, T. D. *Pharm J*, **236**, 578 (1986).
90. Schultz, G. S., Sibbald, R. G., Falanga, V., and Stacey, M. *Wound Repair Regen*, **11** (suppl.1), S1-S28 (2003).
91. Seaman, S. *J. Am Pod Assoc*, **92**, 24–33 (2002).
92. Sharon, B. and Elizabeth, A. A. *The Journal for Prevention and Healing*, **25**(2), 87–92 (2012).
93. Shukla, A. *Biochem Biophys Res Commun*, **244**(2), 434–439 (1998).
94. Singer, A. J. and Clark, R. A. F. *N. Engl J Med*, **341**(10), 738–746 (1999).
95. Steed, D. L. *Surg Clin North Am*, **83**, 547–555 (2003).
96. Stephen, H. J. and Callaghan, R. *Wounds UK*, **7**(1), 54–57 (2011).
97. Sweitzer, S. M., Fann, S. A., Borg, T. K., Baynes, J. W., Yost, M. J *Diabetes Educ*, **32**(2), 197–210 (2006).
98. Thomas, S. *Wound Management and Dressing*. Pharmaceutical Press: London (1990).
99. Tredget, E. E., Shankowsky, H. A., Groeneveld, A., and Burrell, R. *J Burn Care Rehabil*, **19**, 531–537 (1998).

100. Turner, T. D. The development of wound management products. In D. Krasner and D. Kane (eds). *Chronic Wound Care*: A Clinical Source Book for Healthcare Professionals, Second Edition. Health Management Publications, Inc., Wayne, PA, 124–38 (1997).
101. Victoria, J. C., Natasa, M., Martin J. S., John C. M., and Bojana V. Proc. SPIE 6413, Smart Materials IV, 64130X, December 22, 2006, doi:10.1117/12.712573
102. Wagner, F. W. Jr. *Orthopedics.*, **10**(1), 163–172 (1987).
103. Wei, W., Shaoqiang, L., Yechen, X., Yadong, H., Yi, T., Lu, C., Xiaokun L. *Life Sciences*, **82**(3–4), 190–204 (2008).
104. Wetzler, C. *J Invest Dermatol*, **115**(2), 245–253 (2000).
105. White, R. *Nurs Stand*, **20**(10), 57–64 (2005).
106. Wilkinson, L. J., White, R. J., Chipman, J. K. *J. Wound Care*, **20**(11), 543–549 (2011).
107. Winter, G. D. *Nature*, **193**, 293–294 (1962).
108. Yen, H. L., Jung, J. C., Ming C. Y., Chiang T. C, and Wen F. L. *Carbohyd Polym.*, **88**(3), 809–819 (2012).
109. Zykova, S. N. *Diabetes*. **49**(9), 1451–1458 (2000).

CHAPTER 8

RECENT ADVANCES IN DIABETIC FOOT CARE: THE ROLE OF FOOTWEAR AND ORTHOSIS

G. SARASWATHY, GAUTHAM GOPALAKRISHNA, B. N. DAS, and VIJAY VISWANATHAN

CONTENTS

ABSTRACT

Therapeutic footwear has proved for decades as one of the important therapeutic interventions for diabetic foot ulcer. The primary goal of therapeutic footwear is to protect and prevent the foot from the complications, such as calluses and diabetic foot ulcers or even amputations for patients with diabetes. The proper design and customization of therapeutic footwear based on subject's as well as physician's needs is important to increase the patient's compliance of using the therapeutic footwear. The aim of our research is to improve the design and materials of customized therapeutic footwear for patients with diabetes.

The quality function deployment (QFD), which is a quantitative tool that aims at giving, the top most priority to the needs/requirements of the customers into the process of product development, that was used to identify the requirements for therapeutic footwear from patients, doctors, and technicians points of view. The qualitative data used in this study was obtained through anecdotal evidence from groups of patients using therapeutic footwear, doctors prescribing therapeutic footwear, footwear technicians, and related field experts through a range of interviews and surveys. This helped in the identification of the requirements to be used as a reference in the customization of therapeutic footwear for patients with diabetes as well as features that are required to be designed to develop customized therapeutic footwear. By using the QFD method, the user needs are mapped out and integrated in the total product development process. By concentrating on these technical areas, it is therefore expected to increase the satisfaction of patients with diabetes among the users of therapeutic footwear. Also integration of Teoriya Resheniya Izobretatelskikh Zadatch (TRIZ) (Theory of the Solution of Inventive Problems) into QFD helped in obtaining the solution for the negative relationship that is likely to affect the product development process in near future.

The results from QFD analysis revealed that 'Entire material' and attribute, 'density' were most important for meeting the demands of the users. The other important product characteristics were design and porosity. Insole in therapeutic footwear is playing an important role in pressure distribution and offloading at risk areas of ulcer development in diabetic foot. Therefore, density and porosity of materials used as insole and design of insole and midsole were taken as priority area of our research. Types of polyurethane based porous viscoelastic materials were developed and analyzed for application as cushion insole in therapeutic footwear for patients with diabetes. The results of physicomechanical and patient's trial tests were encouraging. Further, new design of therapeutic footwear for low risk category patients and orthosis for high risk category patients were designed and fabricated exclusively for patients with diabetes. The details of advances in design and materials for therapeutic footwear and orthosis for patients with diabetes were discussed in this chapter.

8.1 INTRODUCTION

8.1.1 FOOT COMPLICATIONS OF DIABETES MELLITUS

Regardless of the type of diabetes long duration of diabetes, and failure to achieve optimal glycemic control can cause damage to the body's small and large blood vessels and nerves. Damage to these vessels and nerves can affect all organs in the body: however, the eyes, heart, kidneys, and skin are most commonly affected in patients with diabetes. Early manifestations of diabetes may present initially in the foot. Neuropathy, lesions, ulceration, and amputation are common complications of diabetes involving foot.

PERIPHERAL NEUROPATHY

The most common type of peripheral neuropathy damages are the nerves of the limbs, especially the feet. Nerves on both sides of the body are affected. Common symptoms of peripheral neuropathy are:

- Numbness or insensitivity to pain or temperature
- Tingling, burning, or prickling
- Sharp pains or cramps
- Extreme sensitivity to touch, even light touch
- Loss of balance and coordination.

These symptoms are often worse at night. The damage to nerves often results in loss of reflexes and muscle weakness (Llewelyn, 1998). Due to muscle weakness, the foot often becomes wider and shorter, the gait (walking pattern) and distribution pattern of load (stress) from body weight while walking and running also changes, and foot ulcers appear as pressure is put on parts of the foot that are less protected. In cases of peripheral neuropathy a small inconspicuous break in the skin can become a portal of entry for bacteria (Armstrong, 1996). Because of the loss of sensation, injuries may go unnoticed and often become infected. If ulcers or foot injuries are not treated in time, the infection may involve the bone and require amputation (Levin, 1993; Reiber, 2001) "to protect rest of the foot or limb".

PERIPHERAL ARTERIAL DISEASE (PAD)

The PAD is a condition characterized by atherosclerotic occlusive disease of the lower extremities. It is a major risk factor for lower extremity amputation in patients with diabetes. The abnormal metabolic state accompanying diabetes results changes in the state of arterial structure and function. The initial assessment of PAD in patients with diabetes will begin with a thorough medical history and physical examination to help identify those patients with PAD risk factors, symptoms of claudication, rest pain, and functional impairment. The PAD is one of the risk factor for diabetic foot ulcer occurrence and recurrence (Dubsky, 2012).

DIABETIC FOOT ULCER

The diabetic foot ulcers are the major cause of hospitalization of patients with diabetes (Ghanassia, 2008). Foot ulcers and their subsequent complications are an important cause of morbidity and mortality in patients with diabetes. Annual incidence of foot ulcers is 1% to 4% and prevalence 5% to 10% in patients with diabetes. About 50% of non-traumatic lower limb amputations are due to diabetes. These patients have a high mortality following amputation, ranging from 39% to 80% at 5 year (Moulik, 2003). Once ulcerated, the areas heal with scar tissue that is less vascular and less elastic than the native tissue thus, reulceration at the same site is very common among patients with diabetes and therefore, prevention of ulcerations is essential.

According to the patient's diabetic foot disease status and risk of developing foot ulcers, they can be classified into diabetic foot category. Table 1 shows the disease symptoms for foot ulcers and appropriate recommended treatments for each category. The category is determined by the progress of complications of peripheral neuropathy, PAD, presence and conditions of foot ulcer, history of foot ulcer, and presence of foot deformity.

TABLE 1 Classification of patients with diabetes by risk for developing diabetic foot ulcers

Diabetic foot risk category	Symptoms	Treatments
0	Diabetes mellitus Protective sensation intact Good vascular status No history of previous ulcers	Diabetic education; Correctly fitting and cushioned off the shelf footwear.
1	Diabetes mellitus Loss of protective sensation No history of previous ulcers No evidence of foot deformity present	Diabetic education; Appropriate/ therapeutic footwear.
2	Diabetes mellitus Neuropathy (insensate foot) with apparent foot deformity No previous history of neuropathic ulceration or Charcot joints.	Diabetic education; Appropriate/ therapeutic footwear.
3	Diabetes mellitus Neuropathy (insensate foot) with apparent foot deformity History of pathology including ulceration and / or Charcot joints.	Diabetic education and regular usage of custom made/ prescribed footwear to reduce the risk of recurrence of ulcerations.

TABLE 1 *(Continued)*

4	Insensate injury, that is a neuropathic ulcer, or an acute Charcot's joint. The ankle-brachial index of >0.80 mm Hg is shown, and foot deformity is usually present.	Routine debridement of callous / ulcer to healthy tissue, as well as routine dressings (daily) and irrigation of lesion with saline. Pressure offloading at ulcer site with Ankle foot orthosis or customized therapeutic footwear.
5	Patient with an infected diabetic foot may or may not have intact protective sensation, and an infected lesion is present. Charcot's joint may be evident.	Limb threatening infections should be debrided and sepsis controlled. Antibiotics may be prescribed to aid healing of lesion. Pressure offloading at ulcer site with orthotics.
6	Dysvascular foot. Patients may or may not have intact protective sensation. A non-infected ulcer may or may not be present.	Vascular consultation with the surgeon is considered for possible revascularisation. If the foot is infected antibiotic treatment is proposed. Customized and Prescription footwear for regular use.

LOWER EXTREMITY AMPUTATION (LEA)

The plantar neuropathic ulcer is the condition that most commonly leads to amputation (Sumpio, 2000). Moreover, the risk of amputation increases 10-fold in patients with diabetes and concurrent end-stage renal disease (Eggers, 1999). In industrialized countries, diabetes is the leading cause of non-traumatic and LEAs (ADA, 1999; Foundation for accountability, 1996). According to 1997, hospital discharge data, diabetes accounted for approximately 87,720 LEAs in the United States, representing 67% of all LEAs (CDC, 2001). The LEA rate was highest among men, non-Hispanics/Latinos, African, Americans, and the elderly. Eighty five persent of LEAs are preceded by a foot ulceration that provides a portal for infection (Armstrong, 1998; Reiber, 1995). From these, 14% to 24% will proceed to major amputation (Ramsey, 1999). Another report identified minor trauma, ulceration, and faulty wound healing as precursors to 73% of LEAs, often in combination with gangrene and infection (Litzelman, 1997).

8.1.2 RISK FACTORS FOR LEA IN DIABETIC FOOT

The common risk factors in patients with diabetes that may lead to LEA are:

- Absence of protective sensation due to peripheral neuropathy.
- Arterial insufficiency.
- Foot deformity and callus formation resulting in focal areas of high pressure.
- Autonomic neuropathy causing decreased sweating and dry, fissured skin.
- Limited joint mobility.
- Obesity.
- Impaired vision.
- Poor glucose control leading to impaired wound healing.
- Poor footwear that causes skin breakdown or inadequately protects the skin.
- High pressure and shear forces.
- History of foot ulcer or amputation.

8.2 RISK FACTORS FOR DIABETIC FOOT ULCER

The risk factors for developing diabetic ulcers include the presence of sensory peripheral neuropathy, altered biomechanics, elevated pressure on the sole of the foot, and limited joint mobility. The structural changes discussed along with vascular insufficiency, infection, and uneven plantar pressure predisposes the person with diabetes to develop foot ulceration

(Figure.1). The people with diabetes, who have neuropathy are 1.7 times more likely to develop a foot ulceration, in persons with both neuropathy and foot deformity, the risk is 12 times greater,and in those who also have a history of pathology (prior amputation or ulceration), the risk is 36 times greater (Armstrong et al, 1998). The people with diabetes who have increased risk for lower extremity ulceration are males, people with diabetes for more than 10 years, are the people who use tobacco and those with a history of poor glycemic control or the presence of cardiac, retinal, or renal complications (Boulton et al, 2004).

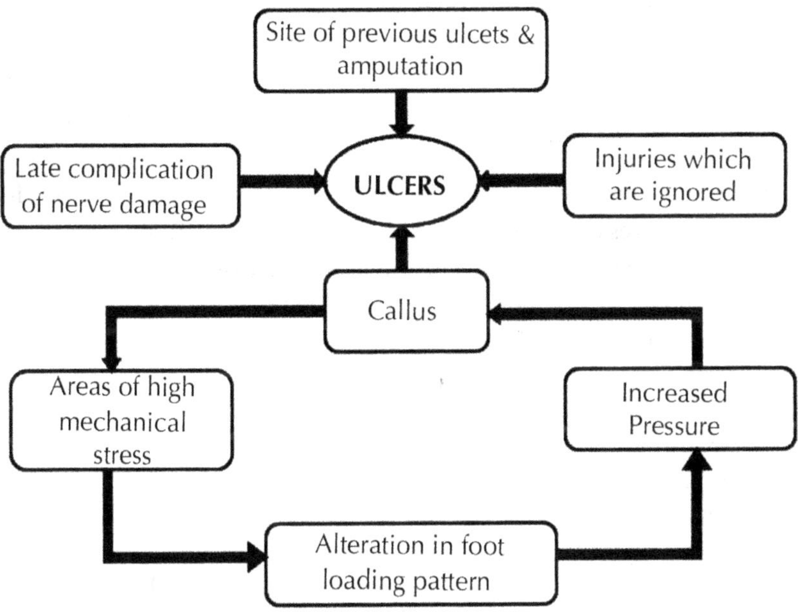

FIGURE 1 Pathway to Diabetic Foot Ulcers.

It should be emphasized that the most common offending agent or cause of traumatic foot ulceration is footwear (Birke, 2000; Tyrrell, 2002; Apelqvist, 1990). If neuropathic ulcers occur elsewhere in the foot, it is usually due to footwear that is too tight. The use of ill-fitting shoes is instrumental in the development of blisters, callus, and corns, which can lead to ulceration in patients with diabetes. Footwear has been implicated as an extrinsic cause of foot ulcers in people with diabetes and high risk foot conditions (Crausaz, 1988). The pathways usually involve injury when a foot with impaired sensation and/or deformity experiences minor trauma or elevated plantar pressure, resulting in tissue damage (Apelqvist, 2000). Foot ulceration has been associated with constant or repetitive pressure from tight shoes over bony prominences on the dorsum of the lesser toes, at the medial aspect of the first metatarsal head, or the lateral aspect of the fifth metatarsal (Lavery, 1998) In a large prospective study, Abbott et al. (2002) found that the main cause (55%) of ulceration was pressure from footwear (Abbott, 2002). When ulceration occurs on the side of the foot, it is most likely due to ill-fitting shoes and ischemic pressure necrosis. When the ulceration is on the dorsum of the foot, it is usually the result of trauma.

The elevated foot pressure is an important risk factor for foot complications. Ninety four percent of diabetic foot ulcers occur at areas of increased pressure (Bus, 2004). The plantar surface of the forefoot is found to be the most common location for the development of an ulcer. Forefoot and rear foot pressure ratios are increased in the severe diabetic neuropathic foot, indicating an imbalance in pressure distribution. The factors that are responsible for abnormal stress on foot are:

- Diminished senses at the foot — this alters gait pattern.
- Weakness of the muscles.
- Thinning of fat pads.
- Bony prominences.
- Limited joint mobility.
- Joint deformity.
- Callus.
- Altered tissue properties.
- Previous foot surgery.
- Over pronation/supination.
- Poor activity level.
- Foot deformity causing areas of high pressure.
- Obesity.
- Poor glucose control.

- Poor footwear.
- History of LEA.
- History of foot ulceration.
- Elevated peak plantar pressure (PPP).

8.3 PREVENTION AND TREATMENT OF DIABETIC FOOT ULCERS

The diabetic foot is the hardest foot to manage, because it has all of the biomechanical challenges that non-diabetic feet have, coupled with the soft tissue challenges related to diabetes. The prevention is considered a key element in avoiding ulcer recidivism and diabetic LEA (Edmonds, as 1986; ADA, 2000; Pecoraro, 1990; Lavery, 1998; LoGerfo, 1984; Armstrong 1998). The prevention and treatment of diabetic foot ulcer is best accomplished with a multidisciplinary approach consisting of a team of professionals committed to this ideal (Apelqvist, 2000). The reduction in pressure at the site of ulceration, usually on a weightbearing site (plantar surface of the foot) is essential for treatment of diabetic foot ulceration. Avoiding foot injury by wearing well-fitted shoes and examining the feet daily can help prevent amputations. Therapeutic shoes with pressure-relieving insoles and high toe box, that protect the high risk foot are an essential element of the prevention program and have been associated with significant reductions in ulcer development (Shaw, 1997; Delmas, 2006; Mueller, 1997). Therapeutic footwear is designed primarily for the prevention of ulcer occurrence (Janisse, 1995). For patients under risk category 0 to 3, appropriate/therapeutic footwear help to prevent ulcer formation and in patients those who have active ulcers in risk category 4 to 6, if they use appropriate /therapeutic footwear ulcer relapsing may be prevented. Therapeutic footwear is helpful both in treatment as will as prevention of diabetic foot ulceration. Footwear constructed with orthotics is also recommended frequently for the diabetic patient. This can be accomplished by the application of a number of external devices. There are recent advances in the field of pressure offloading devices for patients with diabetes.

8.4 PLANTAR PRESSURE OFFLOADING DEVICES

The plantar pressure offloading can be accomplished by the application of a number of external devices. It is important that there is a member of the team skilled in the fabrication and modification of offloading devices, such as a foot care specialist. Foot pressures, shock, and shear can be reduced with appropriately fitted shoes, insoles, and socks. Total non-weight bearing using a wheelchair or crutches is the most effective method of relieving pressure although most patients have difficulty complying with these modalities.

8.4.1 TOTAL CONTACT CASTS

Total contact casts (TCCs) and removal casts are effective in significantly reducing pressure but may cause additional problems when inappropriately applied. The TCCs are used for offloading the plantar aspect of the foot. Caravaggi et al.(2000) had described the effectiveness of fibreglass off-bearing nonremovable cast in the treatment of neuropathic foot ulcer. The bandage was composed of fiber glass imbued with a polyurethane resin of that confers high resistance to loading. A bandage with German cotton and tubular stockinet was placed on the limb. To further protect bony protrusions, such as the malleolus and tibial crista, pieces of protective rubber foam were applied. The structure was reinforced with a stick made of a Scotchcast bandage placed in the middle of the two malleoli, extending beyond them for at least 20 cm to give rigidity to the cast. The same material was used to build a rigid plantar sole. About 3–8 layers was applied to construct the sole depended on the weight of the patient. An aluminum stirrup was anchored to the structure as a support to allow walking. The procedure shows that clinical skill is required for application and still remains a costly and time-consuming process. Patient compliance is necessary to minimize complications. Inappropriate application may result in a new ulceration. Another important issue is the high percentage of patients, such as those with vascular disease, bilateral ulcers, or lower limb amputation, who cannot tolerate TCCs (Brem, 2004). Postural instability may be exacerbated. Additional Contraindications include acute infection ischemia, deep ulcers, and draining wounds, ataxic patients and those who are noncompliant, blind, or morbidly obese (Lavery, 1996). In general, wounds on the posterior heel should not be treated with TCCs. Though TCC offers better pressure offloading and is considered as gold standard for management of neuropathic foot ulcers due to the limitations as mentioned, advanced offloading techniques are emerged to help both patients and doctors.

8.4.2 REMOVABLE WALKER OR ANKLE FOOT ORTHOSIS

A commercially available removable boot that reduces plantar pressures is called as removable walker. An ankle-foot orthosis (AFO) is an orthosis or brace (usually plastic) that surrounds the ankle and at least part of the foot. AFOs are externally applied and intended to control position and motion of the ankle, compensate for weakness, or correct deformities. They control the ankle directly, and can be designed to control the knee joint indirectly as well. AFOs are commonly used in the treatment of disorders affecting muscle function such as stroke, spinal cord injury, muscular dystrophy, cerebral palsy, polio, multiple sclerosis, and peripheral neuropathy. AFO has been used as pressure offloading device for treating neuropathic foot ulcers (Bus, 2008; Spencer, 2008; Boninger, 1996). Pragmatically, removable cast walkers may be preferable to TCCs, as they do not have the same inherent disadvantages. Pressure reduction has been shown to be similar to TCCs with certain types of devices. Removable walking casts facilitate daily wound inspection and wound care. Infection can be readily detected and complications addressed. Faglia et al.(2010) studied the effectiveness of removable walker cast (Stabil-D) in the healing of diabetic plantar foot ulcer in comparison with nonremovable fibre glass off-bearing cast. The results indicated that the use of Stabil-D is as effective as use of a TCC in the treatment of neuropathic plantar forefoot ulcers. The Stabil-D device is composed of a specifically designed rigid, boat-shaped, and fully rocker bottom sole. Unfortunately, while these devices may seem to be equivalent to TCCs, the fact that they are removable often leads to lapses in adherence to care. Also, patients should not drive automobiles while wearing casts or any offloading device. Another disadvantage of this device is high cost.

8.4.3 HALF SHOES

Half shoes offer support only under the rear and mid-foot. The half-shoes were originally designed to protect the forefoot after an elective surgery. The features are:

- Inexpensive.
- Easy to apply.
- Less effective than TCC.
- Hampers gait.

8.4.4 HEALING SANDALS (ROCKER BOTTOM SOLE)

Healing sandals are designed with a rigid rocker to the bottom of a shoe or sandal. Some sandals may have a pressure-reducing insole. Giacalone et al.(1997) compared plantar pressures between custom healing sandals and postoperative shoes using unmodified prescription shoe gear as a control and reported that the healing sandal significantly reduced plantar forefoot pressure in all areas of the forefoot except the fifth metatarsal head. The postoperative shoe did not significantly reduce pressure at any site in the forefoot when compared with unmodified prescription shoe gear. The features of healing sandal are:

- Limit dorsiflexion therefore distributes pressure of metatarsal heads.
- Lightweight and stable.
- Reusable.
- Requires significant amount of time and experience to produce therefore not easily accessible.
- Not as efficient compared to other methods of offloading.

8.4.5 FELTED FOAM

The application of felted foam is a promising method for plantar pressure reduction in the ulcer region of neuropathic diabetic foot. Bilayered felted foam is used a dressing over the plantar surface with opening for the wound. Zimny et al, (2003) assessed the effects of felted foam dressing on the wound healing for plantar pressure reduction in the therapy of neuropathic foot ulcers and reported that the felted foam technique is a useful alternative in the therapy of the neuropathic diabetic foot syndrome, especially in patients who are not able to avoid weight-bearing reliably. This technique is inexpensive and accessible but may produce pressure and shear at wound edges.

8.4.6 CRUTCHES, WALKERS,AND WHEELCHAIRS

The use of consistently crutches, walkers and wheelchairs will offload pressure effectively. But the limitations are:

- Requires upper body strength and endurance,
- May not be used all the time,
- Difficulty in navigating indoors,
- Can increase pressures on contralateral side.

8.4.7 THERAPEUTIC FOOTWEAR

Therapeutic footwear (TFW) plays an important role in diabetic footcare (Vijay et al, 2004). TFW for patients with diabetes is designed for protecting the insensitive diabetic foot and to accommodate pressure "hot spots" by conforming to heat and pressure. By customizing to the foot, orthosis provides the comfort and protection needed in diabetic footcare. Footwear constructed with orthotics is also recommended frequently for the diabetic patient. Therapeutic footwear for patients with diabetes is designed to have the following features:

Adequate width	:	To accommodate broad foot of patients with diabetes
Extra space for toes	:	To avoid callous or corns formation by preventing the toes ribbing on upper material and also to dissipate pressure on forefoot
Cushioned arch	:	To provide uniform plantar pressure distribution on walking
Foam insoles	:	To accommodate bony prominences of metatarsals
Soles for stability & shock absorption	:	To absorb ground reaction force to protect bones of lower extremity.
Upper		To protect from injury and friction
Firm Heel Counter	:	To support the ankle

The TFW have the potential to:

- Relieve high pressure areas,
- Offload high risk areas,
- Support the arch,
- Relieve pain,
- Limit painful range of motion,
- Provide proper shoe fit,
- Assist in wound treatment,
- Prevent ulcers and amputation,
- Enhance stability and balance,
- Increase comfort,
- Improve foot function,
- Increase mobility and performance,
- Correct biomechanical defects,
- Accommodate foot deformity.

TYPES OF THERAPEUTIC FOOTWEAR

CUSTOM-MADE/PRESCRIPTION FOOTWEAR

The most diabetic feet can be managed with off-the-shelf shoes. However, in many cases, including many Charcot conditions, custom molded footwear (either open type sandal or closed type shoe) is the best treatment for the person with diabetes. When severe deformities are present, a custom-made shoe can be constructed from a cast or model of the patient's foot (Saraswathy et al, 2004). People with peripheral neuropathy may choose wrong size footwear because without proper sensation, the correct size seems to be too large. Too small a shoe can cause a blister or abrasion that can result in an ulcer and/or other foot complications. In people with diabetes and a prior foot ulcer, decreased reulceration was reported in several studies comparing patients wearing prescription footwear with those wearing their own footwear (Shaw, 1994). Standard recommendations in the majority of outpatient settings usually consist of a prescription for a post-surgical shoe or over-the-counter athletic shoes. But athletic shoes are not appropriate for the diabetic foot, as they are not designed to reduce pressure or prevent injury in the deformed and insensate foot. Therefore, appropriate custom made footwear which is prescribed by podiatrist based on patient's risk category is necessary to treat or prevent diabetic foot ulcer.

MODIFIED SHOE

This involves modifying the outside of the patient's own shoe in some way, such as modifying the shape of the sole or adding shock-absorbing or stabilizing materials. With extensive modifications of in-depth shoes, even the most severe deformities can usually be accommodated.

HEALING SHOES

Immediately following surgery or ulcer treatment, some type of shoe may be necessary before a regular shoe can be worn. These include custom sandals (open toe), heat-moldable healing shoes (closed toe), and post-operative shoes.

IN-DEPTH SHOES

The in-depth shoe is the basis for most footwear prescriptions. It is generally an oxford-type or athletic shoe with an additional 1/4 to 1/2 inch of depth throughout the shoe, allowing extra volume to accommodate any needed inserts or orthoses, as well as deformities commonly associated with a diabetic foot. In-depth shoes also tend to be light in weight, have shock-absorbing soles, and come in a wide range of shapes and sizes to accommodate virtually any foot.

ORTHOTICS

People with diabetes usually require foot orthoses to balance and protect the foot and to unload and alleviate diabetic foot problems. Orthotics are custom-made shoe inserts which serve to correct or relieve misalignment and pressure areas of the foot and provides shock absorption. Both pre-made/custom-made orthoses are commonly prescribed for patients with diabetes, including a special "total contact orthosis", which is made from a model of patient's foot and offers a high level of comfort and pressure relief.

A systematic review was conducted to assess the effectiveness of pressure relieving interventions in prevention and treatment of diabetic foot ulcers. Spencer (2004) reviewed four randomized controlled trials of pressure relieving interventions and concluded that in-shoe orthotics are of benefit. Orthotic devices come in many shapes and sizes, and materials and fall into three main categories: those designed to change foot function, are primarily protective in nature, and those that combine functional control and protection.

RIGID ORTHOSIS

The rigid orthotic device, designed to control function, is often composed a firm material such as plastic or carbon fiber, and is used primarily for walking or dress shoes. Such orthotics is made from a mold after a podiatrist takes a plaster cast or other kind of image of the foot. Rigid orthotics control motion in two major foot joints that lie directly below the ankle joint and may improve or eliminate strains, aches, and pains in the legs, thighs, and lower back.

SOFT ORTHOSIS

Soft orthotics absorbs shock, increase balance, and offload pressure spots. They are typically made up of soft, cushy materials. Soft orthosis is worn against the sole of the foot, extending from the heel past the ball of the foot, including the toes. Such orthotics are also made from a mold after a podiatrist takes a plaster cast or other kind of image of the foot. Soft orthoses are usually effective for diabetic, arthritic, and deformed feet.

SEMI-RIGID ORTHOSIS

Semi-rigid orthotics provide foot balance for walking or participating in sports. Sometimes, different sports call for different kinds of semi-rigid orthotics. The typical semi-rigid orthotic is made up of layers of soft material, reinforced with more rigid materials. Children are sometimes given orthosis to treat flatfoot or in-toeing or out-toeing disorders. Athletes often are given orthosis to mitigate pain while they train and compete. While over-the-counter orthotic inserts help people with mild symptoms, they normally cannot correct the wide range of symptoms that prescription foot orthosis can since they are made to fit a person with an "average" foot shape.

CUSTOM ORTHOSIS

The custom orthosis can perform a myriad of functions to correct foot abnormalities and prevent future problems. There are several main purposes of orthosis:

- Relieve areas of excessive plantar pressure by evenly distributing pressure over the entire bottom surface of the foot and/or redistributing plantar forces on the foot.
- Reduce shock with shock-absorbing materials.
- Stabilize and support deformities and limit joint motion with the use of more rigid, supportive materials.
- Reduce shear by minimizing horizontal foot movement through shear-reducing materials.
- Accommodate deformities with the use of soft, moldable materials in the shell and top cover.

8.5 MATERIALS USED FOR THERAPEUTIC FOOTWEAR FABRICATION

The materials used to make the custom-molded orthotics need to be sufficiently firm to support the foot and offload the problem area, yet not too firm as to cause other problems or aggravate the pre-existing problem. The material must be able to endure cyclic compression, shear combined with compression and allow for force distribution of plantar pressure throughout the material. No single material satisfies all of these requirements. In healthy individuals, the fat pad beneath the foot acts as a viscoelastic shock absorber. With overuse, or following diabetes mellitus or trauma, changes may occur in the structure of the heel pad/fat pad beneath the foot, including a reduction in thickness, rendering it dysvascular (Jahhs et al, 1992). This results in a loss of shock absorbing capacity, which may lead to diffuse heel pain, plantar fasciitis, and Achilles tendonitis or plantar ulcers in case of diabetes patients. Therefore orthotic materials are expected to perform like a natural fatpad. To achieve this, two layers of different materials of different density are routinely used to make custom-molded orthotics. In a study comparing commercially available materials, medium density crossed linked polypropylene (Pelite TM) was determined (Showers, 1985) to be the most suitable for the base of the orthotics as it can be molded to the shapes of the foot. The materials used for the base of the orthotics must be carefully selected to ensure that they are lightweight, flexible, strong, resilient, and retain their shape despite compression forces. These properties may be achieved with viscoelastic materials. Viscoelastic materials came into widespread clinical use during 1980's for use in footwear. The top cover or the material which comes in contact with the foot is routinely made of an expanded rubber (example, Spenco TM) or polyurethane (PU) foam (example PPTTM) as they provide cushioning, decrease friction, and shear forces (Brodsky JW, 1988; Pratt, 1989). Viscoelastic materials are commonly used as an insole material in the construction of various types of shoes. Like other elastic materials, viscoelastic materials are effective in redistributing the pressure beneath the foot, thereby reducing local pressures and the stresses on foot structure. Viscoelastic material recovers from deformation over a period of time, and the energy, which was used to deform it, is largely converted to heat. The time course of this recovery depends on the formulation of the viscoelastic material; to be effective in the heel of a shoe, most of the recovery needs to occur before the next step is taken. Many different polymers have been used for these purposes, as either elastomer or foams. For example, Polyurethane elastomers *(Sorbothane)*, Polyurethane foams *(Poron)*, Polyethylene foams *(Plastozote)*, Ethylene vinyl acetate *(EVA)*, Synthetic rubber foams *(neoprene)*, and Silicone gel. These materials are viscoelastic to a greater or lesser extent.

Though there are several advancements in therapeutic intervention of diabetic foot ulcer based on plantar pressure offloading methods using footwear or orthotics, there is a great challenge of convincing patients to wear therapeutic footwear and orthotics regularly. The non-use of therapeutic footwear is a common problem among the patients who are suggested or prescribed to use them regularly. Though patients with diabetes, who are falling under risk category 1, 2, and 3, use therapeutic footwear as per the guidance of doctor/podiatrist, they use other pairs of footwear too based on their own willingness. It was found that the patients with diabetes buy this footwear on doctor's recommendation but will not use it; or though they buy and use, not regularly or discontinue using it after some period of time. Non-use rates of various types of therapeutic footwear vary from 20% to 25% for first time users and from 4% to 19% among experienced users who were provided with a subsequent pair of therapeutic footwear (Netten et al, 2009).

Generally, patient compliance on using any therapeutic product requires higher product quality. To be a successful therapeutic intervention, therapeutic footwear must meet the needs and wants of both the patients and doctors. The proper design and customization of therapeutic footwear based on patient's as well as physician's needs is important to increase the patient's compliance of using the therapeutic footwear. Therefore those issues that prevent the patients from using this footwear need to be focused. The main objective of this study is to identify the requirements to be used as a reference in the development of therapeutic footwear and to improve the material properties and design of therapeutic footwear for patients with diabetes by translating the patient's requirements into product requirements.

8.6 IDENTIFICATION OF REQUIREMENT FOR THERAPEUTIC FOOTWEAR

The best method to know about the quality and performance of any product is taking survey from the end users using questionnaires. Preparation of effective and efficient questionnaire which will help analyze both the customers and products is important to achieve the objective. Jannink et al.(2004) have developed questionnaire for usability evaluation of orthopaedic shoes specifically for patients with degenerative disorders of the foot. Herold and Palmer (1992) used questionnaire for usability evaluation of surgical shoes specifically for patients with rheumatoid arthritis. Fisher and McLellan (1989) had assessed patient's satisfaction with lower limb orthosis using questionnaire method. In our study also, the questionnaires were used as the main data-gathering instruments. The requirements for therapeutic footwear from patients, doctors, and footwear technicians will differ according to their point of view. Therefore effort was made to identify their needs and wants separately using different questionnaires which were uniquely prepared for each group. The aim was to give the top most priority to the needs/requirements of the customers into the process of therapeutic footwear development. The user needs are mapped out and integrated in the total therapeutic footwear development process. By concentrating on these technical areas it is therefore expected to increase the satisfaction of patients with diabetes among the users of therapeutic footwear.

Patients those who are visiting Department of Podiatry and Department of Footcare at M. V. Hospital of Diabetes, Diabetes Research Centre, Chennai were included in the study. 102 patients who are using therapeutic footwear as preventive and therapeutic measure for foot ulcer at least for 6 months; 45 to 65 years old, having diabetes for more than 6 years, were participated in this survey after informed consent. The procedure of this study was approved by the medical ethics committee of the M. V Hospital for diabetes and Diabetes Research Centre, Chennai. 12 diabetologist who are expertise in treating diabetic foot ulcer and prescribe therapeutic footwear for their patients were included in the survey. 10 footwear technicians who fabricate therapeutic footwear for patients with diabetes based on prescription from diabetologist were involved in the survey. Researchers (Biomechanist/Biomedical Engineer) from Central Leather Research Institute (CLRI), Chennai who are involved in the research on design and development of therapeutic footwear for plantar pressure offloading, were also participated in the survey.

The filled in questionnaires were critically analyzed and the results from this analysis revealed that aesthetics and durability using QFD of footwear that is entire material used for therapeutic footwear fabrication were most important parameters for meeting the demands of the users. The important product characteristics to achieve these demands are design of footwear and density and porosity of the materials. From the patients and technicians it was found that the insole of the footwear that comes in contact with foot becomes old faster than other materials. Insole in therapeutic footwear is playing an important role in pressure distribution and offloading at risk areas of ulcer development in diabetic foot. Therefore density and porosity of materials used as insole and new design of therapeutic footwear exclusively for patients with diabetes were taken as priority area of our research.

8.7 NEW MATERIALS FOR THERAPEUTIC FOOTWEAR APPLICATIONS

Many viscoelastic materials are used in shoes to replace the shock-absorbing and pressure distributing functions of natural fat pad beneath the foot that was lost due to some conditions such as diabetes, age or overuse. In a series of long term wear tests on a variety of insole materials, Pratt and his coworkers found that when new PU elastomer and PU foams were similar to each other in shock absorbing performance and better than other materials. After prolonged use, however, the elastomer retained most of their properties of shock absorption whereas foams deteriorated (Pratt 1990). Brodsky et al.(1988) compared five different insole materials used for diabetic footwear and found that soft foam materials gave the best pressure redistribution initially, but they suffered from compression set with dynamic compression testing. Insoles are now available which consist of a base layer of PU elastomer covered by a layer of PU foam. The elastomer provides good shock attenuation and pressure distribution but does not feel soft; foam provides some shock attenuation, gives good pressure distribution, feels soft to the touch and is reasonably resistant to compression set. So there is a need for porous viscoelastic materials which possess the mechanical properties of elastomers as well as soft and cushion property of foam materials. The aim of this research work was to prepare viscoelastic materials based on polyurethanes having the highest degree of phase separation that provides for the elastomeric nature of these polymers. The main objectives of the work were:

- To synthesize fiber forming polyurethanes based on an organic aromatic diisocyanate, a polyether polyol and chain extender containing secondary nitrogen group and active hydrogens.
- To provide a process for fabrication of viscoelastic porous PU sheets of 3 to 6 mm thickness, for application as cushion insole in therapeutic footwear.
- To develop viscoelastic porous PU sheets of different thickness by changing the volume of polymer solution.
- To develop viscoelastic porous PU sheets of different density/porosity by changing the composition of polymer solution.

- To develop viscoelastic porous PU sheets of different density/porosity by changing the concentration of polymer solution.
- To develop insole materials using viscoelastic porous PU sheets which obviates the drawbacks of the hitherto known prior art as detailed above.
- To develop therapeutic footwear incorporating the developed insole materials and distributing to patients of risk category 2 and 3.
- To study the efficacy of developed viscoelastic porous PU sheets as insole materials by following up of those patients by measuring the plantar pressure using HR mat systems, Tekscan, USA.

8.7.1 PREPARATION OF PU SHEETS

Polymer structures with a high concentration of amide groups can be made with the addition of hydrazine or a diacid hydrazide to a diisocyanate. Various polyurethanes were prepared by chain extending the isocyanate terminated prepolymer with terepthalic dihydrazide, 5-hydroxy isothalic dihydrazide and 1,4 butane dial. The processing method used to develop PU sheets is phase inversion or coagulation method. Dimethyl formamide was used to prepare PU solution and distilled water was used as nonsolvent or coagulant. PU solution in room temperature was taken in polypropylene tray to a height of 3–6 mm and left for 15–20 min to allow evaporation of the solvent to form a microskin layer over the surface. Then the coagulant, water was sprayed uniformly over the surface to a height of 2 mm and left for 15 min. Then the tray was filled with water at the rate of 10 to 20 mL per min and left for overnight. PU sheets were also prepared with blends of commercial PU and experimental PU in 1:1 ratio. Blends were prepared as homogenous solution in dimethylformamide (DMF) and made into sheets as explained above (Sample 1 to 11). Further PU sheets were prepared with only commercial polyurethane in various concentrations. 15%, 20%, 25%, 30%, 45%, and 50% W/V of PU solutions were prepared with DMF and made into sheets by the same method using water as non-solvent (Figure 2). Figure 3 shows the picture of insoles cut from the PU sheets of sample number 12 to 24 developed with various concentrations of polyesterurethane. The synthesized PU sheets were characterized for physical properties such as thickness, density, hardness, compression set, cushion energy, cushion factor, tensile strength, tear strength, water absorption (% CS) and desorption, and abrasion resistance to find their suitability for application as cushioned insole in TFW and the results were compared to the properties of commercially available insole materials such as Micro cellular rubber (MCR), PU foam, EVA foam, Dr. Scholl's heel pad, Dr. Scholl's Shoe insert, which are currently being used as cushion inserts in conventional shoes or insoles in TFW. Morphological characteristics of PU sheets were also analyzed by scanning electron microscopy (SEM) to study the size and distribution of pores on the surface and inside of the PU sheets (Saraswathy et al, 2008; Saraswathy et al, 2009).

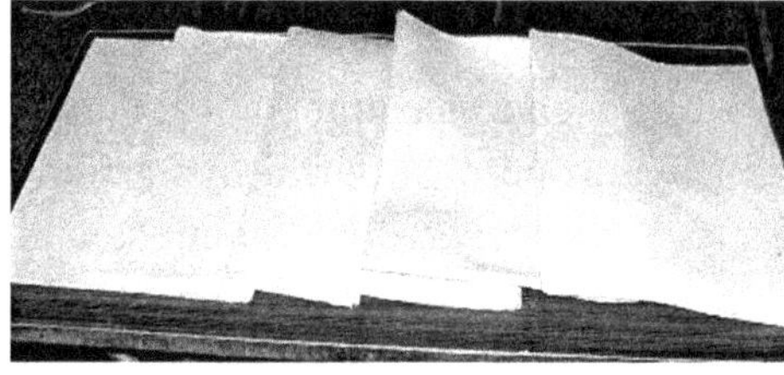

FIGURE 2 Photographs of developed PU sheets with various concentrations.

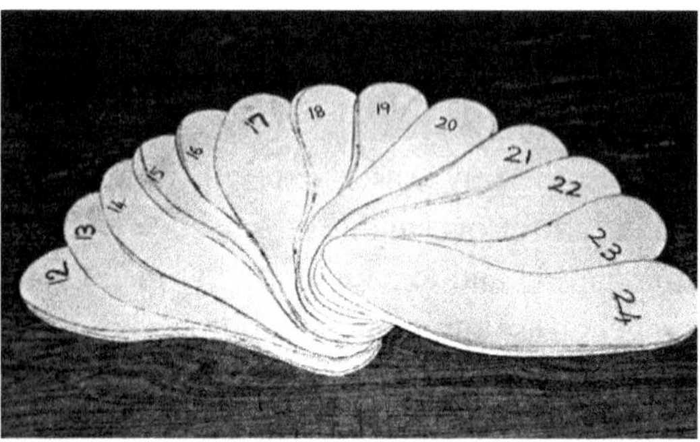

FIGURE 3 Insoles cut from PU sheets of sample number 12 to 24 developed with various concentrations of polyesterurethane.

The ideal range of hardness of insole materials is 18 to 22 shore A because the materials will deform on walking and regain its original thickness before the second step is taken. Therefore PU sheets of sample number 3, 4, 7, 10, 12, 14, 15, 17, and 18 which have hardness in the range of 15 to 22 shore A can be used as insole materials where uniform pressure distribution under the foot is essential. The commercial insoles had shown low range of hardness of 4–10 shore A and microcellular polymer (MP) of 12–14 shore A. Due to low hardness values the commercial insole materials available in the market did not meet the needs of insole for application in therapeutic footwear. On each step the footwear is subjected to the load of 2–3 times of our body weight. If these foam materials are used as insole materials they will deform with low value of load and may be uncomfortable to the wearer. Therefore these sheets are not suitable for application as cushion insole materials. The slightly higher hardness of MCP than other foams may be due to the finishing or modification of surface of the foam.

The density of the material has linear effect on hardness. As the density increases hardness also increases. Therefore, with the same composition of polymer solution the required hardness of the material can be achieved by changing the volume of solvent while preparing the PU solution thus changing the density. Therefore the samples which had lower range of hardness will be improved by increasing the density of the materials by increasing the polymer concentration. Among the commercial samples MCP had lower density of 0.0822 g/cm^3. Due to low density MCP is very light material and preferred as insole than other foams which had given density between 0.1618 and 0.2580 g/cm^3.

All the samples had shown % CS less than 4.2%. The pores (air) inside the sheets make the sheets to deform under load. Since the pores did not collapse on removal of load, the sheets could regain its thickness. The required percentage of CS for insole materials is maximum 5% for better durability. In case of commercial materials only PU foam had given CS of 1.7%, whereas others had shown more than 6% of CS and MCP had shown 65.0% of CS. All the commercial materials having pores are basically foams and the basic material is either synthetic polymer or rubber. As the method of production of foams differs with company the commercial materials had shown different values of compression set. MCP which had given higher value of CS may perform well when new and will suffer compression of its thickness (called “bottom out”) on repeated or long use.

Another important property for insole is cushionability which is analyzed from values of cushion energy and cushion factor. The higher the cushion energy, the greater the cushioning effect of the insole is likely to be in wear. Rigid materials and very weak soft foams both give low results since the former are incompressible and the later 'bottom out'. Insoles giving values greater than 70 N. mm would be expected to reduce underfoot peak pressures in walking considerably. Also a low cushion factor indicates an effective material with typical values ranging from 8 to 4. In our study, PU samples 14, 18, and 19 had given CEw above 70 N.mm for comparable thickness. They also have a better cushion factor. Knowing the cushion factor for a given material makes it possible to determine the thickness of insole needed to achieve a required cushion energy value. Therefore the CEw can be increased by increasing the thickness of the sheets.

The PU based sheets developed by coagulation method have the cushioning and mechanical properties that are needed for an insole material. The sheets developed with only CPU had shown better mechanical properties and those developed with combination of CPU and PUSC had shown better cushion properties than that of commercial materials. Especially the percentage compression set had obtained less for the developed materials which is a major drawback of commercially available foams. The micro and macro pores which were formed from solvent exchange on the surface and inside the polymer helps in cushion and water absorption properties of the materials. The fiber forming property of PUSC had contributed in viscoelastic nature of the sheets. Therefore all the sheets can be as insole material in therapeutic footwear for uniform distribution of pressure used under the foot and to prevent ulcer formation. The required thickness of sheet for better cushion properties varies for each material and the density of the material determines the hardness. Therefore the required mechanical and cushioning properties of insole material for individual patient can be achieved by developing the sheet with required thickness and density by changing the polymer content, polymer concentration, and solvent volume.

8.7.2 THE MAIN ADVANTAGES OF DEVELOPED INSOLE MATERIALS

- New porous viscoelastic sheets developed using polyurethane having fiber forming property and by coagulation method have micro to macro sized pores both on surface as well as inside of the material.
- The PU sheets with different density, hardness, and thickness can be developed by changing the concentration and volume of polymer solution
- The asymmetric PU sheet may act as a dual density material, which is more likely in footwear.
- Pores on surface can help in absorption and desorption of sweat/moisture, and the pores inside of the material helps in cushion and resilience nature of material.
- Since there is no usage of chemicals like plasticizer, blowing agent, pigment, surfactant, filler and mold release agents, and adhesive, it can be used safely in manufacture of therapeutic footwear.
- SEM photographs had showed the presence of upper spongy layer and compact dense lower layer in the same sheet. Therefore, better viscoelastic nature than foam materials, presence of pores and macrovoids for water transmission and presence of different density layers are achieved with the single sheet, by simple fabrication method.
- Since there are no layers of different materials of different thickness of materials or different density of materials used in construction of cushion system, the cost of production would be less while comparing to the currently available cushion systems.

8.7.3 STUDY OF EFFECTIVENESS OF PU INSOLES FOR REDUCING PLANTAR PRESSURE IN PATIENTS WITH DIABETES AT HIGH-RISK FOR FOOT ULCERS

This study evaluated the effectiveness of PU insoles in reducing plantar pressure in patients at high-risk for foot ulcers. Seven patients with diabetes in risk category 1 and 2 (men, women), were selected from M. V Hospital for Diabetes, Chennai, and participated in this study after giving informed consent. Patients with amputation or severe deformity were excluded.

Weight and height were measured to determine their influence on the treatment effect. The mean (SD) age, height, and weight of the subjects were 53.57 ± 8.58 years, 156.85 ± 5.55 cm, and 57.28 ± 9.04 kg, respectively. The body mass index (BMI) was 23.25 ± 3.10 kg/m^2 and the duration of diabetes was 9.57 ± 5.53 years. The clinical data of seven patients who are participated in the study is represented in Table 2. Two subjects had prior plantar ulcers. At the time of the experiment, they had remained healed for at least three months while wearing their prescription footwear. Foot deformity was assessed subjectively. Among the deformities present were claw toes, hammer toes, hallux abducto valgus (HAV), limited joint mobility (LJM) at the first metatarsal– phalangeal joint, valgus, prominent MTHs, and amputation of the toes. Subjects also had to be able to walk independently with only minor assistance, in case of balance problems. All patients were volunteers free of ulceration at the time of testing, and provided informed consent. All participants had peripheral sensory neuropathy. Neuropathy was confirmed by a loss of protective sensation on the plantar surface of the foot, as determined by the inability to feel the 10 g Semmes–Weinstein monofilament on the hallux of both feet. Light touch, pain and vibratory perceptions were assessed. Light touch (monofilament) and pain (pinprick) were tested on 10 predetermined sites. These sites were: 1st, 3rd, and 5th apices of the toes, plantar aspect of the 1st, 3rd, and 5th metatarsophalangeal joints, plantar aspect of the navicular, cuboid and central heel, and dorsal aspect of the navicular. Blood supply to the feet was assessed and was seemed to be adequate for healing.

TABLE 2 Clinical data of 7 patients with diabetes

Patient*	Risk Category of developing ulcers	Age (years)	Duration of Diabetes (years)	Weight (Kg)	Height (cm)	BMI (kg/m2)	B.P (mm Hg)	ABI - RL	ABI - LL
1	2	62	15	52.6	160	20.54	120/80	0.69	0.59
2	1	45	5	50.5	150	22.44	130/80	1.0	1.0
3	1	45	10	60.2	150	26.75	140/80	-	-

TABLE 2 *(Continued)*

4	1	68	15	58.22	160	22.74	140/80	1.0	0.9
5	1	53	4	57.2	155	23.8	140/80	0.9	1.0
6	2	50	3	75	165	27.54	120/80	1.1	1.0
7	2	52	15	47.3	158	18.95	140/80	1.18	1.09
Mean ± SD		53.57 ± 8.58	9.57 ± 5.53	57.28 ± 9.04	156.85 ± 5.55	23.25 ± 3.10			

Sample number 12 to 18, having hardness in the range of 15 to 22 shore A, were selected for developing therapeutic footwear. One pair of insole of standard size 8 was cut from each PU sheet (Figure 2 and 3). Therapeutic footwear of open type were developed using insoles of sample number 12 to 18. Insoles were cut into patients own foot size. One pair of therapeutic footwear of open type incorporating PU insoles was developed using each sample and distributed to patients for regular use (Figure 4). The usual design of footwear was used and no change in material other than insole was made. The PPP and total contact areas were measured on day 1 and after 3 months on walking with therapeutic footwear, using In-shoe F-scan system, Tekscan, USA. There was a significant difference in PPP between with and without therapeutic footwear ($p< 0.0001$). PPP was lower when patients were walking in therapeutic footwear with PU insoles as compared to barefoot. Peak pressures were located under the metatarsal heads or heels. The preorthotic peak pressure under the feet was 482 kPa and the postorthotic pressure was reduced to 185 kPa ($P< 0.001$) (Figure 5). The mean reduction in pressure was 61.6% and ranged from 37.0 to 75.2%. The preorthotic contact area was 6292 mm^2 and the postorthotic contact area was increased to 9054 mm^2 ($P< 0.001$), suggesting a more even pressure distribution (Figure 6). The mean increase in the contact area was 44% and ranged from 9.4% to 77.1%. The changes between preorthotic and postorthotic pressure distribution for patient number 1 and 6 are shown in Figure 7. The PPP were lower and total contact areas were higher in case of therapeutic footwear both on day 1 and after 3 months. This study and patient's reports support the use of developed PU insoles for therapeutic footwear applications and orthosis fabrication in patients with diabetes.

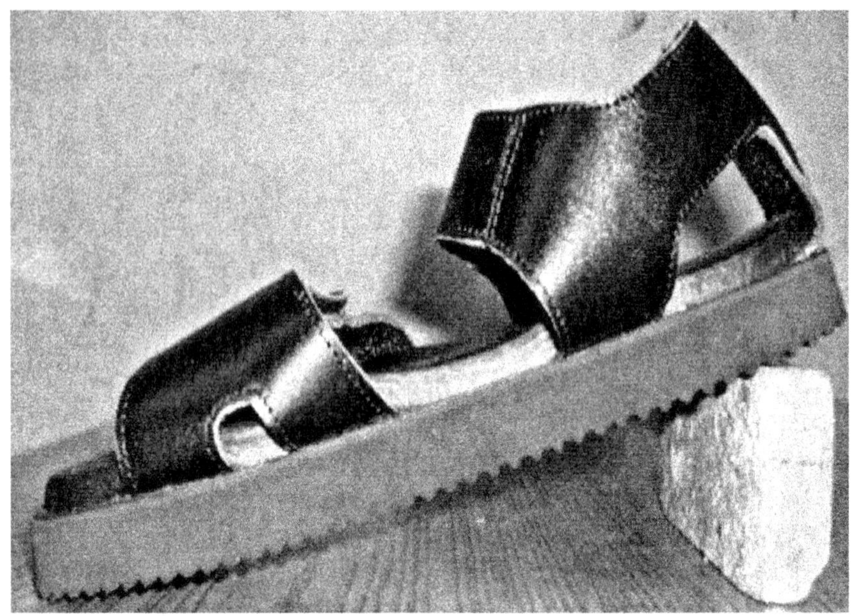

FIGURE 4 Therapeutic custom made footwear developed with new PU insole.

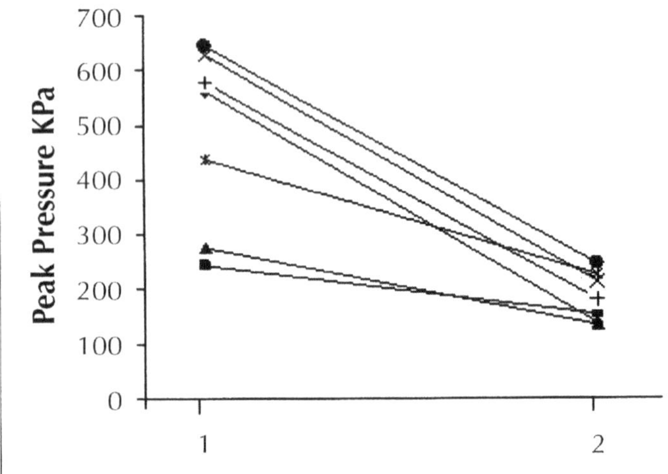

FIGURE 5 The PPP in 7 subjects on walking with 1) Barefoot and 2) Therapeutic footwear.

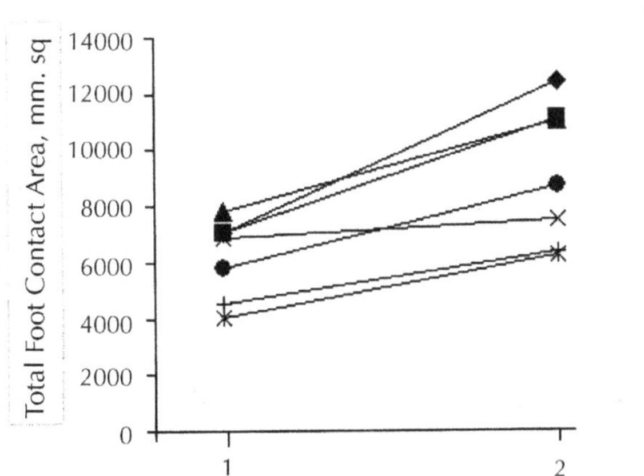

FIGURE 6 Total contact area in 7 subjects on walking with 1) Barefoot and 2) Therapeutic footwear.

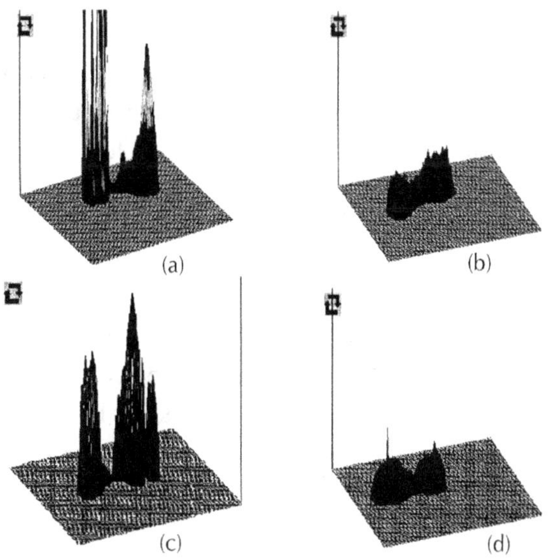

FIGURE 7 3-D view of plantar pressure distribution in patient number 1 (a) on barefoot, (b) on wearing therapeutic footwear; 3-D view of plantar pressure distribution in patient number 6 (c) on barefoot, (d) on wearing therapeutic footwear.

The purpose of this study was to evaluate the amount of pressure reduction achieved at focal areas of the foot with the use of custom-made therapeutic footwear incorporating PU insoles which were designed and developed in this research work. From the F-scan test results, it can be seen that the difference in peak pressure, total contact area and force/time integral reached statistical significance for the barefoot versus therapeutic footwear condition.

The contact area parameter measured was that of the plantar surface of the foot while weight-bearing. This was measured as it is believed that if the contact surface area under the foot is increased, pressure will be more evenly distributed. It appears that this commonly accepted idea is more intuitively driven rather than research-based. The difference in contact area with and without the insole in this study was statistically significant, with the surface area increasing during the wearing of the therapeutic footwear. However, as was noted with the peak pressures, some participants demonstrated large changes in contact area whereas in other instances this was small. There was no trend in contact area increase, with peak pressure decrease with the orthotic measurements; therefore whether a relationship exists between the two is not clear from the results of this research.

This study has looked specifically at the effectiveness of novel porous viscoelastic PU insole in the reduction of plantar pressures in patients with diabetes and a history of previous ulceration. The results indicate that therapeutic footwear incorporated with newly developed insole reduced plantar pressures and increased foot contact area. However, the amount of pressure reduction achieved was variable with patients. In conclusion, the authors recommend the use of porous viscoelastic PU insoles for plantar pressure reduction in combination with other factors in the treatment and prevention of neuropathic foot ulceration to achieve patient's compliance on using therapeutic footwear regularly as this PU insole material has better durability, cushionability, and comfort than the other conventional materials as per the results of our research. But another factor which is required by the patients is better design of the therapeutic footwear to use it for long duration. Therefore a new design of open type TFW was designed and elaborated in this chapter.

8.8 NEW DESIGN OF THERAPEUTIC FOOTWEAR FOR LOW RISK CATEGORY PATIENTS

The therapeutic footwear for patients for risk category 1 and 2 is designed to provide complete footwear for treatment of diabetic foot and prevention of diabetic foot ulcer. This TFW is useful for the treatment of diabetic foot along with other medical treatments. The footwear is selectively made of materials for its topsole, insole and bottom sole, comprising preferably cushioning material like Polyurethane (PU). A full length (PU) foam layer (FLI) inner sole was included in the footwear to cradle and support the foot and a PU molded outer sole. The extra depth PU unit sole has a specially derived angle of slant provided on the sole (USR) to give the 'Rocker' effect that is essentially used to offload pressure from the plantar surface of the foot (Figure 8). The outsole has a specially provided tread pattern for better grip and traction, as illustrated in the Figure 9. The shoe upper is selectively made of cow softy leather with lining material. The back of the shoe upper is also made rigid with a counter stiffener (RCS) for limiting joint mobility. The upper has been specially designed to take care of fluctuations in foot volume and is therefore provided with adjustable velcro fasteners (AVF). The underfoot pressure reduction/dissipation is achieved in therapeutic footwear under this study, by increasing the contact surface area of underfoot and the top sole. The foam layer provided in the sole compresses to accommodate the whole foot within itself and it easily adjusts when shearing takes place, minimizing the effect of shear.

The beneficial effect of this new design of therapeutic footwear was studied by way of actual use and the protocol followed and the results obtained are detailed. The study subjects were carefully selected from male patients with diabetic neuropathy without any present or previous foot ulceration. Protective sensation was assessed for each leg with the calibrated Rydel–Seiffer tuning fork and the 5.07 monofilament. Loss of protective sensation as a result of neuropathy was presumed in the presence of insensitivity to the 5.07 monofilament or a vibration perception of 4/8 or below. A total number of 50 pairs of newly designed footwear as shown in Figure 8, which are basically adjustable sandals fabricated to suit their requirement, being of size 8 were prepared and given to the selected 50 subjects for wearing. The recording and analysis of underfoot pressure distribution was carried out for those subjects wearing the specially designed sandals.

Dynamic plantar pressure was evaluated using the runescape (RS) Scan in-shoe pressure measurement. Data were collected at 250 Hz using 0.7 mm thick capacitance insole with 356 sensors and a spatial sensor resolution dependent on insole size. For each patient, four gait trials were conducted with the RS scan insole kept in direct contact with the sole of the foot. Subjects were asked practice walking wearing the therapeutic footwear until they felt comfortable, so that their gait pattern would be as consistent as possible during each trial. Data obtained from the metatarsal heads only were used as the peak pressure. At the follow up examination done after 3 months, 6 months, and later, the same parameter was measured for all the patients. Further, the patients' foot conditions were monitored for occurrence of problems such as ulceration, shoe bite and so on. The patients were investigated for adherence to the recommended schedule of use/wearing of the prescribed footwear and after getting the confirmation about the correct norm of usage, the inspection of the footwear was carried out for wear pattern of insole.

The record of plantar pressure distribution was observed in ten randomly selected patients from the said example of study with 50 selected subjects (Patients with diabetes under risk category 1 and 2). From the pressure contour patterns of the foot, the dramatic changes in the pressure pattern on wearing the new customized footwear as compared to the barefoot was evident. Table 3 highlight the barefoot pressures as well as in shoe pressures of subjects measured after wearing the specially designed footwear. The pressure has been well distributed and reduced with reduction in plantar pressures resulting in better shock absorption and cushioning. The high pressure areas are well accommodated and adjusted and whole foot has a balanced pressure. The foam layer compresses itself to accommodate the whole foot within itself and it easily adjusts itself when shearing takes place, minimizing the effect of shear.

A further follow up study was conducted for the selected patients at an interval of 3 months to monitor the trend of pressure distribution, and another follow up covering a period of over 6 months to monitor comparative progress of pressure reduction/distribution after recommended further use of footwear corrected to suit the foot of patient after initial period of usage. The plantar pressure was found to have either reduced further or have remained unchanged. The result shows that the methodology adopted for therapeutic application of the specially designed footwear for patients with diabetes and neuropathy has proven to be efficacious in minimizing underfoot pressure resulting in more comfort to the wearer.

TABLE 3 Plantar pressure comparison over six months' time span

Sl. No.	Bare Foot Pressure (KPa)	Fw. Pressure 1 (KPa)	Fw. Pressure 2 (KPa)	Fw. Pres-sure 3 (KPa)	Hrs. of Usage	Ulceration status
1	96.0	52	49	51	6–10 hrs.	No new ulcer
2	78.6	45	42	40	>10 hrs.	No new ulcer
3	77.3	33	29	34	6–10 hrs.	No new ulcer
4	71.7	38	35	39	6–10 hrs.	No new ulcer
5	69.4	40	34	36	6–10 hrs.	No new ulcer
6	68.0	38	33	36	6–10 hrs.	No new ulcer
7	66.5	21	16	18	6–10 hrs.	No new ulcer
8	53.4	33	34	30	6–10 hrs.	No new ulcer
9	49.1	33	35	32	6–10 hrs.	No new ulcer
10	48.6	26	24	29	6–10 hrs.	No new ulcer

The accompanying Figure 10 illustrates the graphical plot of the said data related to trend of pressure reduction pattern for each of selected ten subjects (patients) compared to the barefoot pressure reduction/distribution. The plot reveals drastic plantar pressure reduction which is clearly visible from the initial Barefoot plot and the TFW-follow up-1, TFW-follow up-2, and TFW-follow up-3 plots recorded on first visit wearing customized footwear and then on second and third visits respectively by the patients at intervals of 3 and 6 months of recommended usage.

The developed footwear thus targets specific high pressure areas particularly susceptible to neuropathic ulceration and with the right combination of lasts, materials, and design markedly reduces the pressures in these areas. The pedorthic therapeutic footwear, through use of specially designed rocker bottomed soles and custom molded footbeds, relieves underfoot biomechanical pressures to a very large extent.

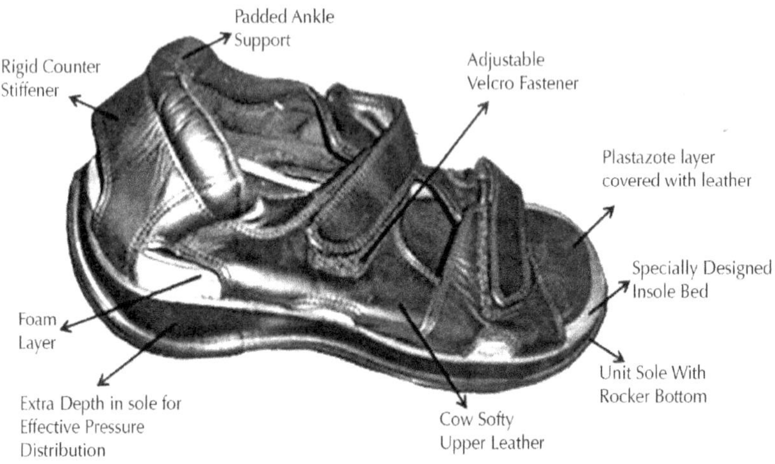

FIGURE 8 The newly developed footwear and its details.

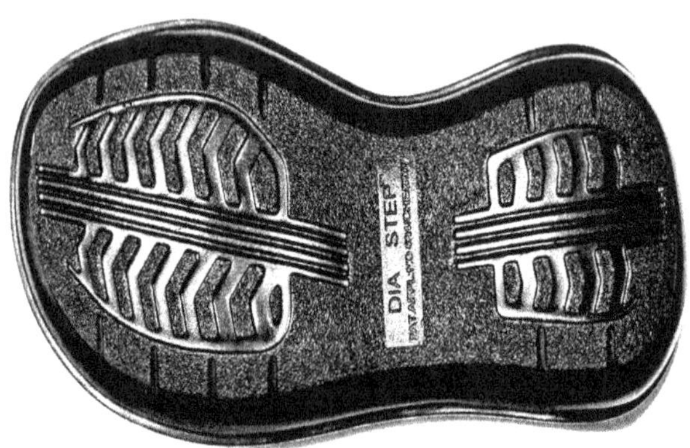

FIGURE 9 The outsole design provided with tread pattern for better grip and traction.

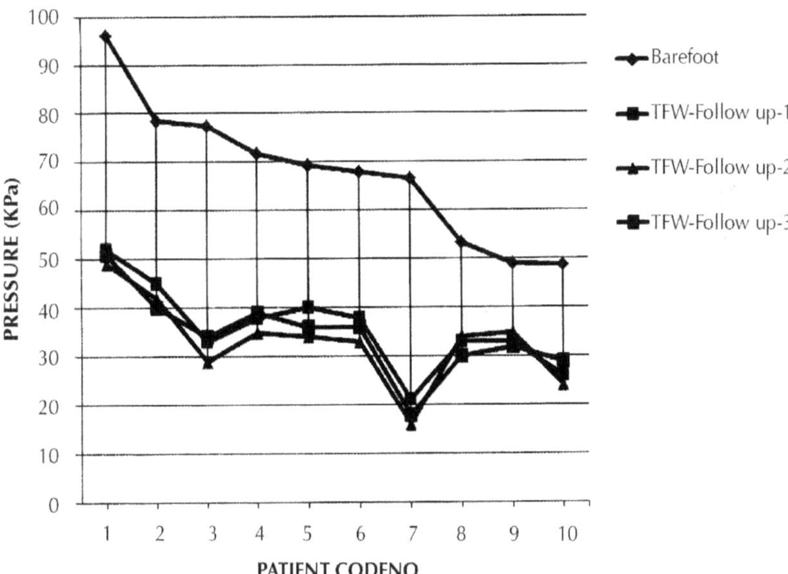

FIGURE 10 Comparison of barefoot pressures and pressures after wearing the specially designed therapeutic footwear at visits 0, 1, and 2.

Prevention and early interventions for foot ulcers are imperative to promote early healing and avoid foot/lower limb amputation. Improving the footwear design, durability, comfort, and the patient's knowledge on benefits of using therapeutic footwear and physician's knowledge on footwear design and material is essential in therapeutic intervention of treating diabetic foot using footwear. The new materials and new design for therapeutic footwear for patients with diabetes, that are developed in our study are the efforts to increase the appearance and performance of footwear for better compliance of wearing therapeutic footwear for regular use to treat and prevent diabetic foot complications. This will help in early healing and prevention of complications from diabetic foot ulcers, improved health, productivity and quality of life for patients with diabetes and reduced costs to patients, the health care system, and society.

KEYWORDS

- **Ankle-foot orthosis (AFO)**
- **Lower extremity amputation (LEA)**
- **Peripheral arterial disease (PAD)**
- **Peripheral neuropathy**
- **Quality function deployment (QFD)**
- **Therapeutic footwear (TFW)**

ACKNOWLEDGMENT

Authors thank all the patients who volunteered in studies with new design and materials for therapeutic footwear application and all supportive staff of CSIR-CLRI and MV hospital for diabetes.

REFERENCES

1. American Diabetes Association (ADA). *Ostomy. Wound Manag.*, **45**, 2–47 (1999).
2. American Diabetes Association. *Diabetes Care.*, **23**, S55–S56 (2000).
3. Abbott, C. A., Carrington, A. L., Ashe, H., Bath, S., Every, L. C., Griffiths, J., Hann, A. W., Hussein, A., Jackson, N., Johnson, K. E., Ryder, C. H., Torkington, R., Van Ross, E. R. E., Whalley, A. M., Widdows, P., Williamson, S., and Boulton, A. J. M. *Diabetic Med.*, **19**, 377–384 (2002).
4. Apelqvist, J., Larsson, J., and Agardh, C. D. *J. Diabetes. Compl.*, 4, 21 (1990).
5. Apelqvist, J. and Larsson, J. *Diabetes-Metab. Res.*, **16**, S75–S83 (2000).
6. Apelqvist, J, Bakker, K., van Houtum, W. H., Nabuurs-Franssen, M. H., and Schaper, N. C. *Diabetes-Metab. Res.*, **16**(1), S84–S92 (2000).
7. Armstrong, D. G., Lavery, L. A., and Harkless, L. B. *J. Am. Podiat. Med. Assn.*, **86**, 311–316 (1996).
8. Armstrong, D. G., Lavery, L. A., and Harkless, L. B. *Diabetes Care.*, **21**, 855–859 (1998).
9. Armstrong, D. G. and Lavery, L. A. *Am. Fam. Phys.*, **57,** 1325–1332 (1998).
10. Bakker, K. and Cavanagh, P. R. *Diabetes Metab. Res.*, **24**, S162–80 (2008).
11. Birke, J. A., Patout, C. A., and Foto, J. G. *J. Orthop. Sport. Phys.*, **30**, 91–97 (2000).
12. Boninger, M. L. and Leonard, J. A. Jr., *J. Rehab. Res. Dev.*, **33**, 16–22 (1996).
13. Brem, H., Sheehan, P., and Boulton, A. J. *Am. J. Surg.*, **187**, S1–S10 (2004).

14. Brodsky, J. W., Kourosh, S., Stills, N., and Mooney, V. *Foot Ankle.*, **9**, 111–116 (1988).
15. Bus, S. A., Ulbrecht, J. S., and Cavanagh, P. R. *Clin. Biomech.*, **9**, 629–638 (2004).
16. Bus, S. A., Valk, G. D., Deursen R. W. V., Armstrong, D. G., Caravaggi, C., Hlavácek, P., and Spencer, S. A. The Cochrane Collaboration. Published by John Wiley & Sons, Ltd. The Cochrane Library, (3) (2008).
17. Caravaggi, C., Faglia, E., Giglio, R. D., Mantero, M., Quarantiello, A., Sommariva, E., Gino, M., Pritelli, C., and Morabito, A. *Diabetes Care.*, **23**, 1746–1751 (2000).
18. Centers for Disease Control and Prevention (CDC). Hospital discharge rates for non-traumatic lower extremity amputation by diabetes status—United States, 1997. MMWR; 2001, 50, 954–958.
19. Chantelau, E. and Haage, P. *Diabet. Med.*, **11**, 114–116 (1994).
20. Crausaz, F. M., Clavel, S., Liniger, C., Albeanu, A., and Assal, J. P. *Diabetic Med.*, **5**, 771–775 (1988).
21. Pratt, D. J. *Clin. Biomech.*, **4**, 51–57 (1989).
22. Delmas, L. *Best Practice in the Assessment and Management of Diabetic Foot Ulcers. Rehabil. Nurs.*, **31**, 228–234 (2006).
23. Dubsky, M, Jirkovska, A, Bem, R, Fejfarova, V, Skibova, J, Schaper, N. C., and Lipsky, B. *A. Int. Wound J.*, doi: 10.1111/j.1742-481X.2012.01022.x (2012).
24. Edmonds, M. E., Blundell, M. P., Morris, M. E., et al. *Q. J. Med.*, **232**, 763–771 (1986).
25. Eggers, P., Gohdes, D., and Pugh, J. *Kidney Int.*, **56**, 1524–1533 (1999).
26. Faglia, E., Caravaggi, C., Clerici, G., Sganzaroli, A., Curci, V., Vailati, W., Simonetti, D., and Sommalvico, F. *Diabetes Care*, **33**, 1419–1423 (2010).
27. Fisher, L. R. and McLellan D. L. *Prosthet. Orthot. Int.*, **13**, 29–35 (1989).
28. Foundation for Accountability. Measuring health care quality: Diabetes. [AHCPR Publication no. 96-N021]. Rockville, MD, Agency for Health Care Policy and Research (1996).
29. Ghanassia, E., Villon, L., Franc, J., Dieudonn′E, O. T. D.; Boegner, C., Avignon, A., and Sultan, A. Long-Term Outcome and Disability of Diabetic Patients Hospitalized for Diabetic Foot Ulcers. *Diabetes Care.*, **31**, 1288–1292 (2008).
30. Giacalone, V. F., Armstrong, D. G., Ashry, H. R., Lavery, D. C., Harkless, L. B., and Lavery, L. A. *J Foot Ankle Surg.*, **36**, 28–30 (1997).
31. Herold, D. C. and Palmer, R. G. *J. Rheumatol.*, 19, 1542–1544 (1992).
32. Jahhs, M. H., Kummer, F., and Michelson, J. D. *Foot Ankle.*, **13**, 227–232 (1992).
33. Janisse, D. J. *Clin. Podiatr Med. Surg.*, **12**, 41–61 (1995).
34. Jannink, M. J., de Vries, J., Stewart R. E., Groothoff J. W., and Lankhorst, G. J. *J. Rehabil. Med.*, **36**, 242–248 (2004).
35. Lavery, L. A., Vela, S. A., Lavery, D. C., and Quebedeaux, T. L. *Diabetes Care.*, **19**, 818–821 (1996).
36. Lavery, L. A., Armstrong, D. G., Vela, S. A., Quebedeaux, T. L., and Fleischli, J. G. *Arch. Intern. Med.*, **158**, 157–162 (1998).
37. Levin, M. E., O'Neal, L., and Bowker, J. H. *The diabetic foot*, 5th edition. Mosby (1993).
38. Litzelman, D. K., Marriott, D. J., and Vinicor, F. *Diabetes Care*, **20**(8), 1273–1278 (1997).

39. Llewelyn, J. G., Thomas, P. K., and King, R. H. *J. Neurol.*, **245**, 159–165 (1998).
40. LoGerfo, F. W.and Coffman J. D. *N. Engl. J. Med.*, **311**, 1615–1619 (1984).
41. Moulik, P. K., Mtonga, R., Geoffrey V., and Gill, G.V. *Diabetes Care.*, **26**, 491–494 (2003).
42. Mueller, M. J. *J. Am. Podiatr. Med. Assoc.*, **87**, 360–364 (1997).
43. Netten, J. J. V. Hijmans, J. M., Jannink, M. J. A., Geertzen, J. H. B., and Postema, K. *J. Rehahil. Med.*, **41**, 913–918 (2009).
44. Pecoraro, R. E., Reiber, G., and Burgess, E. M. *Diabetes Care.*, **13**, 513–521 (1990).
45. Pratt, D. J. *Prosthet. Orthot. Int.*, **14**, 59–62 (1990).
46. Ramsey, S., Newton, K., Blough, D., McCulloch, D. K., Sandhu, N., Reiber, G. et al. *Diabetes Care.*, **22**, 382–387 (1999).
47. Reiber, G. E., Boyko, E. J., and Smith, D. G. Lower extremity foot ulcers and amputations in diabetes. In: National Diabetes Data Group (Ed.), Diabetes in America Washington, DC: DHHS 1995, 2nd ed. pp. 409–428.
48. Reiber, G. E. Epidemiology of foot ulcers and amputation in the diabetic foot. Levin and O'Neal's: The Diabetic Foot. Bowker, J.H.; Pfeifer, M. A(eds). St. Louis, CV Mosby, 6th Ed., 2001; pp 13–32.
49. Saraswathy, G., Gautham, G., and Das, B. N. *The Foot.*, **14**(4), 192–197 (2004).
50. Saraswathy, G., Gautham, G., Das, B. N., Ganga, R., and Pal, P. *J. Appl. Polym. Sci.*, **111**(5), 2387–2399 (2008).
51. Saraswathy, G., Gautham, G., Das, B. N., Ganga, R., Pal, S. *Polym. Plast. Tech. Engg.*, **48**, 239–250 (2009).
52. Shaw, J. E. and Boulton, A. J. M. *Diabetes*, **46** (suppl.), S58–S61 (1997).
53. Spencer, S. Pressure relieving interventions for preventing and treating diabetic foot ulcers. The Cochrane Database of Systematic Reviews. In: The Cochrane Library, Issue 1, 2003. The Cochrane Collaboration, 2004.
54. D.C. and Strunk, M. L. Orthot. Prosthet., 38(4), 41 - 48.
55. Sumpio, B. E. *N. Engl. J. Med.*, **343**, 787–793 (2000).
56. Tyrrell, W. *Nursing Standard*, **16**(30), 52–62 (2002).
57. Vijay, V., Sivagami, M., Saraswathy, G., Gautham, G., Das, B. N., Seena, R., Ambady, R. *Diabetes Care.*, **27**, 474–477 (2004).
58. Zimny, S, Schatz, H, and Pfohl, U. *Diabet Med.*, **20**(8),622–625 (2003).

CHAPTER 9

TEMPORAL EFFECT OF REPEATED STRESS ON TYPE-2 EXPERIMENTAL DIABETES

DEBAPRIYA GARABADU and SAIRAM KRISHNAMURTHY

CONTENTS

ABSTRACT

Type-2 diabetes mellitus patients are susceptible to stressors. The study evaluates the temporal effect of repeated stress in the pathophysiology of T2DM. The T2DM was induced in rats by streptozotocine (STZ, 45 mg/kg, i.p.) and nicotinamide (110 mg/kg, i.p.). Two exposures of cold restraint stress (CRS) were given 24 hr apart, before STZ injection (pre-diabetes) and after STZ injection (post-diabetes) to separate groups. The stress control group was exposed to two exposures of CRS. Repeated stress potentiates the pathobiogenesis of T2DM and T2DM aggravates the effect of repeated stress. Further, repeated stress after diabetes induction aggravates diabetes-induced metabolic parameters compared to before diabetes induction. Monoaminergic system, mitochondrial function, and integrity were evaluated in discrete brain regions such as, hippocampus (HIP), hypothalamus (HYP), prefrontal cortex (PFC), striatum (STR), amygdala (AMY), and nucleus accumbens (NAC). Diabetes, repeated stress and stress exposed diabetic rats showed region-specific changes in brain monoaminergic system, mitochondrial dysfunction and loss of integrity. Consequently, brain region-specific changes in oxidative damage and attenuated antioxidant defense system were observed. Temporal differences in brain monoaminergic system, mitochondrial dysfunction, integrity, oxidative damage, and reduced antioxidant defenses were found in both pre and post-diabetes stress exposed rodents. Thus, even though repeated stress exacerbates the physiological consequences of T2DM, it reported differences in the pattern of monoaminergic system, mitochondrial dysfunction in different brain regions. Hence, there are differences in the pathophysiology of stress, diabetes, and stress exposed diabetic conditions. Thus, different treatment paradigms may have to be developed other than conventional therapies to treat these conditions.

9.1 INTRODUCTION

Diabetes mellitus is the leading metabolic disorder prevalent both among the developed and developing countries. However, a majority of the patients belong to the T2DM. Recently, it has been reported that the changes in life style lead to an exponential growth of T2DM among young work force (Li et al., 2013). Further, it has been documented that the psychosocial, a chronic low level stress, increases the prevalence of T2DM apart from other predisposing factors (Faulenbach et al., 2011; Davila et al., 2011). Stress which alters both neuroendocrine and neurotransmitter levels in circulation and in various brain regions is considered to be an important factor in spurt of diabetes mellitus causes worldwide (Whitford et al., 2003). Hence, stress may have an important role in the pathogenesis of T2DM. However, there is no experimental report on the temporal effect of stress on the development of T2DM.

Tissues with high energy demands, such as brain, contain a large number of mitochondria, is more susceptible to the reduction in the aerobic energy metabolism. Increasing data support the idea that brain mitochondrial function declines in both diabetes and stress alone (Moreira et al., 2003; Gong et al., 2011; Cardoso et al., 2013), indicating that mitochondrial dysfunction is common to both disorders. Hence, we presume that in cases of co-occurring diabetes and stress, stress can aggravate brain mitochondrial dysfunction leading to alteration in diabetogenesis.

Mitochondria are produced in the cell body and transported to specific cellular locations of increased energy demands such as synapses. It is evident that synaptic transmission and remodeling require localized mitochondria to generate adenosine triphosphate (ATP) as well as to control local Ca^{2+} concentrations (Tang and Zucker, 1997; Schuman and Chan, 2004). While mitochondria are known to accumulate at the presynaptic terminal for neurotransmitter release (Chang et al., 2006), localization of mitochondria to the postsynaptic terminals has also been demonstrated (Li et al., 2004). Further, it has been established that neurotransmitters such as dopamine (DA) inhibit (Chen et al., 2008) and serotonin 5-hydroxytryptamine (5-HT) promote (Chen et al., 2007) axonal mitochondrial trafficking in the neurons, suggesting that mitochondrial activity plays an important role in the neuronal activity pertinent to specific neurotransmitter. Moreover, individual exposure to either diabetes or stress leads to alteration in brain monoamine metabolism which is not generalized but region-specific to both disorders (Kino et al., 2004). Hence, region-specific mitochondrial activity has to be explored to elaborate the mechanism for region-specific neuronal activity relevant to specific neurotransmitters.

Both hyperglycemia (Fiorentino et al., 2013) and stress (Volkova and Davydov, 2009) are reported to elicit an increase in reactive oxygen species (ROS) production in brain. Increased mitochondrial biogenesis is part of the cellular response to oxidative stress (Rasbach and Schnellmann, 2007). Mitochondrial biogenesis attenuates oxidative stress by increasing mitochondrial capacity to metabolite reducing equivalents. Cells undergoing mitochondrial biogenesis consume less oxygen, maintain mitochondrial membrane potential (MMP), and produce fewer ROS which together decrease cellular damage and increase survival (Karpińska and Gromadzka, 2013). Therefore, lipid oxidative damage may partly explain the mitochondrial biogenesis in different brain regions.

Hence, the present proposal explores the temporal effect of repeated CRS relative to the induction of T2DM. As mitochondria are the common substrate both in diabetes and stress, we aim to establish the mitochondrial basis as a consequence of aberrant neurotransmitter levels in different brain regions. Further, the oxidative stress is correlated with the mitochondrial biogenesis in different brain regions in comorbid diabetes and stress condition.

9.2 MATERIALS AND METHODS

9.2.1 ANIMALS

All experiments were conducted in compliance with the principles of laboratory animal care (NIH publication number 85–23, revised 1985) guidelines. Male Charles Foster strain albino rats (200–250 g) purchased from the Central Animal House, Institute of Medical Sciences, Banaras Hindu University, and were housed in polypropylene cages under controlled environmental conditions (25 ± 1°C, 45–55% relative humidity and 12:12 hr light/dark cycle). The animals had free access to commercial rat feed (Doodh dhara Pashu Ahar, India) and water ad libitum unless stated otherwise during the experiment. Animals were acclimatized for at least 1 week before using them for experiments and exposed only once to every experiment.

9.2.2 CHEMICALS

STZ, thiobarbituric acid (TBA), tetra methyl rhodamine methylester (TMRM), and dexamethasone were procured from Sigma (St. Louis, MO, USA). All other chemicals and reagents were available commercially from local suppliers and were of analytical grade.

9.2.3 INDUCTION OF T2DM

T2DM was induced in overnight fasted rats by a single injection of STZ (45 mg/kg, i.p.), 15 min after nicotinamide (110 mg/kg, i.p.) administration. The STZ was dissolved in 0.1 M citrate buffer (pH 4.5) and nicotinamide was dissolved in physiological saline (Masiello et al., 1998).

9.2.4 INDUCTION OF REPEATED CRS PROCEDURE

Two stress sessions 24 hr apart were performed during the early phase of the light cycle and consisting of a 1 hr restraint period (rat restrainers were transparent plastic tubes 15 cm long × 6.5 cm width) in a 4°C room (Sullivan and Szechtman, 1995).

9.2.5 THE EXPERIMENTAL DESIGN

The animals were acclimatized for 7 days and were randomly divided into five groups *viz*: control, diabetic (T2DM), stress, stress exposure before diabetes induction (pre-diabetes), and stress exposure after diabetes induction (post-diabetes). The day animals received the first exposure of stress was considered as day 1. The experimental protocol was followed for 9 days. The day-wise treatment of all groups is depicted in Table 1. The T2DM was induced in the pre-diabetes group after 24 hr of last episode of CRS, while post-diabetes group animals were killed after 24 hr of last episode of stress session. On day 4, two animals in T2DM group and one animal each in pre-diabetes and post-diabetes group were found dead. Two rats died on day 8 in the post-diabetes group. All the animals were killed on day 9 of the experimental protocol by cervical dislocation and, the brains were removed and were microdissected (Palkovits and Brownstein, 1988) into HIP, HYP, PFC, STR, AMY, and NAC and stored immediately at 80°C till further study.

9.2.6 ESTIMATION OF PLASMA GLUCOSE AND TRIGLYCERIDE (TG) LEVEL

In type-2 diabetes there is increase in the levels of glucose and TG in the plasma due to aberration in the metabolism of glucose and lipid respectively. Thus, the plasma glucose and TG were estimated in this experiment to observe the extent of abnormality in glucose and lipid metabolism respectively. Therefore, on the day 1, 3, 5, and 9 of the experimental protocol, 1 mL of blood was collected through retro-orbital puncture and centrifuged at 3000 g for 5 min at 4°C (Toleikis and Godin, 1995) to obtain plasma for measuring the glucose, TG and corticosterone (CORT) levels. The plasma glucose and TG were determined spectrophotometrically (Beckman Coulter DU 7400 UV–VIS Spectrophotometer; Fullerton, CA) in triplicate using the glucose (GOD PAP) kit (Priman Instrument Pvt. Ltd., India) and TG GPO-PAP kit (Span Diagnostics Ltd., India) respectively.

TABLE 1 Experimental protocol indicating day-wise exposure of stress and T2DM in rats

Groups	Day 1	Day 2	Day 3	Day 4	Day 5	Day 6	Day 7	Day 8	Day 9
Control	-	-	-	-	-	-	-	-	Killed
T2DM	-	-	STZ	-	-	-	-	-	Killed
Stress	CRS	CRS	-	-	-	-	-	-	Killed
Pre-diabetes	CRS	CRS	STZ	-	-	-	-	-	Killed
Post-diabetes	-	-	STZ	-	-	-	CRS	CRS	Killed

9.2.7 ESTIMATION OF PLASMA CORT LEVEL

The secretion of CORT to plasma is considered as a peripheral measure of hypothalamic–pituitary–adrena (HPA) axis function. Thus, the extent of effect of either CRS or type-2 diabetes or their combination on HPA axis activity was evaluated by assessing the level of CORT in the plasma. The plasma CORT was quantified in a High Performance Liquid Chromatography (HPLC) with Ultraviolet (UV) detector system (Waters, USA, Garabadu et al., 2011). The chromatogram was recorded and analyzed with Empower software (Version 2.0).

9.2.8 ESTIMATION OF ULCER INDEX

It is well accepted that the gastric ulcers are predominant in psychologically stressed animals and the gastric ulcers are considered as the markers of deleterious effect of stress. Thus, in this experiment, we had estimated the ulcer index as a measure of stress. The stomach was cut through greater curvature and a blind observer calculated the ulcer index by following standard protocol (Sairam et al., 2002).

9.2.9 ASSESSMENT OF MITOCHONDRIAL FUNCTION, INTEGRITY, AND OXIDATIVE STRESS

MITOCHONDRIA ISOLATION PROCEDURE

Mitochondria were isolated by following standard procedure of Pedersen et al., (1978). Briefly, the brain regions were homogenized in (1:10, w/v) ice cold isolation buffer (250 mM sucrose, 1 mM EGTA, and 10 mM HEPES–KOH, pH 7.2) followed by centrifugation at 600 × g/5 min. The resultant supernatant was centrifuged at 10,000 × g/15 min. The resultant pellets were suspended in 1 mL medium (250 mM sucrose, 0.3 mM EGTA, and 10 mM HEPES–KOH, pH 7.2) and again centrifuged at 14,000

× g/10 min. All centrifugation procedures were performed at 4°C. The final mitochondrial pellet was resuspended in medium (250 mM sucrose and 10 mM HEPES–KOH, pH 7.2) and used within 3 hr. The mitochondrial protein content was estimated using the method of Lowry et al., 1951.

ESTIMATION OF MITOCHONDRIAL SUCCINATE DEHYDROGENASE (SDH) ACTIVITY

During energy metabolism in the cytoplasm of the cell, a number of electron carriers such as nicotinamide adenine dinucleotide (NADH), nicotinamide adenine dinucleotide phosphate (NADPH), and so on are formed in the cytoplasm. They enter into the mitochondrial matrix and move through the electron transport chain to generate ATP. The mitochondrial SDH enzyme is the complex-II enzyme of the electron transport chain. The mitochondrial SDH activity was evaluated to assess the function of mitochondria. The mitochondrial SDH was determined by following standard protocol (Sally and Margaret, 1989) based on the progressive reduction of nitro blue tetrazolium (NBT) to an insoluble colored compound diformazan (dfz) which was used as a reaction indicator. The reaction of NBT was mediated by H^+ released in the conversion of succinate to fumarate. The concentration of NBT–dfz produced was measured at 570 nm. The mean SDH activity of each region was expressed as micromole formazan produced per min per milligram of protein.

ESTIMATION OF MMP

During ATP generation in the mitochondria, a potential difference is observed across the inner mitochondrial membrane due to the movement of hydrogen ion. The TMRM is bound to the hydrogen ion and gets excited and thus exhibits fluorescence. The TMRM uptake was directly proportional to the potential across the inner mitochondrial membrane. The Rhodamine dye taken up by mitochondria was measured with spectrofluorometer (Hitachi, F-2500, Japan; Huang, 2002). Briefly, the mitochondrial suspension was mixed with TMRM solution and incubated for 5 min at

25°C followed by frequent washings (four times) to remove any unbound TMRM. The florescence emission was read at an excitation λ of 535 ± 10 nm and emission λ of 580 ± 10 nm using slit number 10. The peak fluorescence intensity recorded was around 570 ± 5 nm. The intensity of fluorescence was recorded which was considered to be proportional to MMP.

ESTIMATION OF MITOCHONDRIAL MALONDIALDEHYDE (MDA)

The lipid peroxidation (LPO) has been established as a major mechanism of cellular injury in most biological systems. The mechanism involves a process where unsaturated lipids are oxidized to form reactive radical species as well as toxic by products that can be harmful to the host system. Polyunsaturated lipids are especially susceptible to this type of damage and they can react to form lipid peroxides. The LPO are themselves unstable, and undergo additional decomposition to form a complex series of compounds including reactive carbonyl compounds. Polyunsaturated fatty acid peroxides further react to form MDA. Therefore, mitochondrial MDA content was measured described by Uchiyama and Mihara (1978) and modified by Sunderman et al., (1985) to explore the extent of oxidative damage. Briefly, the chromophore MDA formed from TBA in the reaction was measured at 532 nm. The MDA concentrations were expressed as micromoles of MDA per milligram of protein.

ESTIMATION OF MITOCHONDRIAL SUPEROXIDE DISMUTASE (SOD) ACTIVITY

The SOD enzyme catalyzes the dismutation of peroxide radicals into hydrogen peroxide and water, and thus minimizes oxidative damage. The mitochondrial SOD activity was evaluated to assess the extent of antioxidant activity. The activity of SOD was assayed by the method of Kakkar et al, (1984) based on the formation of NADH–phenazine methosulphate measured at 560 nm against butanol as blank. A single unit of the enzyme was expressed as 50% inhibition of NBT reduction per minute per milligram of protein under the assay conditions.

ESTIMATION OF MITOCHONDRIAL CATALASE (CAT) ACTIVITY

The CAT enzyme converts hydrogen peroxides into water and thus exhibits antioxidative activity. Thus, the extent of antioxidative activity of mitochondrial CAT enzyme was measured in this experiment. The decomposition of hydrogen peroxide in presence of CAT was followed at 240 nm (Beers and Sizer, 1952). The results were expressed as units (U) of CAT activity/min/mg of protein.

ESTIMATION OF BRAIN SEROTONIN (5-HT), NOREPINEPHRINE (NE), DOPAMINE (DA), AND THEIR METABOLITES

The level of 5-HT, NE, DA and their metabolites were estimated in distinct brain regions using HPLC/ electrochemical detection (ECD) to understand the neurochemical basis of stress and diabetes interaction (Garabadu et al., 2011).

9.2.10 DATA ANALYSIS

The results are expressed as mean ± standard error of the mean (SEM). The statistical significance for time-course effects on plasma glucose, TG and CORT levels were analyzed by two-way analysis of variance (ANOVA) followed by *post hoc* Bonferroni test. All other data sets were analyzed by one-way ANOVA followed by *post hoc* Student–Newman–Keuls test. $P < 0.05$ was considered to be statistically significant throughout the experimental data analysis.

9.3 DISCUSSION

The basic objective of the present investigation was to evaluate the temporal effect of repeated CRS in the pathobiogenesis of experimentally-induced type-2 diabetes in rats. Presently, we report that repeated stress potentiated diabetogenesis and complimentarily, type-2 diabetes aggravated the consequences of repeated CRS. Interestingly, post-diabetes stress exposure was more precarious than pre-diabetes stress exposure. Mitochondrial dysfunction, loss of mitochondrial integrity and mitochondrial oxidative damages were observed in all most all brain regions in post-diabetes stressed animals. Further, overall monoaminergic changes in different brain regions were more significant in post-diabetes stressed rats than pre-diabetes stressed animals. Thus, we for the first time show the temporal effect of stress on diabetogenesis, which may have important implications in treatment of co-occurring type-2 diabetes and stress.

Both clinical and preclinical studies indicate that stress can also induce hyperglycemia as observed in type-2 diabetes (Faulenbach et al., 2011; Davila et al., 2011). In the present study, we for the first time report that pre- and post-diabetes stress exposure caused significant hyperglycemia during the course of diabetogenesis. However, hyperglycemia was higher in post-diabetes than pre-diabetes stress exposure on day 9. This shows that not only stress significantly aggravates diabetogenesis but is also dependent on the time of stress exposure relative to diabetes induction. Moreover, we also found that stress had a time variable effect on diabetes with respect to the level of TG similar to that of hyperglycemia. Earlier studies have reported that diabetes and stress alone leads to hypertriglyceridaemia (Reaven et al., 1975; Kushnerova et al., 2007). Therefore, stress altered the metabolic consequences of type-2 diabetes which was however time-dependent.

The CRS is a well established psychological stress model where ulcer index is used as a marker for severity of stress (Garabadu et al., 2011; Krishnamurthy et al., 2011). Similarly, gastric ulcers are reported in diabetic subjects (Hanson et al., 1990). In the present study, significant gastric ulcers were observed with repeated CRS in contrast to type-2 diabetes. Interestingly, gastric ulcers in post-diabetes stress condition were comparatively higher in numbers and severity than pre-diabetes stress condition, indicating the temporal effect of stress on type-2 diabetes. Therefore, diabetogenesis could aggravate the consequences of stress, the severity depending upon the timing of exposure of stress.

Hypercorticosteronemia is commonly observed in both stress and diabetes (Wang et al., 2004; Kumar et al., 2007; de Oliveira et al., 2011), a result of over-activation of HPA axis (Krishnamurthy et al., 2013). In the present study, both type-2 diabetes and repeated CRS caused significant increase in CORT level on day 9 signifying the exaggerated activation of HPA axis. There was significant increase in the level of CORT in the plasma in the post-diabetic stressed animals on day 9 than all other group rats. These results indicate that repeated stress can influence the outcome of hypercorticosteronemia in T2DM depending upon the time of exposure. As hypercortisolemia is a cardinal metabolic disturbance observed in type-2 diabetic patients (Chiodini et al., 2007), it can be assumed that the hyperglycemia and hypertriglyceridaemia may be due to hypercorticosteronemia. The exact plausible mechanism has to be further investigated.

It has been suggested that CORT has significant diabetogenic effect upon biochemical functions of liver mitochondria in diabetic rats (Brignone et al., 1991). Further, hyperglycemia and hypertriglyceridaemia can lead to ROS production which can compromise mitochondrial function (Cardoso et al., 2010; Benani et al., 2007). The activity of SDH is considered as a marker for electron transport chain (ETC) and mitochondrial function (Reddy et al., 2011). The present study reveals that both T2DM (except HYP) and stress increased the SDH activity in all the brain regions. This indicates that stress and T2DM increases mitochondrial function and produce region-specific SDH activity independently. These results are similar to those observed by other studies, where brain mitochondrial SDH activity has been increased both in diabetic and stress conditions (Patel and Katyare, 2006; Ceretta et al., 2010). Diabetes-induced increase in SDH activity was further augmented in all the brain regions when stress exposed to type-2 diabetic rats either before or after STZ injection. Hence, there exist regional differences in brain mitochondrial function in terms of SDH activity in co-occurring diabetes and stress conditions. This shows that brain mitochondrial bioenergetics is different in stress, T2DM and in stressed diabetic rats.

The activity of ETC and MMP, a marker for mitochondrial integrity are closely associated (Reddy et al., 2011). Moreover, cells undergoing mitochondrial biogenesis maintain MMP (Cohen et al., 2004). In the present study, both T2DM and stress decreased the MMP in all the brain regions, indicating loss of mitochondrial integrity and decrease in mitochondrial biogenesis (Cardoso et al., 2010 and Gong et al., 2011). Further, the magnitude of loss in MMP was higher in post-diabetes than pre-diabetes stress exposure. Therefore, the loss of mitochondrial integrity and decrease in mitochondrial biogenesis were influenced by stress and its timing of exposure in diabetic rats.

The role of oxidative lipid and protein damage in the pathogenesis of the diabetic state and stress conditions has been studied extensively (Fukui et al., 2001). The current observations indicate that diabetes elevated MDA level especially in HIP, HYP and STR. Repeated stress caused oxidative damage in all the brain regions except AMY. These results suggest that both diabetes and stress can cause region-specific oxidative damage which is similar to the earlier findings (Tuzcu and Baydas, 2006; Menabde et al., 2011). It is interesting to note that HIP, HYP and STR share a common target for oxidative damage induced by either diabetes or stress condition. The magnitude of mitochondrial oxidative damage in co-occurring diabetes and stress condition was higher than type-2 diabetic rats in all the brain regions except NAC. Further, post-diabetes stress exposure caused significant increase in oxidative damage in all the brain regions than pre-diabetes stressed rats. Considering both LPO and MMP, mitochondrial biogenesis is severely attenuated in all the brain regions of post-diabetes stressed rats as mitochondrial biogenesis is part of the cellular response to oxidative stress (Rasbach and Schnellmann, 2007). Furthermore, mitochondrial lipid oxidative damage also follows a temporal pattern as observed with loss of mitochondrial function and integrity relative to timing of stress in diabetic rats. In the present study, stress during diabetes increased the SDH activity (except HYP and STR) even though; this did not translate to loss of MMP in all the brain regions, indicating that other mechanisms may be involved apart from SDH activity in the ETC (Singer et al., 1973).

Several reports have suggested that there is decrease in the activities of anti-oxidant enzymes in diabetic as well as stress conditions (Preet et al., 2005; Siddiqui et al., 2005; Menabde et al., 2011). Here, the diabetes and stress-induced attenuation in antioxidant defense system (in terms of SOD and CAT activity) was common to HYP and STR. The diabetes-induced attenuation of antioxidant defense system was further aggravated by pre-diabetes stress exposure in HYP, PFC and NAC. However, post-diabetes stress exposure aggravated diabetes-induced loss in antioxidant enzyme activities in all the brain regions. Comparatively, the extent of loss in antioxidant enzymes activity was more significant during post-diabetes stress exposure than pre-diabetes stress exposure. The decreased activities of SOD and CAT may be in response to increased production of hydrogen peroxide and superoxide by the auto-oxidation of excess glucose in hyperglycemic condition (Aragno et al., 1997). Therefore, the region-specific loss in antioxidant defense mechanism also follows temporal pattern as observed with mitochondrial lipid oxidative damage, loss in mitochondrial function and integrity.

In the present study, the level of 5-HT, 5-HIAA and their turnover were changed region-specifically in all the brain regions in both type-2 diabetes and stressed rodents which are similar to that of earlier reports (Kino et al., 2004; Barber et al., 2003). The present study explores the fact that the extent of loss of 5-HT level was more in all the brain regions in post-diabetes stressed animals compared to pre-diabetes stressed rats suggesting that stress after type-2 diabetes induction may further exaggerate serotonergic system. Furthermore, both prediabetes and post-diabetes stressed rats showed increase in 5-HIAA level in all the brain regions except HIP compared to type-2 diabetic animals. While only post-diabetes stressed rats showed significant increase in 5-HIAA level in HIP compared to type-2 diabetic animals. However, the level of 5-HIAA was more in all the brain regions in post-diabetes stressed rats compared to pre-diabetes stressed animals indicating that the excess metabolite of 5-HT may be due to over activity of either 5-HT neurons or metabolizing enzymes. Similarly, both pre and post-diabetes stressed rats showed increase in 5-HIAA/5-HT ratio in all the brain regions except HIP compared to type-2 diabetic animals. In HIP only post-diabetes stressed animals showed increase in 5-HIAA/5-HT ratio compared to type-2 diabetic rats. Further, the 5-HIAA/5-HT ratio was higher in all the brain regions in post-diabetes stressed rats compared to pre-diabetes stressed animals, suggesting that stress after T2DM induction may hyper activate the serotonergic system in all the brain regions.

Earlier reports have suggested that the change in the level of NE is region-specific in both type-2 diabetes and stress condition separately which is similar to our present findings (Kino et al., 2004; Barber et al., 2003). When stress was associated with T2DM, both pre- and post-diabetes stressed rats showed significant increase in the level of NE in HIP and PFC compared to type-2 diabetic animals. However, the level of increase in NE was higher in STR, AMY, and NAC in post-diabetes stressed rats compared to type-2 diabetic animals, but the pre-diabetes stressed rats showed significant increase in NE level compared to type-2 diabetic animals. Further, post-diabetes stressed rats showed significant increase in NE level in all the brain regions except HYP (decrease) suggesting that repeated CRS after T2DM induction led to over activity of noradrenergic system in almost all brain regions.

Both T2DM and repeated CRS caused region-specific changes in the levels of DA, DOPAC and HVA, and ratios of DOPAC/DA and HVA/DA individually in the present study which are similar to earlier reports (Kino et al., 2004; Barber et al., 2003). Both pre- and post-diabetes stress exposure caused significant decrease in the level of DA in HYP and STR compared to type-2 diabetes. Moreover, the level of DA was decreased significantly in PFC of post-diabetes stressed rats only compared to type-2 diabetic animals. Further, the extent of decrease in the level of DA was more in PFC only in post-diabetes stressed animals compared to pre-diabetes stressed rats, suggesting that stress after T2DM induction specifically affects PFC though stress and type-2 diabetes showed region-specific changes in the level of DA in more than one brain regions when considered alone. Only post-diabetes stressed rats showed increase in both DOPAC and HVA level in all the brain regions compared to type-2 diabetic and pre-diabetes stressed animals. However, the ratio of DOPAC/DA was higher in HYP and NAC in both pre and post-diabetes stressed rats compared to type-2 diabetic animals. But, only post-diabetes stressed rats showed significant increase in the ratio of DOPAC/DA in PFC, STR, and AMY compared to type-2 diabetic animals. Further, the extent of increase in the ratio of DOPAC/DA was higher in all the brain regions except HIP in post-diabetes stressed rats compared to pre-diabetes stressed animals. Furthermore, the ratio of HVA/DA was more in HYP, PFC and STR in both pre and post-diabetes stressed animals compared to type-2 diabetic rodents. But, there was significant increase in the ratio of HVA/DA in AMY and NAC in post-diabetes stressed rodents compared to type-2 diabetic rats. The extent of increase in the ratio of HVA/DA was higher in all the brain regions except HIP in post-diabetes stressed rats compared to pre-diabetes stressed animals, indicating that stress after T2DM induction led to region-specific over activity of dopaminergic system.

The neuronal activity relevant to specific neurotransmitter is strongly modulated by mitochondrial activity (Kino et al., 2004). We have reported that post-diabetes stress caused increase in serotonergic turnover in almost all the brain regions except STR. This effect could be due to either decrease in neuronal activity or increased activity of metabolizing enzymes of serotonergic system. Further, as 5-HT promotes axonal mitochondrial trafficking in serotonergic neurons (Chen et al., 2007), decrease in mitochondrial biogenesis and integrity may underlie the neuronal activity of serotonergic neurons. Similarly, the change in noradrenergic system was observed in all the brain regions of both pre- and post-diabetes stressed animals. The present study revealed that the NE level was higher in all the brain regions of post-diabetes stressed rats than pre-diabetes stressed animals with the exception that in HYP the level of NE was significantly lower in post-diabetes stress group animals than prediabetes stress group rats. Though there is no report on mitochondria trafficking of noradrenergic system, the present study shows that the noradrenergic system follows similar trend of serotonergic system with axonal mitochondrial trafficking which has to be clarified in the future studies. Likewise serotonergic and noradrenergic system, the changes in dopaminergic system were observed in all the brain regions of diabetic rats those exposed to repeated stress temporally relative to diabetes induction. Pre- and post-diabetes stressed animals showed increase in DA turnover in all the brain regions, and the increase in DA turnover was higher in post-diabetes stress exposure than pre-diabetes stress exposure in all the brain regions. Therefore, the increased DA turnover may underlie the decreased mitochondrial biogenesis and integrity as DA inhibits axonal mitochondrial trafficking (Chen et al., 2008). Studies in animal models of diabetes demonstrate cognitive, structural, neurochemical and psychobiologic alterations, besides cellular apoptotic activity on central nervous system (CNS); however, the mechanisms are not well elucidated (Biessels et al., 1994). In the present study, comorbid diabetes and stress condition shows the changes in neurochemical levels and mitochondrial function in different brain regions which may lead to behavioral abnormalities, which has to be evaluated in the future studies.

In conclusion, we report the effect of repeated stress and its temporal effect on type-2 experimental diabetes. Repeated stress potentiates the pathobiogenesis of type-2 diabetes and type-2 diabetes aggravates the effect of repeated stress. Hence, there seem to be a bi-directional relationship between diabetes and repeated stress. Interestingly, we observe that timing of stress relative to diabetes induction produce differential effects. Repeated stress after diabetes induction aggravates diabetes-induced metabolic parameters than before diabetes induction. Similarly, the effects of stress are exacerbated in post-diabetes stress exposure than pre-diabetes stress exposure. Diabetes, repeated stress and stress exposed diabetic rats show region-specific changes in brain monoamine system, mitochondrial dysfunction and loss of integrity in different regions of the brain. Consequently to mitochondrial dysfunction the brain region-specific changes in oxidative damage and attenuated antioxidant defense system are observed. Temporal differences in mitochondrial dysfunction, integrity, oxidative damage and reduced antioxidant defenses are found in both pre- and post-diabetes stress exposed rodents. Thus, even though repeated stress exacerbates the physiological consequences of type-2 diabetes, we report differences in pattern of mitochondrial dysfunction in different brain regions. Thus, due differences in mitochondrial bioenergetics in different brain regions the pathophysiology of stress; diabetes and stress during diabetes may be different. This may require different treatment paradigms other than conventional therapies to treat these conditions. Nevertheless, drugs targeting mitochondria may be useful in the treatment of co-occurring type-2 diabetes and stress conditions.

9.4 RESULTS

9.4.1 THE ALTERATION IN BIOCHEMICAL PARAMETERS SUCH AS PLASMA GLUCOSE, TG, AND CORT LEVEL IN TEMPORALLY TREATED REPEATED STRESS ON TYPE-2 DIABETIC RATS

Table 2 shows the alteration in the plasma glucose, TG, and CORT levels in rats at different time points of STZ induction. Two-way ANOVA revealed that there were significant differences for plasma glucose, TG and CORT levels among group ([$F(4, 12) = 2.32$, $P < 0.05$], [$F(4, 12) = 1.99$, $P < 0.05$] and [$F(4, 12) = 4.16$, $p < 0.05$] respectively) and time

([F (3, 12) = 6.89, P< 0.05], [F (3, 12) = 7.80, P< 0.05] and [F (3, 12) = 4.36, p< 0.05] respectively). *Post hoc* analysis revealed that on day 5 (3rd day of STZ injection); diabetes was induced in all STZ injected groups as observed from increase in plasma glucose level to more than 250 mg/dl. Even though stress caused hyperglycemia, the increase in glucose level was below the normal diabetes range on day 5. However, introduction of repeated two days stress before diabetic induction significantly increased glucose level on day 5 even significantly higher than the diabetes group. There was significant increase in glucose level on day 9 compared to day 5 in T2DM, pre and post-diabetes groups. However, in the stress group there were no significant changes in glucose level between day 5 and day 9. On day 9 (7th day of STZ injection), the glucose level was significantly higher in both prediabetes and postdiabetes groups compared to T2DM group. However, the extent of hyperglycemia was more in case of post-diabetes than pre-diabetes group. Similarly, the plasma TG profile followed the same pattern as that of glucose level indicating that metabolic parameters were altered profoundly with the temporal treatment of repeated stress on diabetes especially in post-diabetes stress condition.

TABLE 2 The time-dependent changes in the level of plasma glucose, TG and CORT in stress, diabetes and stress exposed diabetic rats at different time point of the experimental protocol

Group	Day	Glucose (mg/dl)	Triglyceride (mg/dl)	Corticosterone (μg/dl)
Control	1	75.05 ± 0.95	87.88 ± 2.56	16.6 ± 0.35
	3	74.95 ± 0.99	88.13 ± 2.99	16.38 ± 0.39
	5	76.01 ± 0.73	88.46 ± 1.81	16.73 ± 0.41
	9	76.09 ± 0.66	87.37 ± 1.64	16.58 ± 0.33
T2DM	1	71.90 ± 1.23	81.34 ± 1.77	16.56 ± 0.35
	3	75.97 ± 1.14	89.81 ± 1.30	16.56 ± 0.29
	5	268.09 ± 7.13a,b,*	189.31 ± 1.49a,b,*	23.27 ± 0.19a,b,*
	9	512.79 ± 2.93a,b,c,*	393.67 ± 11.64a,b,c,*	43.55 ± 0.29a,b,c,*

TABLE 2 *(Continued)*

Stress	1	71.68 ± 1.11	88.89 ± 2.92	16.65 ± 0.48
	3	80.44 ± 1.87	95.20 ± 1.48	122.15 ± 0.29a,*,@
	5	116.67 ± 3.40a,b,*,@	150.98 ± 1.77a,b,*,@	133.18 ± 0.45a,b,*,@
	9	124.13 ± 4.69a,b,*,@	156.25 ± 1.59a,b,*,@	144.25 ± 1.61a,b,c,*,@
Pre-diabetes	1	76.86 ± 1.16	86.36 ± 1.83	16.70 ± 0.22
	3	123.61 ± 0.73a,*,@,$	103.16 ± 0.91a,*,@,$	122.38 ± 0.23a,*,@
	5	283.37 ± 5.37a,b,*,@,$	232.28 ± 4.46a,b,*,@,$	122.44 ± 0.42a,*,@,$
	9	471.69 ± 3.52a,b,c,*,@,$	381.19 ± 3.22a,b,c,*,@,$	138.30 ± 0.71a,b,c,*,@,$
Post-diabetes	1	74.87 ± 1.71	89.39 ± 2.98	16.65 ± 0.29
	3	77.81 ± 3.84	92.57 ± 1.73	16.25 ± 0.19
	5	251.77 ± 3.05a,b,*,$,#	209.68 ± 1.79a,b,*,$,#	25.72 ± 0.72 a, b,*,$,#
	9	578.66 ± 0.68a,b,c,*,@,$,#	466.67 ± 12.10 a, b, c,*,@,$,#	193.37 ± 1.11 a, b, c,*,@,$,#

All values are Mean ± SEM. [a]$P< 0.05$ compared to Day-1, [b]$P< 0.05$ compared to Day-3, [c]$P< 0.05$ compared to Day-5, *$P< 0.05$ compared to control, [@]$P< 0.05$ compared to T2DM, [$]$P< 0.05$ compared to stress and [#]$P< 0.05$ compared to prediabetes.

Stress caused significant increase in plasma CORT level on day 5 (3rd day after last episode of repeated CRS) compared to control. There was significant hypercorticosteronemia in diabetes compared to control. However, the extent of hypercorticosteronemia in stress was relatively higher compared to diabetes. Pre-diabetes showed higher hypercorticosteronemia compared to diabetes. However, the increase in plasma CORT level was still higher in stress group compared to pre-diabetes group, indicating that diabetes interferes with the stress response. Further on day 5, the repeated stress exposure was not performed in post-diabetes group and therefore the pattern of plasma CORT level was similar to that of T2DM group. Interestingly, the magnitude of increase in the plasma CORT level in all the experimentally manipulated groups was significantly higher on day 9 compared to day 5. Moreover, the extent of hypercorticosteronemia was significantly higher in post-diabetes group compared to pre-diabetes group, suggesting that diabetes is more prone to stress exposure.

9.4.2 THE EFFECT OF REPEATED CRS ON DIABETIC RATS RELATIVE TO STZ-INDUCTION ON ULCER INDEX

The result of CRS exposed diabetic rats at different time point of STZ induction in terms of ulcer index is depicted in Figure 1. Statistical analysis by One-way ANOVA showed that the ulcer index was significantly different among groups [F (4, 19) = 52.73, P< 0.05]. *Post hoc* analysis revealed that in contrast to diabetes group, stress caused significant gastric ulcer compared to control. There was significant increase in ulcer index in both pre and post-diabetes stress exposure compared to diabetes control. Moreover, post-diabetes group showed increased ulcer index compared to pre-diabetes group, indicating that diabetes facilitates the stress response.

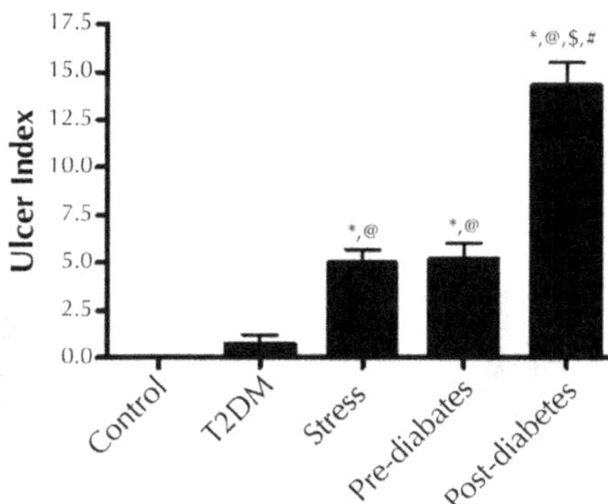

FIGURE 1 The effect of diabetes, stress and their combinations on ulcer index. All values are Mean ± SEM. **P*< 0.05 compared to control, @*P*< 0.05 compared to T2DM, $*P*< 0.05 compared to stress and #*P*< 0.05 compared to prediabetes.

9.4.3 TEMPORAL EFFECT OF REPEATED CRS CHALLENGED DIABETIC RATS ON MITOCHONDRIAL FUNCTION AND INTEGRITY IN DIFFERENT BRAIN REGIONS

The alterations in the SDH activity (A) and MMP (B) in different brain regions is depicted in Figure 2. Statistical analysis revealed that there was significant difference among groups in percentage activity of complex-2 enzyme SDH in HIP [F (4, 19) = 301.46, P< 0.05], HYP [F (4, 19) – 60.510], PFC [F (4, 19) = 99.586, P< 0.05], STR [F (4, 19) = 228.46, P< 0.05], AMY [F (4, 19) = 174.37, P< 0.05] and NAC [F (4, 19) = 115.13, P< 0.05]. Diabetes increased the SDH activity in all brain regions except HYP compared to control. Stress significantly increased SDH activity in all brain regions compared to control. Pre and post-diabetes groups showed increased SDH activity in all the brain regions compared to control and diabetes groups. However, the SDH activity of post-diabetes group was higher in all brain regions except HYP and STR compared to pre-diabetes group.

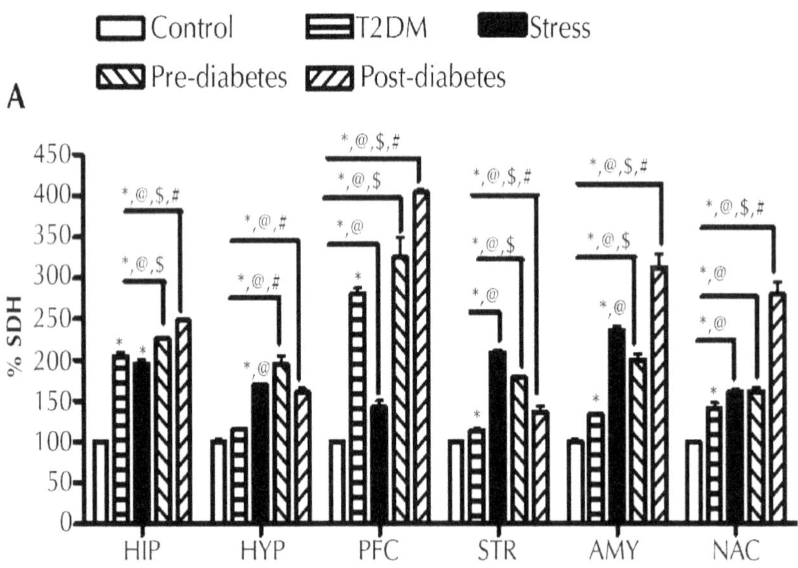

FIGURE 2 *(Continued)*

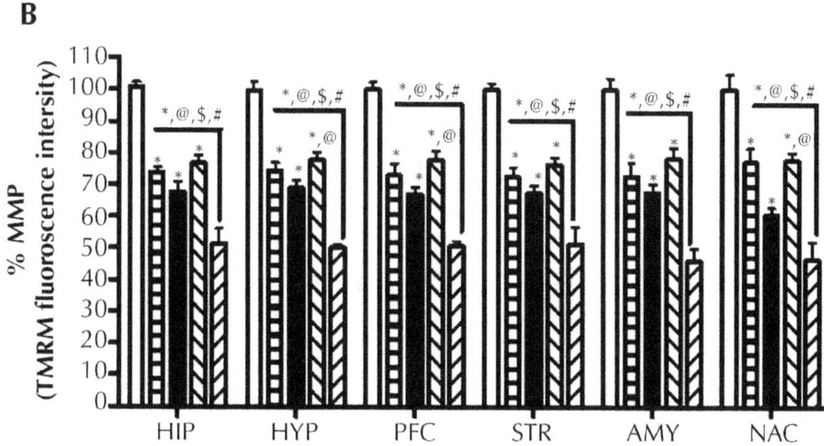

FIGURE 2 The changes in mitochondrial function in terms of SDH (A) activity and MMP (B) in different brain regions of stress, diabetes and their combinations are depicted. All values are Mean ± SEM. **P*< 0.05 compared to control, @*P*< 0.05 compared to T2DM, $*P*< 0.05 compared to stress and #*P*< 0.05 compared to prediabetes.

Similarly, statistical analysis revealed that there was significant interactions among groups in percentage of MMP in HIP [F (4, 19) = 38.24, P< 0.05], HYP [F (4, 19) = 46.65, P< 0.05], PFC [F (4, 19) = 49.36, P< 0.05], STR [F (4, 19) = 34.71, P< 0.05], AMY [F (4, 19) = 28.76, P< 0.05] and NAC [F (4, 19) = 26.54, P< 0.05]. *Post hoc* analysis revealed that the MMP was decreased in all the brain regions of T2DM, stress, pre and post-diabetes compared to control. However, post-diabetes group caused a significant loss in MMP in all the brain regions compared to all other experimental manipulations.

9.4.4 MITOCHONDRIAL OXIDATIVE STRESS IN DIFFERENT BRAIN REGIONS IS MODULATED BY THE REPEATED CRS TREATMENT TO DIABETIC RATS AT DIFFERENT TIME POINT OF DIABETES INDUCTION

Figure 3 depicts the effect of CRS challenged diabetic rats at different time point of STZ induction on mitochondrial LPO (A), SOD (B) and

CAT (C) activities. Statistical analysis revealed that there were significant differences in percentage of MDA level among groups in HIP [F (4, 19) = 20.54, P< 0.05], HYP [F (4, 19) = 61.85, P< 0.05], PFC [F (4, 19) = 153.7, P< 0.05], STR [F (4, 19) = 31.40, P< 0.05], AMY [F (4, 19) = 24.94, P< 0.05] and NAC [F (4, 19) = 28.07, P< 0.05]. *Post hoc* analysis revealed that the increase in the MDA level was restricted to HIP, HYP and STR in T2DM group. However, stress significantly increased the MDA level in all the brain regions except AMY compared to control rats. The diabetes-induced oxidative damage in terms of increased MDA level was extended to PFC and AMY in pre-diabetes group, but post-diabetes group showed significant oxidative damage in all the brain regions. Further, the extent of oxidative damage in post-diabetes group was higher compared to pre-diabetes group in all the brain regions, suggesting that stress after diabetes increase the severity of oxidative damage in more brain areas than before diabetes.

One-way ANOVA revealed that the percentage of SOD activity in HIP [F (4, 19) = 9.0, P< 0.05], HYP [F (4, 19) = 51.92, P< 0.05], PFC [F (4, 19) = 117.1, P< 0.05], STR [F (4, 19) = 62.342, P< 0.05], AMY [F (4, 19) = 130.79, P< 0.05] and NAC [F (4, 19) = 47.675, P< 0.05] was significantly altered among groups. Similar statistical analysis revealed that there was significant interactions in the CAT activity in HIP [F (4, 19) = 29.696, P< 0.05], HYP [F (4, 19) = 79.407, P< 0.05], PFC [F (4, 19) = 36.552, P< 0.05], STR [F (4, 19) = 36.280, P< 0.05], AMY [F (4, 19) = 27.183, P< 0.05] and NAC [F (4, 19) = 111.59, P< 0.05] among the groups. *Post hoc* analysis revealed that the attenuation of antioxidant defense system (SOD and CAT) was limited to HYP and STR by both diabetes and stress conditions compared to control. Pre-diabetes group showed further decrease in SOD as well as CAT activity in HYP, PFC and NAC compared to T2DM group. However, the reduced activity of both the antioxidant enzymes was higher in all the brain parts of post-diabetes group compared to T2DM group. Moreover, post-diabetes group showed further loss in activity of both antioxidant enzymes in all the brain regions compared to pre-diabetes group, indicating that stress after diabetes attenuates antioxidant defense mechanism more profoundly than before diabetes.

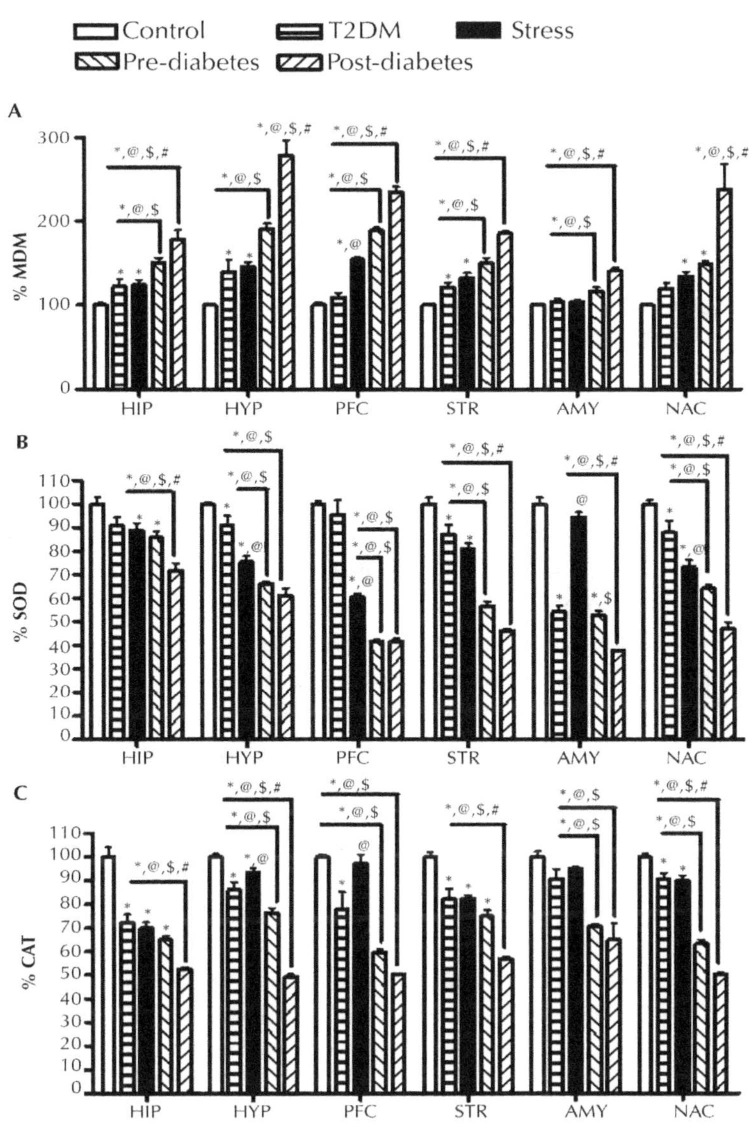

FIGURE 3 The alterations in the mitochondrial oxidative stress profile in terms of LPO (A), SOD (B) and CAT (C) activities in different brain regions of stress, diabetes and their combinations. All values are Mean ± SEM. *P< 0.05 compared to control, [@]P< 0.05 compared to T2DM, [$]$P$< 0.05 compared to stress and [#]P< 0.05 compared to prediabetes.

9.4.5 SEROTONERGIC SYSTEM IN DIFFERENT BRAIN REGIONS OF DIABETIC RATS IS ALTERED BY THE TEMPORAL EFFECT OF REPEATED CRS

The figure 4 depicts the changes in the levels of 5-HT (A), 5-HIAA (B) and ratios of 5-HIAA/5-HT (C) in different brain regions. Statistical analysis by one-way ANOVA revealed that there was significant interactions among groups in percentage level of 5-HT in HIP [F (4, 19) = 36.77, p< 0.05], HYP [F (4, 19) = 7.87, p< 0.05], PFC [F (4, 19) = 42.10, p< 0.05], AMY [F (4, 19) = 42.24, p< 0.05] and NAC [F (4, 19) = 58.11, p< 0.05]. However, there was no significant interactions among groups in percentage level of 5-HT in STR [F (4, 19) = 0.57, p >0.05]. *Post hoc* analysis revealed that T2DM led to significant decrease in 5-HT level in HIP and PFC compared to control. The level of 5-HT was significantly lower in all the brain regions except HYP and STR in repeated stressed rats compared to control. Pre and post-diabetes stress exposure caused decrease in 5-HT level in all the brain regions except HYP and STR compared to control and T2DM group animals. Moreover, post-diabetes stressed animals showed significant decrease in 5-HT level in all the brain regions except STR compared to pre-diabetes stressed rats.

Similarly, statistical analysis revealed that there was significant interactions among groups in percentage level of 5-hydroxyindoleacetic acid (5-HIAA) in HIP [F (4, 19) = 22.30, p< 0.05], HYP [F (4, 19) = 15.76, p< 0.05], PFC [F (4, 19) = 9.56, p< 0.05], STR [F (4, 19) = 18.79, p< 0.05], AMY [F (4, 19) = 37.17, p< 0.05] and NAC [F (4, 19) = 24.27, p< 0.05]. *Post hoc* analysis revealed that the level of 5-HIAA in T2DM group was significantly higher in all the brain regions except HIP and PFC compared to control. CRS caused significant increase in 5-HIAA level in all the brain regions compared to control. Pre and post-diabetes stress exposure caused significant increase in 5-HIAA level in all the brain regions except HIP compared to control and T2DM group animals. Post-diabetes stress exposure led to significant increase in 5-HIAA level in HIP compared to control and T2DM group rats. Moreover, Post-diabetes group showed significant increase in 5-HIAA level in all the brain regions compared to pre-diabetes group.

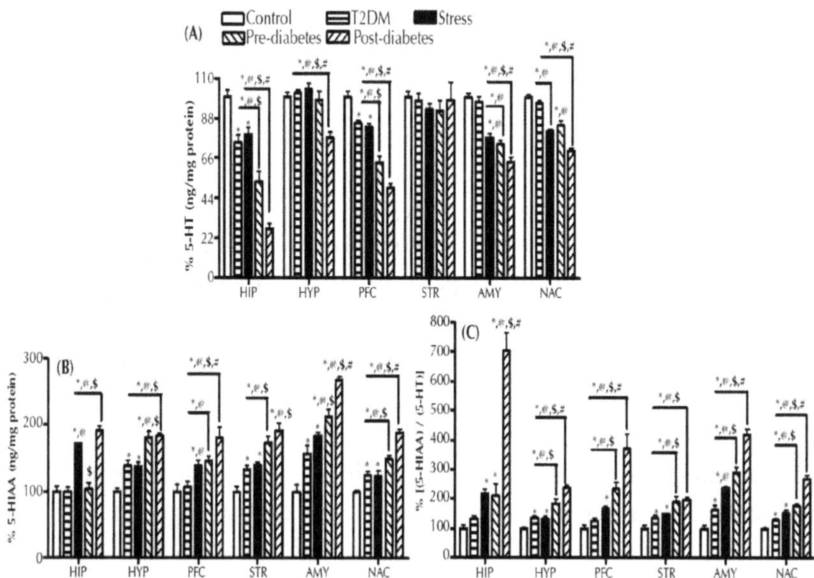

FIGURE 4 The changes in levels of 5-HT (A), 5-HIAA (B) and ratio of 5-HIAA/5-HT in different brain regions of stress, diabetes and their combinations are depicted. All values are Mean ± SEM. **P*< 0.05 compared to control, @*P*< 0.05 compared to T2DM, $*P*< 0.05 compared to stress and #*P*< 0.05 compared to pre-diabetes.

Statistical analysis revealed that there was significant interactions among groups in percentage ratio of 5-HIAA/5-HT in HIP [F (4, 19) = 59.83, p< 0.05], HYP [F (4, 19) = 29.06, p< 0.05], PFC [F (4, 19) = 24.47, p< 0.05], STR [F (4, 19) = 12.55, p< 0.05], AMY [F (4, 19) = 67.95, p< 0.05] and NAC [F (4, 19) = 41.96, p< 0.05]. Post hoc analysis revealed that the ratio of 5-HIAA/5-HT was significantly higher in all the brain regions except HIP and PFC in T2DM animals compared to control rats. Repeated CRS caused significant increase in the ratio of 5-HIAA/5-HT in all the brain regions compared to control. Pre and postdiabetes stress exposure caused significant increase in 5-HIAA level in all the brain regions except HIP compared to control and T2DM group animals. Only, postdiabetes stress exposure led to significant increase in the ratio of 5-HIAA/5-HT in HIP compared to control and T2DM group rats. Moreover, Postdiabetes group showed significant increase in the ratio of 5-HIAA/5-HT in all the brain regions except in STR compared to prediabetes group.

9.4.6 MODULATION OF NORADRENERGIC (NE) SYSTEM IN DIFFERENT BRAIN REGIONS OF DIABETIC RATS BY THE TEMPORAL EFFECT OF REPEATED CRS

The level of NE in different brain regions is illustrated in Figure 5. Statistical analysis by one-way ANOVA revealed that there was significant interactions among groups in percentage level of NE in HIP [$F(4, 19) = 31.61$, $p < 0.05$], HYP [$F(4, 19) = 49.06$, $p < 0.05$], PFC [$F(4, 19) = 55.28$, $p < 0.05$], STR [$F(4, 19) = 14.10$, $p < 0.05$], AMY [$F(4, 19) = 11.62$, $p < 0.05$] and NAC [$F(4, 19) = 34.40$, $p < 0.05$]. Post hoc analysis revealed that T2DM led to significant increase in the level of NE in all the brain regions except HYP and AMY compared to control. The level of NE was significantly lower in HYP and no change was observed in AMY in T2DM rats compared to control animals. Stress caused significant increase in NE level in all the brain regions compared to control. Pre and postdiabetes stress exposure caused significant increase in the level of NE in all the brain regions except HYP and AMY compared to control. The level of NE was significantly higher in HYP of prediabetes group while the similar finding was observed in AMY of postdiabetes group compared to control. Prediabetes stress exposure led to further increase in the level of NE in HIP, HYP and PFC only compared to T2DM rats. The level of NE was significantly higher in all the brain regions except HYP in postdiabetes stressed animals compared to T2DM rats. Further, postdiabetes stressed animals showed significant increase in the level of NE in all the brain regions except HYP (decrease) compared to prediabetes stressed rats.

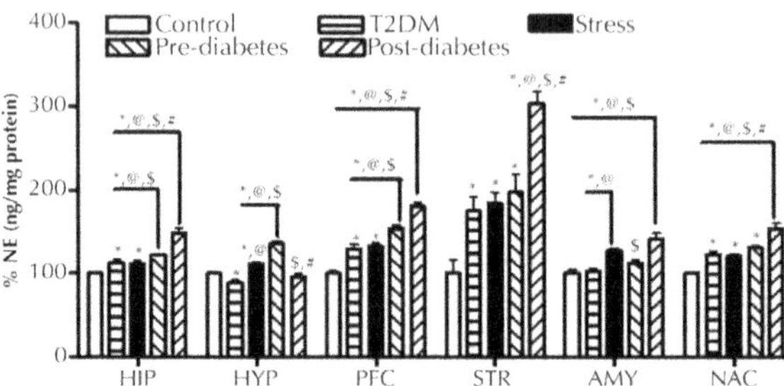

FIGURE 5 The changes in level of NE in different brain regions of stress, diabetes and their combinations are depicted. All values are Mean ± SEM. $*P < 0.05$ compared to control, $^{@}P < 0.05$ compared to T2DM, $^{\$}P < 0.05$ compared to stress and $^{\#}P < 0.05$ compared to prediabetes.

9.4.7 TEMPORAL EFFECT OF REPEATED CRS ON DOPAMINERGIC SYSTEM IN DIFFERENT BRAIN REGIONS OF DIABETIC RATS

The figure 6 depicts the changes in the levels of DA (A), 3,4-dihydroxyphenylacetic acid (DOPAC) (B), homovanillic acid (HVA) (D) and ratios of DOPAC/DA (C) and HVA/DA (E) in different brain regions. Statistical analysis by one-way ANOVA revealed that there was significant interactions among groups in percentage level of DA in HIP [$F (4, 19) = 10.61$, $p< 0.05$], HYP [$F (4, 19) = 41.08$, $p< 0.05$], PFC [$F (4, 19) = 7.81$, $p< 0.05$], STR [$F (4, 19) = 36.82$, $p< 0.05$], AMY [$F (4, 19) = 9.31$, $p< 0.05$] and NAC [$F (4, 19) = 8.13$, $p< 0.05$]. Post hoc analysis revealed that the level of DA in T2DM rats was increased in HIP, STR and NAC, but decreased in HYP and AMY compared to control animals. Repeated CRS exposure decreased the level of DA in all the brain regions compared to control. Stress before and after STZ injection prevented the diabetes-induced increase in DA level in NAC. However, the increase and decrease in DA level was maintained in HIP and AMY of both pre and postdiabetes stresses animals respectively. Both pre and postdiabetes stress exposure did not lead to significant increase in DA level in STR compared to control but showed significant decrease in DA level in STR compared to T2DM. The decrease in DA level was more pronounced in HYP of diabetic rats exposed to stress either before or after STZ injection compared to control diabetic animals. Though the level of DA was not significantly altered in PFC due to diabetes, stress either before or after T2DM induction led to decrease in the level of DA in PFC. Further, the decrease in the level of DA in PFC was higher in postdiabetes stressed animals compared to prediabetes stressed rats.

Similar statistical analysis revealed that there was significant differences among groups in percentage level of DOPAC in HIP [$F (4, 19) = 9.49$, $p< 0.05$], HYP [$F (4, 19) = 9.48$, $p< 0.05$], PFC [$F (4, 19) = 12.01$, $p< 0.05$], STR [$F (4, 19) = 9.40$, $p< 0.05$], AMY [$F (4, 19) = 7.61$, $p< 0.05$] and NAC [$F (4, 19) = 12.29$, $p< 0.05$]. Post hoc analysis revealed that T2DM significantly increased the level of DOPAC in HYP and PFC compared control. Stress significantly increased the level of DOPAC in all the brain regions except PFC and NAC compared to control. The T2DM-induced increase in the level of DOPAC in HYP and PFC were maintained in prediabetes stress exposure. However, diabetes after stress exposure inhibited the stress-induced increase in the level of DOPAC in HIP, STR and AMY. Although the level of DOPAC was not altered in NAC in either T2DM or stress, but the stress exposure before diabetes induction caused significant increase in the level of DOPAC in NAC compared to control. Further, the increase in the level of DOPAC in NAC in prediabetes stress group animals was insignificant compared to T2DM rats. Stress after diabetes induction caused significant increase in the level of DOPAC in all the brain regions compared to control. Further, the increase in the level of DOPAC was higher in postdiabetes stress exposed rats compared to T2DM and prediabetes stress exposed animals.

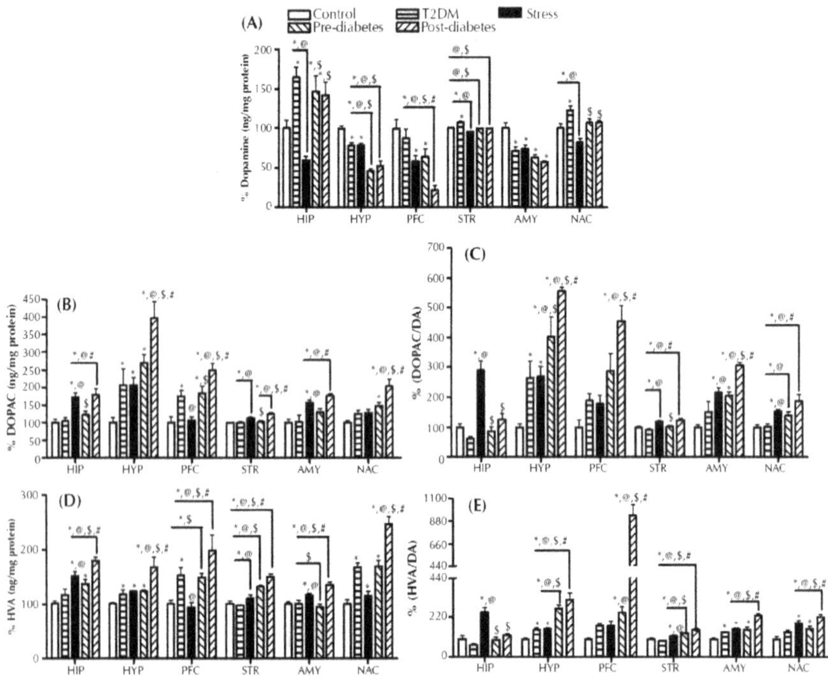

FIGURE 6 The changes in levels of DA (A), DOPAC (B), HVA (D) and ratios of DOPAC/DA (C), HVA/DA (E) in different brain regions of stress, diabetes and their combinations are depicted. All values are Mean ± SEM. $*P< 0.05$ compared to control, $^{@}P< 0.05$ compared to T2DM, $^{\$}P< 0.05$ compared to stress and $^{\#}P< 0.05$ compared to prediabetes.

Similarly, there was significant interaction among groups in percentage ratio of DOPAC/DA in HIP [F (4, 19) = 20.48, p< 0.05], HYP [F (4, 19) = 37.12, p< 0.05], PFC [F (4, 19) = 18.70, p< 0.05], STR [F (4, 19) = 12.64, p< 0.05], AMY [F (4, 19) = 15.42, p< 0.05] and NAC [F (4, 19) = 9.44, p< 0.05]. Post hoc analysis revealed that T2DM led to significant increase in DOPAC/DA ratio only in HYP compared to control. Repeated CRS exposure increased the ratio of DOPAC/DA in all the brain regions except PFC compared to control. The ratio of DOPAC/DA in HIP was not altered in T2DM rats and the ratio was unchanged in HIP in diabetic rats exposed to repeated stress either before or after diabetes induction. The ratio of DOPAC/DA in the HYP was increased significantly in diabetic rats exposed to stress either before or after diabetes induction compared to both control and T2DM animals. Further, the ratio of DOPAC/DA was augmented in HYP in postdiabetes condition compared to prediabetes condition. Stress before T2DM induction extended the diabetes-induced increase in the ratio of DOPAC/DA to AMY and NAC compared to control. However, the increase in the ratio of DOPAC/DA in NAC of prediabetes rats was significantly higher compared to T2DM animals. On contrary, stress after diabetes induction extended the diabetes-induced increase in the ratio of DOPAC/DA to all the brain regions except HIP compared to control, T2DM and prediabetes condition.

Similar statistical analysis revealed that there was significant interaction among groups in percentage level of HVA in HIP [F (4, 19) = 14.60, p< 0.05], HYP [F (4, 19) = 13.83, p< 0.05], PFC [F (4, 19) = 11.55, p< 0.05], STR [F (4, 19) = 16.09, p< 0.05], AMY [F (4, 19) = 8.66, p< 0.05] and NAC [F (4, 19) = 26.74, p< 0.05]. Post hoc analysis revealed that T2DM caused significant increase in the level of HVA in HYP, PFC and NAC compared to control. Stress increased the level of HVA in all the brain regions except PFC compared to control. Prediabetes stress exposure significantly increased the level of HVA in all the brain regions except AMY compared to control. Prediabetes stress exposure led to further increase in the level of HVA only in STR compared to T2DM rats. The level of HVA in all the brain regions was increased significantly in postdiabetes stressed animals compared to control, T2DM and prediabetes stressed rats.

Similarly, there was significant interaction among groups in percentage ratio of HVA/DA in HIP [$F(4, 19) = 13.54$, $p < 0.05$], HYP [$F(4, 19) = 42.13$, $p < 0.05$], PFC [$F(4, 19) = 64.63$, $p < 0.05$], STR [$F(4, 19) = 22.01$, $p < 0.05$], AMY [$F(4, 19) = 21.85$, $p < 0.05$] and NAC [$F(4, 19) = 7.83$, $p < 0.05$]. Post hoc analysis revealed that T2DM significantly increased the ratio of HVA/DA in HYP and AMY compared to control. Repeated CRS exposure increased the ratio of HVA/DA in all the brain regions except PFC compared to control. Pre and postdiabetes stress exposure significantly increased the ratio of HVA/DA in all the brain regions except HIP compared to control. Prediabetes stress exposure caused significant increase in ratio of HVA/DA in HYP, PFC and STR compared to T2DM. The ratio of HVA/DA was increased in all the brain regions except HIP in postdiabetes stress compared to T2DM. Further, the ratio of HVA/DA was significantly increased in all the brain regions except HIP in postdiabetes stressed rats compared to prediabetes stressed animals.

KEYWORDS

- **Brain; monoamine**
- **Hypercorticosteronemia**
- **Hyperglycemia**
- **Mitochondria**
- **Stress**
- **Type-2 diabetes**

ACKNOWLEDGMENT

DG (Senior Research Fellow) is thankful to Council of Scientific and Industrial Research (CSIR), New Delhi, India, for the financial assistantship.

REFERENCES

1. Aragno, M., Brignardello, E., Tamagno, E., Gatto, V., Danni, O., and Boccuzzi, G. Dehydroepiandrosterone administration prevents the oxidative damage induced by acute hyperglycemia in rats. *J. Endocrinol.*, **155**(2), 233–240 (1997).
2. Barber, M., Kasturi, B. S., Austin, M. E., Patel, K. P., MohanKumar, S. M., and MohanKumar, P. S. Diabetes-induced neuroendocrine changes in rats: role of brain monoamines, insulin, and leptin. *Brain Res.*, **964**(1), 128–135 (2003).
3. Beers, R. F. and Sizer, I. W. A spectrophotometric method for measuring the breakdown of hydrogen peroxide by catalase. *J. Biol. Chem.*, **195**, 133–140 (1952).
4. Benani, A., Troy, S., Carmona, M. C., Fioramonti, X., Lorsignol, A., Leloup, C., Casteilla, L., and Pénicaud, L. Role for mitochondrial reactive oxygen species in brain lipid sensing: redox regulation of food intake. *Diabetes*, **56**(1), 152–160 (2007).
5. Biessels, G. J., Kappelle, A. C., Bravenboer, B., Erkelens, D. W., and Gispen, W. H. Cerebral function in diabetes mellitus. *Diabetologia*, **37**(7), 643–650 (1994).
6. Brignone, J. A., Campos de Brignone, C. M., Rebagliati de Mignone, I. R., Ricci, C. R., Susemihl, M. C., and Rodríguez, R. R. Effects of withdrawal of glucocorticoids on improving the function and enzymatic activities of liver mitochondria in female diabetic rats. *Acta Physiol. Pharmacol. Ther. Latinoam.*, **41**(3), 309–323 (1991).
7. Cardoso, S., Santos, M. S., Seiça, R., and Moreira, P. I. Cortical and hippocampal mitochondria bioenergetics and oxidative status during hyperglycemia and/or insulin-induced hypoglycemia. *Biochim. Biophys. Acta*, **1802**(11), 942–951 (2010).
8. Cardoso, S., Santos, M. S., Moreno, A., and Moreira, P. I. UCP2 and ANT differently modulate proton-leak in brain mitochondria of long-term hyperglycemic and recurrent hypoglycemic rats. *J. Bioenerg. Biomembr.*, [Epub ahead of print] (2013).
9. Ceretta, L. B., Réus, G. Z., Rezin, G. T., Scaini, G., Streck, E. L., and Quevedo, J. Brain energy metabolism parameters in an animal model of diabetes. *Metab. Brain Dis.*, **25**(4), 391–396 (2010).
10. Chang, D. T., Honick, A. S., and Reynolds, I. J. Mitochondrial trafficking to synapses in cultured primary cortical neurons. *J. Neurosci.*, **26**, 7035–7045 (2006).
11. Chen, S., Owens, G. C., Crossin, K. L., and Edelman, D. B. Serotonin stimulates mitochondrial transport in hippocampal neurons. *Mol. Cell Neurosci.*, **36**(4), 472–483 (2007).
12. Chen, S., Owens, G. C., and Edelman, D. B. Dopamine inhibits mitochondrial motility in hippocampal neurons. *PLoS One*, **3**(7), e2804 (2008).
13. Chiodini, I., Adda, G., Scillitani, A., Coletti, F., Morelli, V., Di Lembo, S., Epaminonda, P., Masserini, B., Beck-Peccoz, P., Orsi, E., Ambrosi, B., and Arosio, M. Cortisol secretion in patients with type 2 diabetes: relationship with chronic complications. *Diabetes Care*, **30**(1), 83–88 (2007).
14. Cohen, H. Y., Miller, C., and Bitterman, K. J. Calorie restriction promotes mammalian cell survival by inducing the SIRT1 deacetylase. *Science*, **305**, 390–392 (2004).
15. Davila, E. P., Florez, H., Trepka, M. J., Fleming, L. E., Niyonsenga, T., Lee, D. J., and Parkash, J. Long work hours is associated with suboptimal glycemic control among US workers with diabetes. *Am. J. Ind. Med.*, **54**(5), 375–383 (2011).

16. de Oliveira, C., de Mattos, A. B., Biz, C., Oyama, L. M., Ribeiro, E. B., and do Nascimento, C. M. High-fat diet and glucocorticoid treatment cause hyperglycemia associated with adiponectin receptor alterations. *Lipids Health Dis.*, **10**, 11 (2011)
17. Faulenbach, M., Uthoff, H., Schwegler, K., Spinas, G. A., Schmid, C., and Wiesli, P. Effect of psychological stress on glucose control in patients with Type-2 diabetes. *Diabet. Med.*, doi: 10.1111/j.1464-5491.2011.03431.x (2011).
18. Fiorentino, T. V., Prioletta, A., Zuo, P., and Folli, F. Hyperglycemia-induced Oxidative stress and its Role in Diabetes Mellitus related Cardiovascular Diseases. *Curr Pharm Des.* [Epub ahead of print] (2013).
19. Fukui, K., Onodera, K., Shinkai, T., Suzuki, S., and Urano, S. Impairment of learning and memory in rats caused by oxidative stress and aging, and changes in antioxidative defense systems. *Ann. N.Y. Acad. Sci.*, **928**, 168–175 (2001).
20. Garabadu, D., Shah, A., Ahmad, A., Joshi, V. B., Saxena, B., Palit, G., and Krishnamurthy, S. Eugenol as an anti-stress agent: modulation of hypothalamic-pituitary-adrenal axis and brain monoaminergic systems in a rat model of stress. *Stress*, **14**(2), 145–155 (2011).
21. Gong, Y., Chai, Y., Ding, J. H., Sun, X. L., and Hu, G. Chronic mild stress damages mitochondrial ultrastructure and function in mouse brain. *Neurosci. Lett.*, **488**(1), 76–80 (2011).
22. Hanson, C. L., Rodrigue, J. R., Burghen, G. A., Henggeler, S. W., and Onikul-Ross, S. R. Peptic ulcer disease in youths with insulin-dependent diabetes mellitus: a prospective study. *J. Pediatr. Psychol.*, **15**(5), 595–604 (1990).
23. Huang, S. G. Development of a high throughput screening assay for mitochondrial membrane potential in living cells. *J. Biomol. Screen.*, **7**(4), 383–389 (2002).
24. Kakkar, P., Das, B., and Viswanathan, P. N. A modified spectrophotometric assay of superoxide dismutase. *Indian J. Biochem.*, **21**, 130–132 (1984).
25. Karpińska, A. and Gromadzka, G. Oxidative stress and natural antioxidant mechanisms: the role in neurodegeneration. From molecular mechanisms to therapeutic strategies. *Postepy Hig Med Dosw (Online)*, **67**(0), 43–53 (2013).
26. Kim, C., Speisky, M. B., and Kharouba, S. N. Rapid and sensitive method for measuring norepinephrin, dopamine, 5-hydroxytryptamine and their major metabolites in rat brain by high performance liquid chromatography. *J. Chromatogr.*, **386**, 25–35 (1987).
27. Kino, M., Yamato, T., and Aomine, M. Simultaneous measurement of nitric oxide, blood glucose, and monoamines in the hippocampus of diabetic rat: an in vivo microdialysis study. *Neurochem. Int.*, **44**(2), 65–73 (2004).
28. Krishnamurthy, S., Garabadu, D., Reddy, N. R., and Joy, K. P. Risperidone in ultra low dose protects against stress in the rodent cold restraint model by modulating stress pathways. *Neurochem. Res.*, **36**(10), 1750–1758 (2011).
29. Krishnamurthy, S., Garabadu, D., and Reddy, N. R. Asparagus racemosus modulates the hypothalamic-pituitary-adrenal axis and brain monoaminergic systems in rats. *Nutr. Neurosci.*, [Epub ahead of print] (2013).
30. Kumar, A., Aravamudhan, S., Gordic, M., Bhansali, S., and Mohapatra, S. S. Ultrasensitive detection of cortisol with enzyme fragment complementation technology using functionalized nanowire. *Biosens. Bioelectron.*, **22**(9–10), 2138–2144 (2007).

31. Kushnerova, N. F., Rakhmanin, Iu. A., Fomenko, S. E., Chizhova, T. L., and Sheparev, A. A. Impact of the working environment on metabolic reactions in operating pilots. *Gig. Sanit.*, **6**, 34–36 (2006).
32. Li, Z., Okamoto, K., Hayashi, Y., and Sheng, M. The importance of dendritic mitochondria in the morphogenesis and plasticity of spines and synapses. *Cell*, **119**, 873–887 (2004).
33. Li, L., Li, X., Zhou, W., and Messina, J. Acute Psychological Stress Results in the Rapid Development of Insulin Resistance. *J Endocrinol.* [Epub ahead of print] (2013).
34. Lowry, O. H., Rosenborough, N. J., Farr, A. L., and Randall, R. J. Protein measurement with folin phenol reagent. *J. Biol. Chem.*, **193**, 265–275 (1951).
35. Masiello, P., Broca, C., Gross, R., Roye, M., Manteghetti, M., Hillaire-Buys, D., Novelli, M., and Ribes, G. Experimental NIDDM: development of a new model in adult rats administered streptozotocin and nicotinamide. *Diabet.*, **47**, 224–229 (1998).
36. Menabde, K. O., Burdzhanadze, G. M., Chachua, M. V., Kuchukashvyly, Z. T., and Koshorydze, N. I. Tissue specificity of lipid peroxidation under emotional stress in rats. *Ukr. Biokhim. Zh.*, **83**(3), 85–90 (2011).
37. Moreira, P. I., Santos, M. S., Moreno, A. M., Seiça, R., and Oliveira, C. R. Increased vulnerability of brain mitochondria in diabetic (Goto-Kakizaki) rats with aging and amyloid-beta exposure. *Diabetes*, **52**, 1449–1456 (2003).
38. Palkovits, M. and Brownstein, M. J. *Maps and guide to microdissection of the rat brain*. New York, Elsevier (1988).
39. Patel, S. P. and Katyare, S. S. Effect of Alloxan Diabetes and Subsequent Insulin Treatment on Temperature Kinetics Properties of Succinate Oxidase Activity in Rat Kidney Mitochondria. *J. Membrane Biol.*, **213**, 31–37 (2006).
40. Pedersen, P. L., Grenawalt, J. W., Reynafarje, B., Hullihen, J., Decker, G. L., Soper, J. W., and Bustamente, E. Preparation and characterization of mitochondria and submitochondrial particles of rat liver-derived tissues. *Methods Cell Biol.*, **20**, 411–481 (1978).
41. Preet, A., Gupta, B. L., Yadava, P. K., and Baquer, N. Z. Efficacy of lower doses of vanadium in restoring altered glucose metabolism and antioxidant status in diabetic rat lenses. *J. Biosci.*, **30**(2), 221–230 (2005).
42. Rasbach, K. A. and Schnellmann, R. G. Signaling of mitochondrial biogenesis following oxidant injury. *J. Biol. Chem.*, **282**, 2355–2362 (2007).
43. Reaven, G. M., Javorski, W. C., and Reaven, E. Diabetic hypertriglyceridemia. *Am. J. Med. Sci.*, **269**(3), 382–389 (1975).
44. Reddy, N. R., Krishnamurthy, S., Chourasia, T. K., Kumar, A., and Joy, K. P. Glutamate antagonism fails to reverse mitochondrial dysfunction in late phase of experimental neonatal asphyxia in rats. *Neurochem. Int.*, **58**(5), 582–590 (2011).
45. Sairam, K., Rao, Ch. V., Babu, M. D., Kumar, K. V., Agrawal, V. K., and Goel, R. K. Antiulcerogenic effect of methanolic extract of Emblica officinalis: an experimental study. *J. Ethnopharmacol.*, **82**(1), 1–9 (2002).
46. Sally, L. O. and Margaret, A. J. Methods of micro photometric assay of succinate dehydrogenase and cytochrome-C oxidase activities for use on human skeletal muscle. *Histochem. J.*, **21**, 545–555 (1989).
47. Schuman, E. and Chan, D. Fueling synapses. *Cell*, **119**, 738–740 (2004).

48. Siddiqui, M. R., Taha, A., Moorthy, K., Hussain, M. E., Basir, S. F., and Baquer, N. Z. Amelioration of altered antioxidant status and membrane linked functions by vanadium and Trigonella in alloxan diabetic rat brains. *J. Biosci.*, **30**(4), 483–490 (2005).
49. Singer, T. P., Gutman, M., and Massey, V. Succinate dehydrogenase. W. Lovenbarg (Ed.) *Iron-Sulfur Proteins*, Academic Press, New York, **1**, 227–254 (1973).
50. Sullivan, R. M. and Szechtman, H. Asymmetrical influence of mesocortical dopamine depletion on stress ulcer development and subcortical dopamine systems in rats: implications for psychopathology. *Neuroscience*, **65**(3), 757–766 (1995).
51. Sunderman, F. W., Marzouk, A., Hopfer, S. M., Zaharia, O., and Reid, M. C. Increased lipid peroxidation in tissues of nickel chloride-treated rats. *Ann. Clin. Lab Sci.*, **15**, 229–236 (1985).
52. Tang, Y. and Zucker, R. S. Mitochondrial involvement in post-tetanic potentiation of synaptic transmission. *Neuron*, **18**, 483–491 (1997).
53. Toleikis, P. M. and Godin, D. V. Alteration of antioxidant status in diabetic rats by chronic exposure to restraint stressors. *Pharmacol. Biochem. Behav.*, **52**, 355–366 (1995).
54. Tuzcu, M. and Baydas, G. Effect of melatonin and vitamin E on diabetes-induced learning and memory impairment in rats. *Eur. J. Pharmacol.*, **537**(1–3), 106–110 (2006).
55. Uchiyama, M. and Mihara, M. Determination of malonaldehyde precursor in tissues by thiobarbituric acid test. *Anal. Biochem.*, **86**, 271–278 (1978).
56. Volkova, Iu. V. and Davydov, V. V. Effect of stress on the content of free radical oxidation products in subcellular brain fractions in rats of pubertal age. *Ukr. Biokhim. Zh.*, **81**(2), 102–106 (2009).
57. Wang, T. Y., Chen, X. Q., Du, J. Z., Xu, N. Y., Wei, C. B., and Vale, W. W. Corticotropin-releasing factor receptor type 1 and 2 mRNA expression in the rat anterior pituitary is modulated by intermittent hypoxia, cold and restraint. *Neuroscience*, **128**(1), 111–119 (2004).
58. Whitford, D. L., Griffin, S. J., and Prevost, A. T. Influences on the variation in prevalence of Type 2 diabetes between general practices: Practice, patient or socioeconomic factors? *Br. J. Gen. Pract.*, **53**, 9–14 (2003).

CHAPTER 10

SUGAR RICH DIET INDUCED INSULIN RESISTANCE AND ALTERATION IN GUT MICROFLORA

PRASANT KUMAR JENA, SHILPA SINGH, and SRIRAM SESHADRI

CONTENTS

ABSTRACT

The obesity, diabetes, and cardiovascular diseases like metabolic abnormalities are became major health and public health issues worldwide. Obesity and insulin resistance is associated with significant changes in composition and metabolic function of gut microbiota but the pathophysiological processes having this bidirectional association have not been fully elucidated. In the present investigation, we modulated gut microbiota by giving site-specific delivery of gram positive, gram negative, and broad spectrum antibiotics coated with pH-sensitive polymer. Following high fructose rich diet for the Type II diabetes induction, the gram positive removal showed more profound effect on total fat pad, total cholesterol, and triglyceride and had higher tendency to develop insulin resistance or diabetes in these animals. From the findings, it could be concluded that changes in gut microbiota by partial removal of gram negative bacteria may control metabolic endotoxemia, inflammation, and associated disorders by a mechanism that could increase intestinal permeability. It would thus been useful to develop strategies for changing gut microbiota to control, intestinal permeability, metabolic endotoxemia, and associated disorders.

10.1 INTRODUCTION

Sugar rich diet such as high fructose, sucrose fat rich diet has been associated with a higher endotoxemia in humans. There are definitive accepted role of a high fat rich meal and development of metabolic endotoxemia in healthy human subjects (Erridge et al., 2007). In humans, plasma endotoxin levels are associated with sepsis and many inflammatory diseases, which reported that in healthy subject's the plasma endotoxin concentrations range from 1 to 200 pg/mL (Wiedermann et al., 1999; Bolke et al., 2007; Goto et al., 1994; Hasday et al., 1999).

The metabolic endotoxemia following a high fat meal was clearly evident in human aortic endothelial cells, which was likely to be due to the release of soluble inflammatory mediators, such as tumor necrosis factor alpha (TNF-α), from monocytes (Erridge et al., 2007). There was a study that found a link between energy (food) intake and metabolic endotoxemia (Amar et al., 2008) Furthermore, a similar metabolic endotoxemia has been shown to increase adipose TNF-α and Interleukin 6 (IL-6) concentrations and insulin resistance in healthy subjects (Anderson et al., 2007). Human studies suggest that diet induced changes in endotoxemia and it may bridge the gap between food intake behavior and metabolic abnormalities in humans.

The metabolic endotoxemia might act as a gut microbiota related factor involved in the development of type II diabetes and obesity in humans (Dumas et al., 2007). The fasting insulin significantly correlated with metabolic endotoxemia in the non diabetic population, and this correlation persisted when it controlled for sex, age, and body mass index (BMI) (Dumas et al., 2007).

Obesity can be coupled with an altered gut microbiota (Taurnbaugh et al., 2008). The observed alterations in community may be a contributing factor partitioning between lean and obese subjects (Taurnbaugh et al., 2006). It was observed that obese people had lower bacteroidetes and more firmicutes than lean control subjects (Ley et al., 2006). It was suggested that the characteristics of gut microbiota of obese mice take part per se to the addition of fat and body weight gain.

High fat diet fed mice gained significantly more weight and fat mass than the germ free, which were also protected against the high fat diet induced glucose intolerance and insulin resistance. The gut microbiota involved in the regulation of 5' adenosine monophosphate-activated protein kinase (AMPK) activity and fatty acids oxidation. In the absence of gut microbiota, AMPK activity is constitutively higher in muscle, which promotes mitochondrial fatty acid oxidation by higher phosphorylation of its specific target acetyl-CoA carboxylase (ACC) and reduction of malonyl-CoA production (Backhed et al., 2007).

Antibiotic treatment changed the gut microbiota drastically, resulting in significant reduction in the *Lactobacillus* spp., *Bifidobacterium* spp., and *Bacteroides-Prevotella* spp. This drop in antibiotic-treated mice resulted in significant decline in metabolic endotoxemia and inflammatory response (Cani et al., 2008). Macrophages infiltration, oxidative stress, and certain inflammatory markers were reduced in the visceral adipose depots and to a lesser extent in the subcutaneous fat.

The antibiotics are a subgroup of organic anti-infective agents, derived from bacteria or moulds that are toxic to other bacteria. There are various kind of antibiotics present and they are used as per their mechanism of action which were classified may be according to their spectrum and mechanism of action or chemical structure. Antibiotics targeted to bacterial cell wall are penicillins and cephalosporins groups or the cell membrane (polymixins), or obstructions with certain crucial bacterial enzymes (quinolones and sulfonamides) have bactericidal activities. Those that target protein synthesis (macrolides, tetracyclines, oxazolidinones, and aminoglycosides) usually have bacteriostatic action (Finberg et al., 2004). Further classification depends on their target specificity. “Narrow-spectrum” antibiotics generally target specific types of bacteria like gram-negative or gram-positive bacteria; however broad-spectrum antibiotics affect a wide range of the bacteria.

Antibiotics are designed only to target pathogenic organisms but certain related members of the microbiota are also get affected, leaving a print on the gut community long even after the removal of antibiotics (Jakobsson et al., 2010; Jernberg et al., 2007). Antibiotic application also promotes the expansion of antibiotic resistant strains, which can act as a lasing reservoir for resistance genes in the gut microenvironment (Lofmark et al., 2006).

Antibiotic treatment decreased the incidence and delayed the onset of diabetes in a diabetes-prone rat model. The gut bacterial composition of rats that developed diabetes differed from that of those that did not. Specifically, rats that did not develop diabetes displayed a lower number of *Bacteroides* species. Thus, the antibiotic-induced alteration in the gut microbiota led to a reduction in the antigenic load and subsequent inflammation that usually leads to pancreatic β-cell destruction. This study opened newer venues of potentially modulating the intestinal microbiota as a therapeutic strategy (DiBaise et al., 2008).

Antibiotic therapy alters the metabolic profiles of some intestinal contents and faeces, as well as of the blood and urine (following absorption of metabolites through the gut). Metabolic profiles of mice have been studied under different antibiotic regimens (Yap et al., 2008). Decreased production of short-chain fatty acids (SCFA) is the common feature observed in metabolic profile of antibiotic treated mice and human which is important with regard to intestinal health and immunity (Hoverstad et al., 1986).

The SCFAs are rapidly absorbed in the colon, providing a favoured energy source for colonocytes and regulating cell proliferation, differentiation, growth, and apoptosis. Butyrate is the main SCFA with the strongest effect on the cell cycle and has also been involved in regulating many aspects of intestinal immunity. Effects of butyrate on mucosal junctions include improved tight junction permiability, antimicrobial secretion, and mucin expression (Gaudier et al., 2009; Peng et al., 2009).

Gut microbiota facilitate the extraction of calories from ingested dietary substances through their metabolic activity and help to store these calories in host adipose tissue for later use. Furthermore, the gut microflora of obese mice and humans include fewer *Bacteroidetes* and correspondingly more *Firmicutes* compared to their lean subjects, which suggest that differences in caloric extraction of ingested food substances may be due to the composition of the gut microbiota (DiBaise et al., 2008).

Diet is known to be a considerably stronger contributor for structural microbial changes compared with the genetic alteration in this study (Zhang et al., 2010)). In addition to regulating insulin sensitivity, the presence or absence of the microbiota may regulate cholesterol metabolism (Robot et al., 2010). Some evidence indicates that type 2 diabetic, irrespective of obesity, might affect the structural composition of the microbiota as with differences noted between obese and type 2 diabetic patients (Wu et al., 2010; Larsen et al., 2010; Cani et al., 2007).

Type II diabetes might be associated with the dominance of gram-negative bacteria in the gut, such as *Bacteroidetes (*Gerard et al., 2004) and reduction in *Bacteroides-Prevotella* spp. has been associated with improvement in metabolic endotoxemia and decreased systemic inflammatory markers in diabetic mice. Certain prebiotics such as oligofructose might affect the structural composition of the gut microbiota upon high-fat/high sugar diet feeding with improvement in parameters of metabolic inflammation (Gerard et al., 2004).

In this study, an attempt was be made to modulate gut microbiota by administering target specific antibiotic to correlate the effect of diet and antibiotic targeting specifically to small and large intestine of rats.

10.2 MATERIALS

POLYMERS AND REAGENTS:

Acetone, span 80, and paraffin light liquid were purchased from Sigma-Aldrich (Ahmedabad, India). Eudragit L-100-55 and Eudragit S-100, pH-sensitive polymer for the delivery of antibiotic in large intestine [LI] and small intestine [SI] respectively, was kindly gifted by Corel Pharma chem. Pvt. Ltd (Ahmedabad, India). Cefdinir (gram negative [GN] specific antibiotic), linezolid (gram positive [GP] specific antibiotic), and gemifloxacin (broad spectrum [BS] antibiotic) were obtained as a gift sample from Macleods Pharma, Mumbai.

ANIMALS

Wistar rats of female sex weighing 200–300 g were procured from the central animal facility of the Institute of Pharmacy, Nirma University (Ahmedabad). The animals were maintained at controlled temperature as well as humidity and fed with standard diet and water provided *ad libitum*. The care and the use of these animals were in accordance with the guidelines of the CPCSEA (committee for the purpose of control and supervision of experiments on animals). Experimental protocol was approved by Institutional Animal Ethics Committee (IAEC) (protocol no. IS/BT/PhD 11-12-1004). A one-week adaptive period was given to rats and *ad libitum* diet will be provided.

10.3 EXPERIMENTAL PROTOCOL AND DESIGN

Rats (n = 56) were randomized into the following groups:

- CD: Control Normal Control Diet group administered with saline for 30 days.
- CD-GN-LI: Normal Control fed diet administered with dosage of 10 mg/kg cefdinir (Eudragit S100 coated) daily.

- CD-GN-SI: Normal Control fed diet administered with dosage of 10 mg/kg cefdinir (Eudragit L100-55 coated) daily.
- CD-GP-LI: Normal Control fed diet administered with dosage of 10 mg/kg linezolid (Eudragit S100 coated) daily.
- CD-GP-SI: Normal Control fed diet administered with dosage of 10 mg/kg linezolid (Eudragit L100-55 coated) daily.
- CD-BS-LI: Normal Control fed diet administered with dosage of 5.33 mg/kg gemifloxacin (Eudragit L100-55 coated) daily.
- CD-BS-SI: Normal Control fed diet administered with dosage of 5.33 mg/kg gemifloxacin (Eudragit L100-55 coated) daily.
- HFD: High Fructose Diet group administered with saline for 30 days.
- HFD-GN-LI: High Fructose fed diet administered with dosage of 10 mg/kg cefdinir (Eudragit S100 coated) daily.
- HFD-GN-SI: High Fructose fed diet administered with dosage of 10 mg/kg cefdinir (Eudragit L100-55 coated) daily.
- HFD-GP-LI: High Fructose fed diet administered with dosage of 10 mg/kg linezolid (Eudragit S100 coated) daily.
- HFD-GP-SI: High Fructose fed diet administered with dosage of 10 mg/kg linezolid (Eudragit L100-55 coated) daily.
- HFD-BS-LI: High Fructose fed diet administered with dosage of 5.33 mg/kg gemifloxacin (Eudragit L100-55 coated) daily.
- HFD-BS-SI: High Fructose fed diet administered with dosage of 5.33 mg/kg gemifloxacin (Eudragit L100-55 coated) daily.

All the formulations were administered orally using a feeding tube attached to a hypodermic syringe at respective doses. Dosage for each antibiotic was selected as per the Drug Usage guidelines of food and drug administration (FDA).

10.3.1 PREPARATION OF HIGH FRUCTOSE DIET

TABLE 1 Composition of experimental diets given to the rats

Constituents *	Standard** (Normal Control Diet)	High Fructose Diet
Corn starch	65	00

TABLE 1 *(Continued)*

Wheat bran	5	5
Groundnut oil	5	5
Casein	20	20
D. Methionine	0.3	0.3
Salt mixture #	3.5	3.5
Vitamin mixture #	1	1
Choline chloride	0.2	0.2
Fructose	00	65

*: Prepared and mixed according to the method of the association of official analytical chemists

#: Salt mixture (AIN-93-G-MX) and vitamin mixture (AIN-93-VX) from M P. Biomedical. Remaining food items were purchased from Central Drug house Pvt. Ltd (India).

**: Standard diet purchased from Amrut Agrofoods, Mumbai.

PREPARATION OF MICROSPHERE:

Antibiotics (cefdinir, linezolid, gemifloxacin) were taken in different drug polymer ratio (1:2 and 1:1) and were added in an 5 mL acetone organic phase (internal aqueous phase) having 10% w/v Eudragit S-100 and Eudragit L 100–55 and sonicated in an ultrasonicator (JY92-11DN, Syclon, Japan) for 10 min .This solution was then added drop by drop through a disposable syringe into an external aqueous phase containing paraffin light liquid and was emulsified containing the emulsifier and sorbitan sesquioleate 80 (2% v/v). The system was stirred continuously using a mechanical stirrer at 1000 rpm and 38 ± 0.5°C for 5 hr to allow the complete evaporation of the solvent. The paraffin was decanted off, the microspheres were washed repeatedly three times with petroleum ether (40–60°C), collected by filtration and finally dried at 40°C for 1 hr. (Basu and Adhiyaman, 2008; Majumdar et al., 2005).

10.3.2 DETERMINATION OF PHYSIOLOGICAL CHANGES BY SELECTIVE MODULATION OF GUT MICROBIOTA WITH ANTIBIOTICS

Rats were administered respective doses of antibiotic cefdinir, gemifloxacin, and linezolid with specific polymer coating sacrificed at different time point post-administration of drug-laden microspheres.

10.3.3 PARAMETERS ASSESSED

ESTIMATION OF PHYSICAL PARAMETERS

Body weight was recorded daily during the entire study period in each group. Daily food intake for each group was measured and expressed as mean of daily food intake. Body fat was also measured after sacrificing the animals in 15 day intervals.

10.3.4 ESTIMATION OF BIOCHEMICAL PARAMETERS

COLLECTION OF SERUM

The blood samples were withdrawn from retro-orbital plexus under light ether anesthesia without any anticoagulant and allowed to clot for 10 min at room temperature. It was centrifuged at 5000 rpm for 10 min. The serum obtained was kept at 4°C until used.

COLLECTION OF PLASMA

The blood samples were withdrawn from retro-orbital plexus under light ether anesthesia with Acid Citrate Dextrose (ACD) anticoagulant (9 volume blood in 1 volume ACD). It was centrifuged at 5000 rpm for 10 min.

The plasma obtained was kept at 4 °C until it was used. A fraction of whole blood samples were used for determination of DNA isolation. The remaining samples were centrifuged at 4000 g for 10 min at 4 °C and serum was used to determine levels of insulin, glucose, lactate dehydrogenase (LDH), and billirubin. The animals were sacrificed on 30th day at the end of the study by cervical dislocation. The liver, small and Large intestine were excised, rinsed with chilled 0.2 M phosphate buffer and was stored at –20 °C.

10.3.5 MEASUREMENT OF PLASMA AND SERUM PARAMETERS

The plasma triglyceride, cholesterol, high-density lipoprotein (HDL) cholesterol levels, and serum glucose level was measured using commercial kits (Lab Care diagnostics, India). Serum, such as serum glutamic-pyruvic transaminase (SGPT) and serum glutamic oxaloacetic transaminase (SGOT) was also performed for checking liver dysfunction for renal and kidney damage urea, protein and billirubin tests were also done by using commercial kits (Membrez et al., 2008).

10.3.6 LIVER GLYCOGEN CONTENT

The liver glycogen was determined as described by Vander-Vries (1954). Liver tissue (200 mg) was finely ground with 20 mL of 5% trichloroacetic acid in a homogenizer. The protein precipitate was filtered and the clear filtrate was taken for analysis. Liver filtrate (2 mL) was pipetted into a 20 mL calibrated test tube and then 2 mL of 10 N KOH was added before placing it in a boiling water bath for 1 hr. After cooling, 1 mL acetic acid was added to neutralize the excess of alkali and fluid was brought up to the mark with water. Slowly, 2 mL of solution from the previous step was added to 4 mL of anthrone reagent in a separate test tube, which was placed in cold water to prevent excessive heating. After thorough shaking, the test tube was placed in a boiling water bath for exactly 10 min for the development of color and cooled with running tap water. The OD was read within 2 hr at 650 nm.

10.3.7 ASSAY FOR LIVER TOTAL CHOLESTEROL

After euthanasia, rat livers will be removed, rinsed with physiological saline solution, blotted dry, and weighed. The middle lobe will be standardized as the sampling region. A portion of the tissues will be sectioned and soaked in 10% (volume/volume) formaldehyde for 24 hr for subsequent staining, while the remainder was stored at -20°C for further testing. Liver TCH contents was determined after homogenization with Folch solution (chloroform/methanol ratio = 2:1) (Xie et al., 2011).

10.3.8 DETERMINATION OF LIVER TRIGLYCERIDE

The lipids in 200 mg frozen liver will be extracted according to Folch et al. triglyceride will be first hydrolyzed in a basic solution (0.5N KOH in ethanol) and will be then measured using commercial enzymatic triglyceride analysis kit (Membrez et al., 2008).

10.3.9 ORAL GLUCOSE TOLERANCE TEST

The oral glucose tolerance tests were performed between 09:00 to 11:00 hr. The food and fructose were removed from animal cages for 12 hr before the administration of an oral glucose load (2 g/kg of body weight) by oral gavage. Blood samples were collected from the tail vein at 0, 15, 30, 60, 90, and 120 min after glucose administration (Yadav et al., 2006).

10.3.10 STATISTICAL ANALYSIS

The results are presented as mean ± standard error of the mean (SEM). Statistical differences between the means of the various groups were analyzed using one way analysis of variance (ANOVA). Data were considered statistically significant at $P< 0.05$. Statistical analysis was performed using biostat statistical software. The control groups were considered as the standard.

10.4 DISCUSSION AND RESULTS

10.4.1 GUT MICROBIOTA MODULATION AND ITS EFFECT ON ADIPOSITY IN ANTIBIOTIC TREATED MICE

The body weight and food intake did not show any significant difference among the various treatment groups.

The body weight of CD-GP-LI were not identical in weight as compared to control rat initially, but after 30 days treatment their weight was almost similar and was having higher fat pad weight indicating that the gram negative bacteria were most dominantly present in the gut which are responsible for extracting energy from diet. The total fat pad, which is the sum of ependymal, mesenteric, and retroperitoneal was higher in the treatment group as compared to that of the control. In CD-BS-LI the body weight was almost similar to control rats and was slightly lower adipose tissue weight. But, these results are in contradiction to earlier data reported by Cani et al., (2008). The Cani et al., (2008) used broad spectrum antibiotic, which may be responsible for reduction in body weight and based on their finding they hypothesized that the amount of food intake rather than modulation of gut microbiota is responsible for adiposity. In the present investigation, the effects observed were contractory especially in case of high fructose fed group (Graph 1–2).

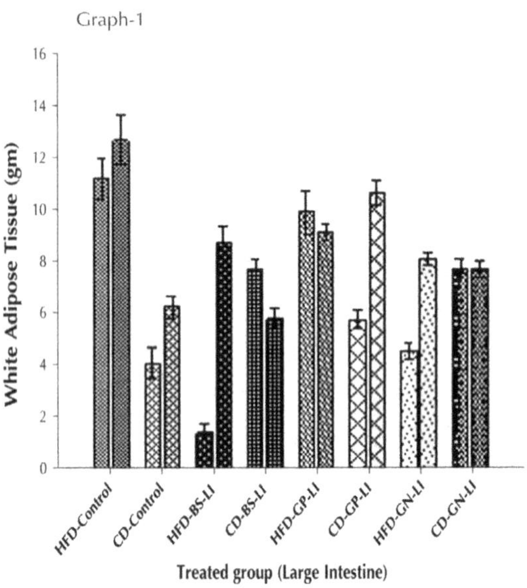

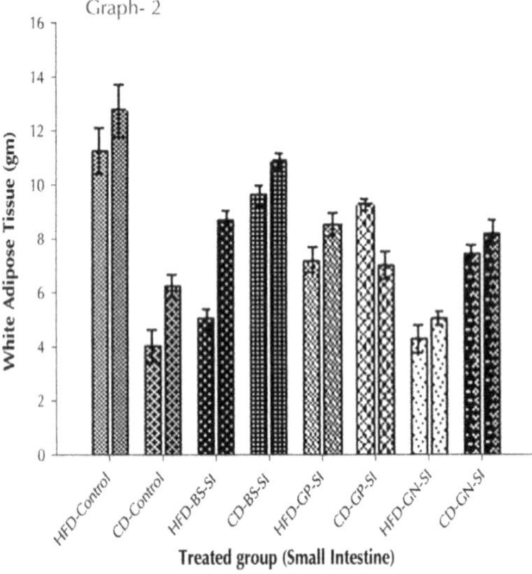

GRAPH 1-2 White Adipose tissue weight in various treatment groups coated with Eudragit L100-55 in graph 1 and Eudragit S100 in graph 2. Data are expressed as Mean ± SE of 3 animals.

10.4.2 INCREASED LEVELS OF LIVER GLYCOGEN AND HDL-C

The liver glycogen levels of CD-GN-LI and CD-GN-SI group rats are higher as compared to the control fed rats, this may be due to partial removal of gram negative bacteria and presence of predominately useful gram positive bacteria like *lactobacilli* and *bifidobacteria* which may be responsible for accumulation of glycogen as reported previously (Cani et al., 2008) (Graph 3–4).

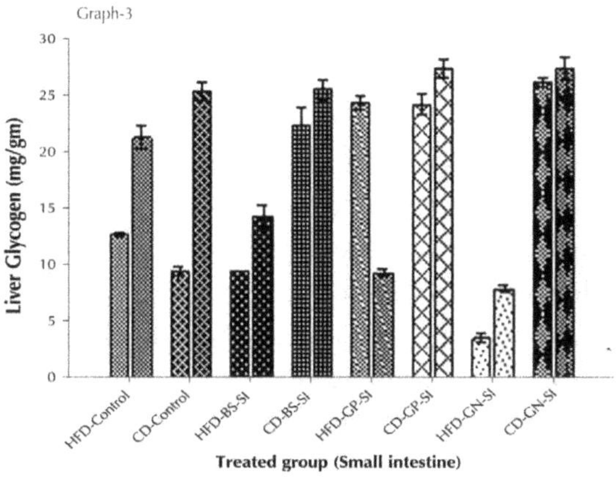

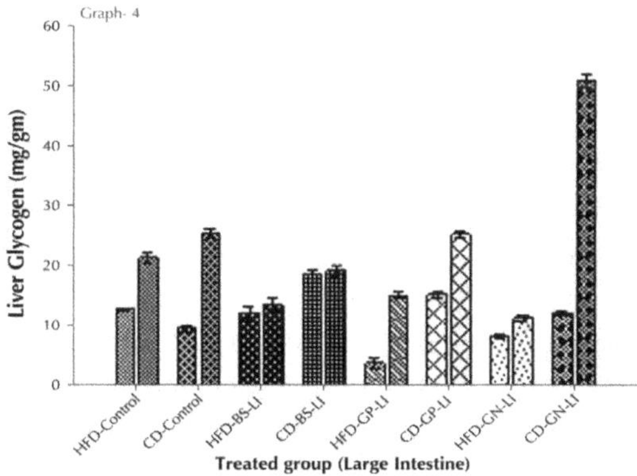

GRAPH 3–4 Assessment of Liver glycogen in various treatment groups coated with Eudragit L100-55 (graph 3) and Eudragit S100 (graph 4). Data are expressed as Mean ± SE of 3 animals.

But there is no significant increase in HFD-GP-SI, CD-GP-SI, HFD-GP-LI and CD-GP-LI compared to the control rats which could be the attributed to the fact that there is partial removal of gram positive bacteria, while in case of CD-BS-SI glycogen level is slightly increased and for HFD-BS-SI, HFD-BS-LI and CD-BS-LI is slightly lower than control fed rats but the mechanism is still unknown.

The liver is a very important organ for regulation of the blood glucose and lipid homeostasis. Fructose is a potent regulator of glycogen synthesis and liver glucose uptake (McGuinness and Cherrington, 2003). The results of present study showed that administration of antibiotics to rats for four weeks inhibited the disturbance in glucose metabolism in the liver by reducing the accumulation of glycogen in liver, which might be due to induced glycogenolysis and/or inhibited gluconeogenesis.

The exposure of the liver to large quantities of fructose leads to rapid stimulation of lipogenesis and triacylglycerol (TG) accumulation due to the ability of fructose to bypass the main regulatory step of the glycolytic pathway, the conversion of glucose-6-phosphate to fructose 1,6 phosphate, controlled by phosphofructokinase.

Thus, the glucose metabolism is negatively regulated by phosphofructokinase and fructose can continuously enter the glycolytic pathway, and fructose can uncontrollably produce glucose, lactate, and pyruvate providing glycerol and acyl portions of acyglycerol molecules, which result in high productions of TG, free fatty acids (FFA), cholesterol, very low density lipoprotein (VLDL), and low density lipoprotein (LDL)-cholesterol (Mayes, 1993). The liver produces excess FFA and TG which migrate through VLDL to skeletal muscles and peripheral tissues to make them insulin resistant and results in hyperinsulinemia (Reaven et al., 1993).

Antibiotic treatment had the protective effect on HDL-C as in HFD-GN-SI and CD-GN-SI on 15 days treatment it was lower than the control rats but after 30 days HDL-C value increased indicating the positive effect of gram positive bacteria. But, HFD-GP-SI values were lower after 30 days treatment indicating the negative impact of gram negative bacteria and in CD-GP-SI, no significant difference was observed compared to control rats after 30 days treatment (Graph 5–6).

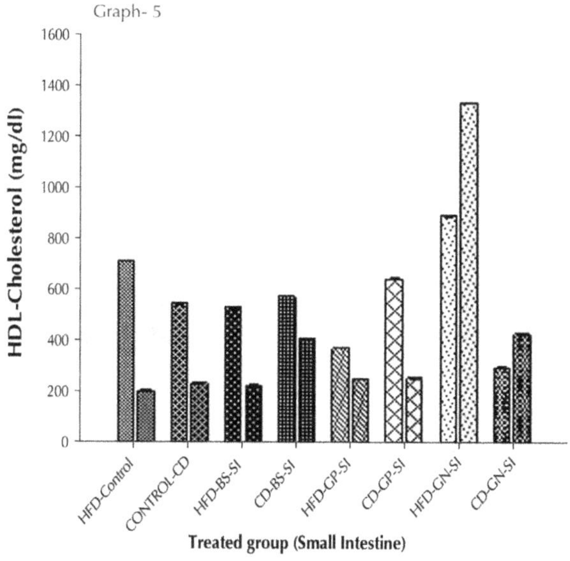

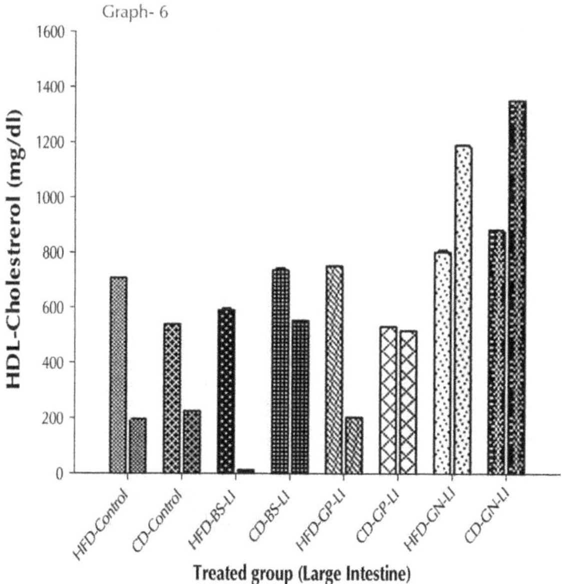

GRAPH 5–6 Assessment of HDL-Cholesterol in various treatment groups coated with Eudragit L100-55 (graph 5) and Eudragit S100 (graph 6). Data are expressed as Mean ± SE of 3 animals.

Similar effect was seen in case of HFD-GN-LI and CD-GN-LI, as there HDL-C values were significantly higher then compared to control rats. While values of HDL-C were lower in case of HFD-GP-LI, indicating the predominance of gram negative bacteria and for CD-GP-SI, not much difference was observed.

While, HFD-BS-SI and HFD-BS-LI were significantly lower than control rats these may be due to high fructose diet given to rats because in case of CD-BS-SI and CD-BS-LI the values were larger than the control fed rat proving that antibiotic modulation could decrease the levels of LDL and VLDL while, increase the values of HDL-C in spite of giving high fructose diet to rats.

The total cholesterol levels of HFD-GP-SI and CD-GP-SI were significantly higher than the control rat which is expected due to the presence of gram negative bacteria but, levels of CD-GN-SI and HFD-GN-SI were also higher compared to the control rats and the reason for this is unknown.

While cholesterol levels of HFD-BS-SI were significantly much higher compared to control rats while that of CD-BS-SI were slightly higher than control rats. Cholesterol levels of CD-GN-LI (Graph 7–8).

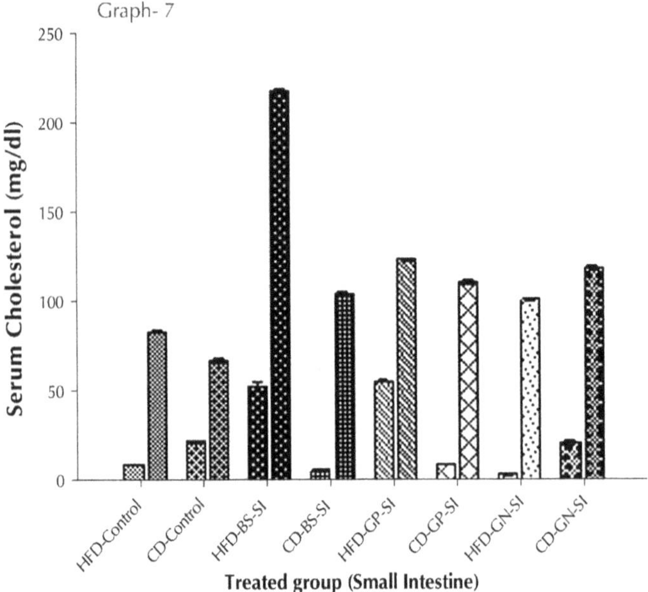

GRAPH *(Continued)*

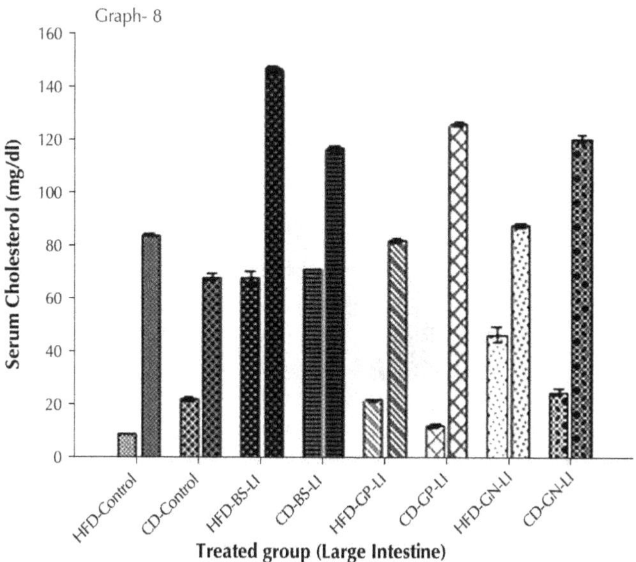

GRAPH 7–8 Assessment of serum cholesteron in various treatment groups coated with Eudragit L100-55 (graph 7) and Eudragit S100 (graph 8). Data are expressed as Mean ± SE of 3 animals.

CD-GP-LI and CD-BS-LI were much higher than control fed rats and HFD-BS-LI were much higher than control fed rats (Gerard et al., 2004).

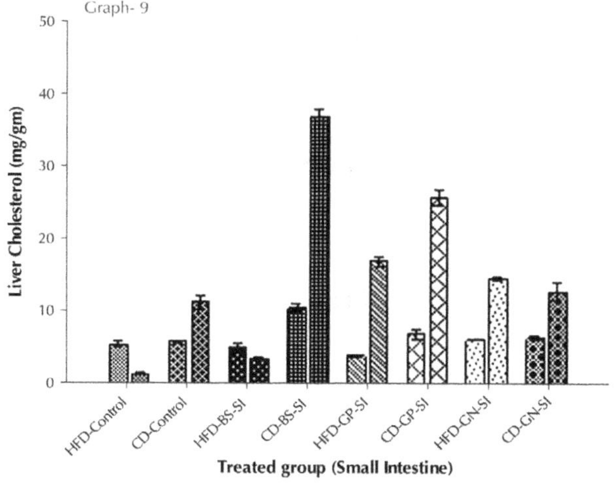

GRAPH *(Continued)*

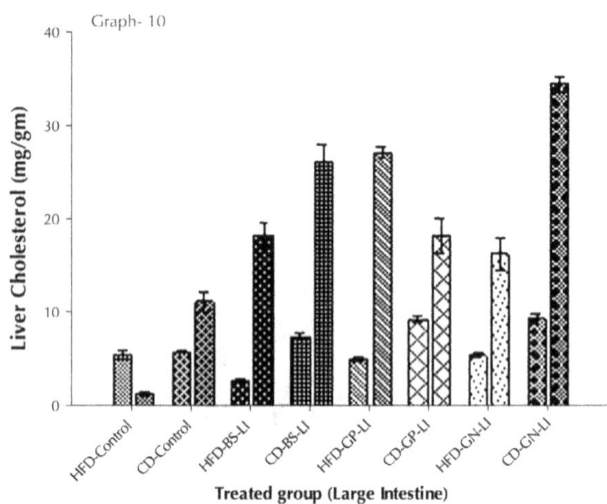

GRAPH 9–10 Assessment of Liver cholesteron in various treatment groups coated with Eudragit L100-55 (graph 9) and Eudragit S100 (graph 10). Data are expressed as Mean ± SE of 3 animals.

While value of liver cholesterol HFD-GN-LI and CD-GN-LI were slightly higher or equal to control rats because of the predominance of gram positive bacteria and values of CD-GP-SI and HFD-GP-SI were much higher compared to the control rats and this may be due to predominance of gram negative bacteria. Similarly values of CD-GP-LI and HFD-GP-LI were significantly higher than control rats (Gerard et al; 2004). But, values of HFD-GN-LI and CD-GN-LI were also higher and reason of higher level of cholesterol in these two groups is unknown (Graph 9–10).

10.4.3 EFFECT ON LIVER AND KIDNEY FUNCTION TESTS

In all treated group of small intestine urea level is higher than control rats. High urea levels suggest impaired kidney function. This may be due to acute or chronic kidney disease. However, there are many things besides kidney disease that can affect urea levels such as decreased blood flow to the kidneys as in congestive heart failure, shock, stress, and recent heart attack or severe burns; bleeding from the gastrointestinal tract; conditions that cause obstruction of urine flow, or dehydration (Clarkson et al., 2008).

All these may occur due to the antibiotic doses targeted to the small and large intestine and modified drug release from the pH sensitive microspheres.

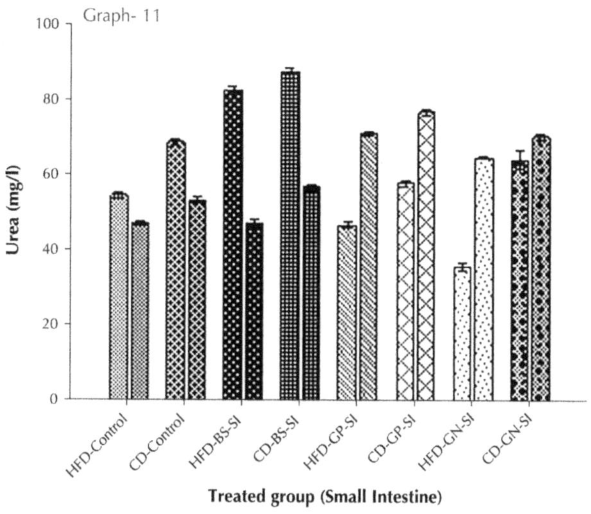

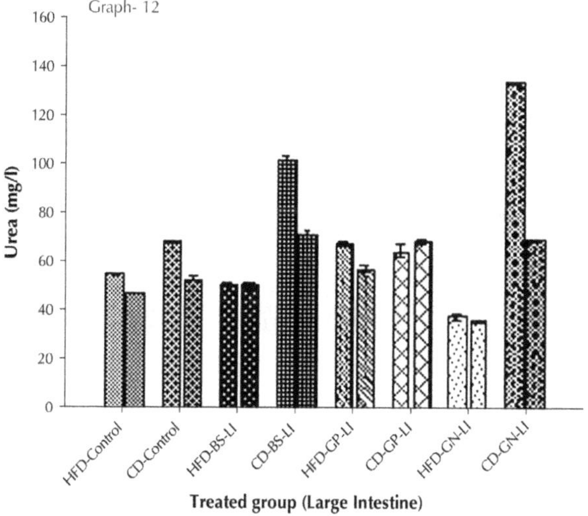

GRAPH 11–12 Assessment of serum Urea in various treatment groups coated with Eudragit L100-55 (graph 11) and Eudragit S100 (graph 12). Data are expressed as Mean ± SE of 3 animals.

In total protein test of treated groups of large intestine that is, CD-GN-LI were slightly lower than control rats. Low total protein levels can suggest a liver disorder, a kidney disorder, or a disorder in which protein is not digested or absorbed properly (Klein et al., 2007; Snanoudj et al., 2008).

Low levels may be seen in severe malnutrition and with conditions that cause malabsorption, such as Celiac or inflammatory bowel disease (IBD) (Heatedly, 1986) while for HFD-GN-LI protein levels are much higher than control rats and high protein level suggests chronic inflammation (Bazari et al., 2007) While, HFD-GP-LI and CD-GP-SI were slightly higher than control rats, similarly broad spectrum antibiotics showed the same results. The treated group of large intestine showed higher levels of protein.

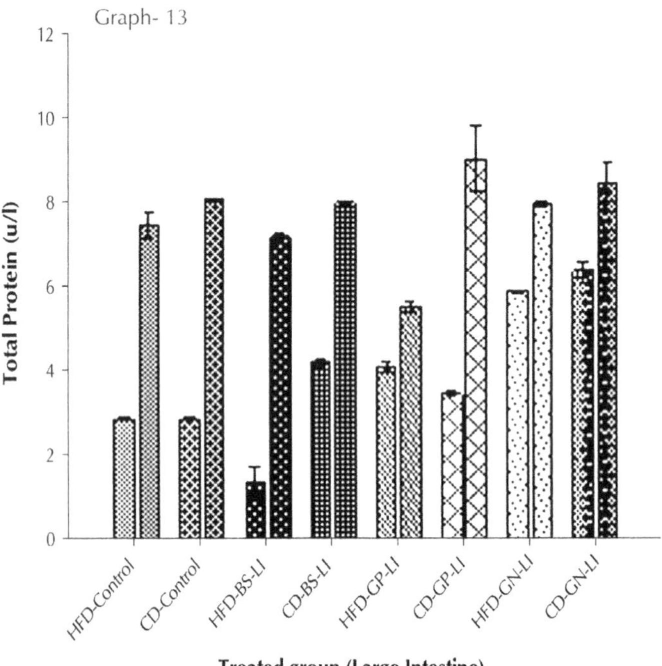

GRAPH *(Continued)*

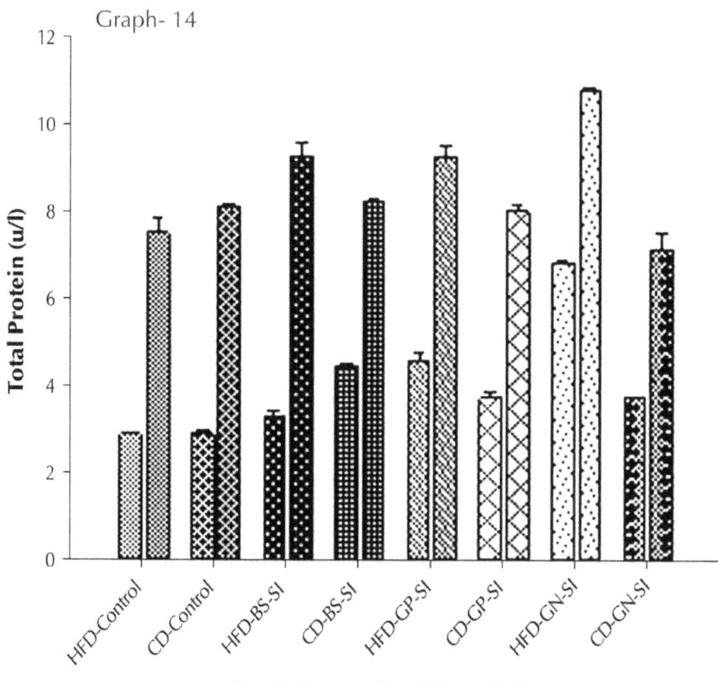

GRAPH 13–14 Assessment of Total Protein in various treatment groups coated with Eudragit L100-55 (graph 13) and Eudragit S100 (graph 14). Data are expressed as Mean ± SE of 3 animals.

The SGOT and SGPT tests values showed that small and large intestine treated group targeted against gram positive bacteria were much higher compared to the control rats indicating liver damage due to inflammation caused by gram negative bacteria. While treated group targeted against gram negative bacteria they, showed comparatively less damage while broad spectrum treated group of rats also showed higher values than control this may be due to continuous administration of broad spectrum antibiotic as shown in graph 15–18 (Berk et al., 2007; Pratt et al., 2007).

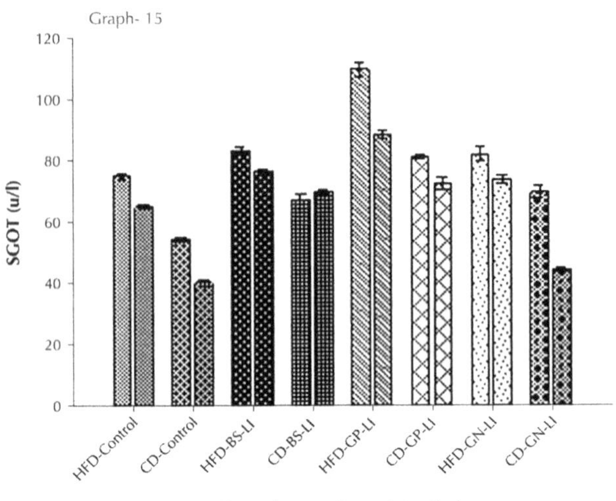

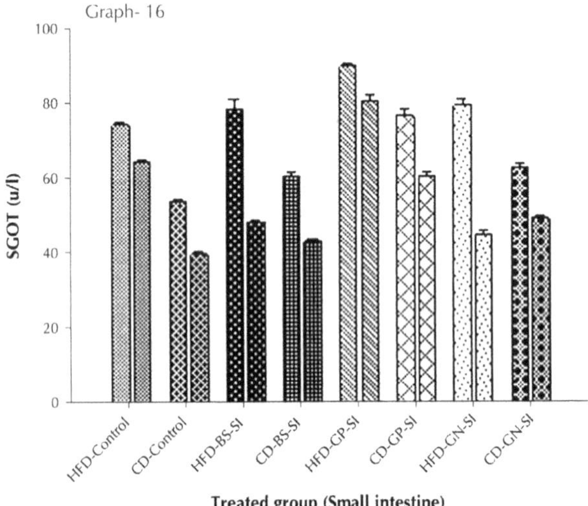

GRAPH 15–16 Assessment of Serum SGOT n in various treatment groups coated with Eudragit L100-55 (graph 15) and Eudragit S100 (graph 16). Data are expressed as Mean ± SE of 3 animals.

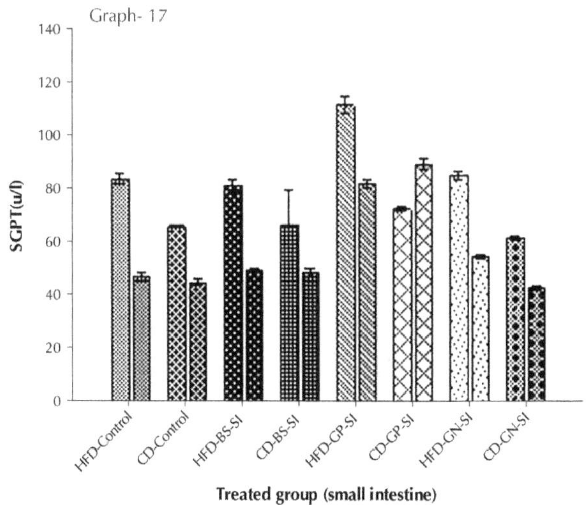

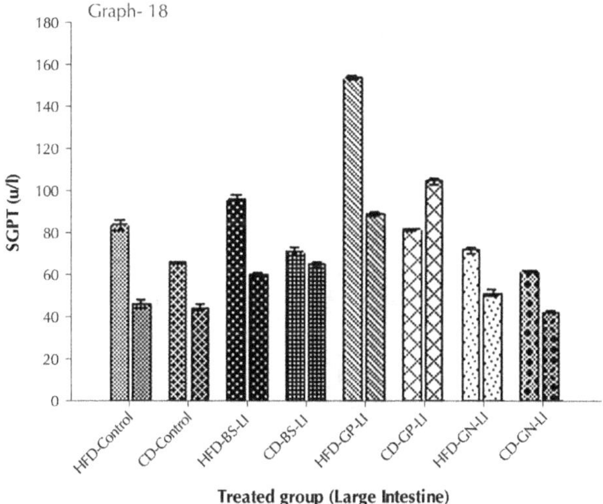

GRAPH 17–18 Assessment of Serum SGPT n in various treatment groups coated with Eudragit L100-55 (graph 17) and Eudragit S100 (graph 18). Data are expressed as Mean ± SE of 3 animals.

Bilirubin levels of CD-BS-LI, HFD-GP-LI, CD-GP-LI and HFD-GN-LI are higher compared to control rats indicating liver damage. Similarly, for HFD-GN-SI, HFD-GP-SI and HFD-BS-SI are higher than the control rats indicating liver damage (Berk et al., 2007; Pratt et al., 2007).

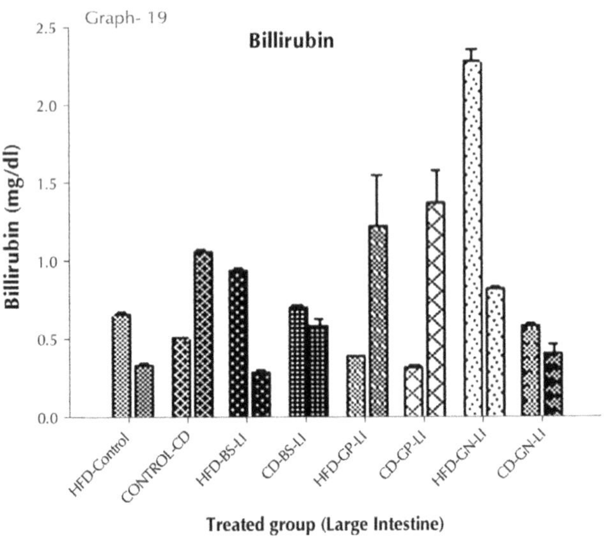

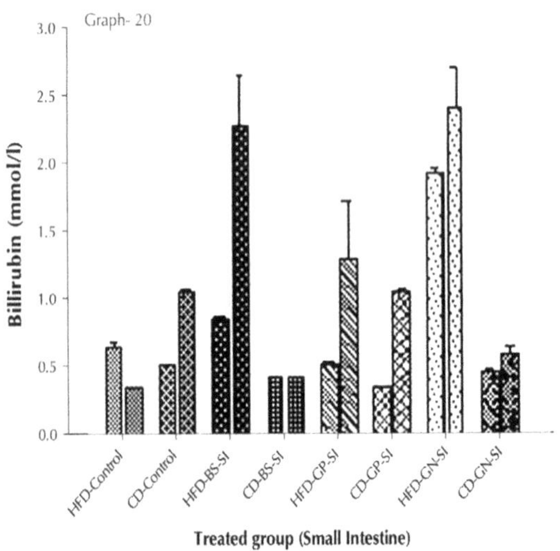

GRAPH 19–20 Assessment of Serum Bilirubin in various treatment groups coated with Eudragit L100-55 (graph 19) and Eudragit S100 (graph 20). Data are expressed as Mean ± SE of 3 animals.

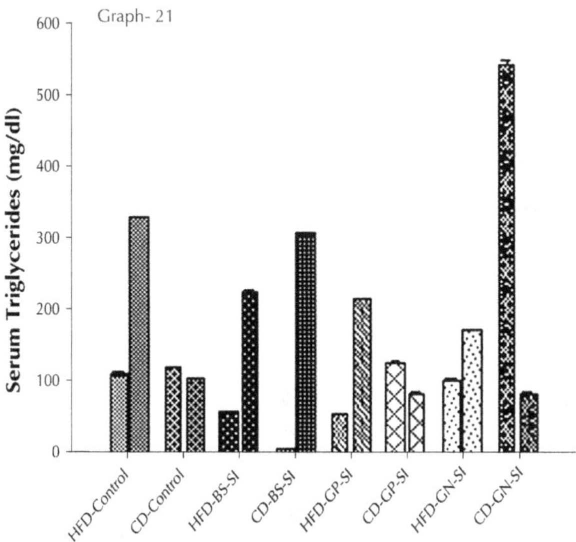

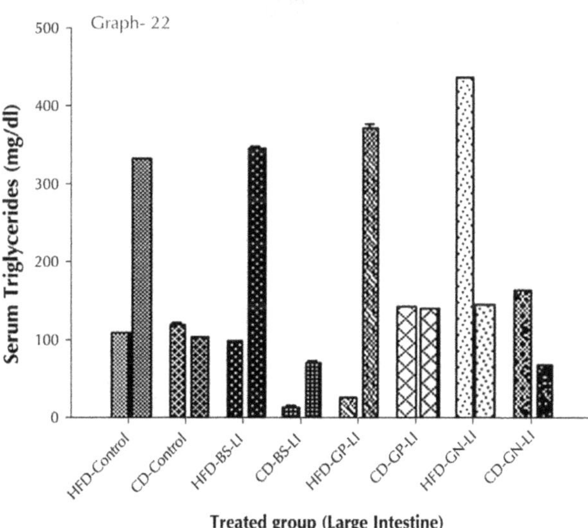

GRAPH 21–22 Assessment of Serum Tryglycerides in various treatment groups coated with Eudragit L100-55 (graph 21) and Eudragit S100 (graph 22). Data are expressed as Mean ± SE of 3 animals.

Levels of serum triglycerides of HFD-GN-LI, CD-GN-LI, HFD-GN-SI, and CD-GN-SI are lower than the control rats these may be due to predominance of gram positive bacteria and HFD-GP-LI, CD-GP-LI, HFD-GP-SI, and CD-GP-SI were higher than the control rats may be due to predominance of gram negative bacteria. While HFD-BS-LI, CD-BS-LI, and HFD-BS-SI were at par or slightly lower than control rats (Chou et al., 2008).

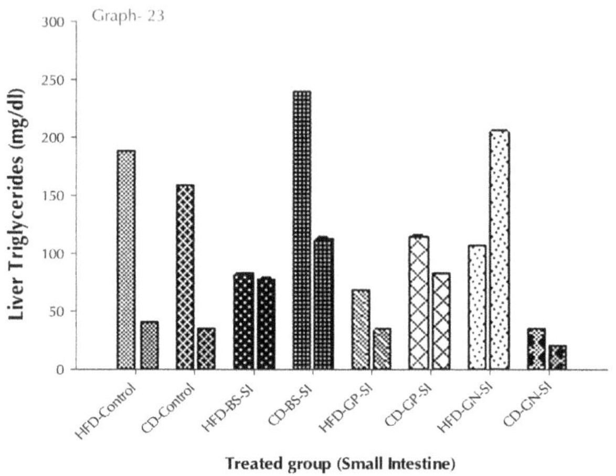

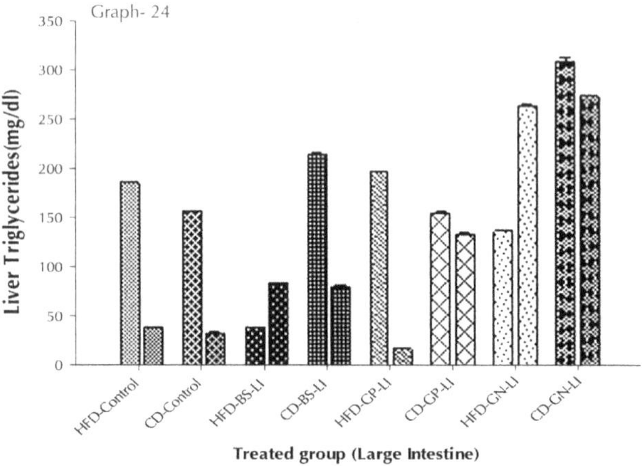

GRAPH 23–24 Assessment of Liver Tryglycerides n in various treatment groups coated with Eudragit L100-55 (graph 23) and Eudragit S100 (graph 24). Data are expressed as Mean ± SE of 3 animals.

While in case of liver triglyceride level only CD-GN-SI showed lower triglyceride level than control rats may be due to gram positive bacteria. And CD-GP-LI and CD-GP-SI is higher than control rats indicating the predominance of gram negative bacteria.

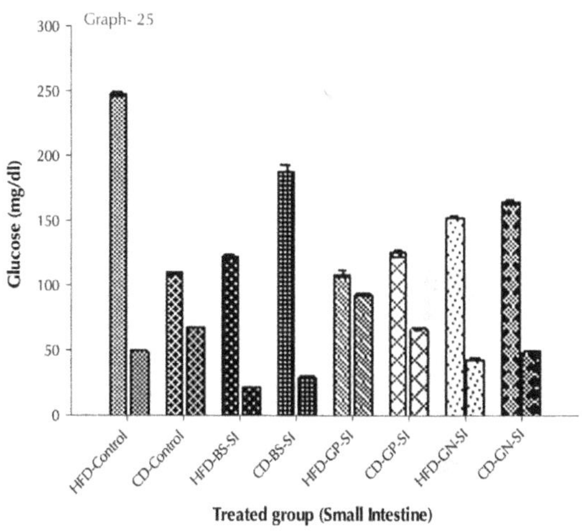

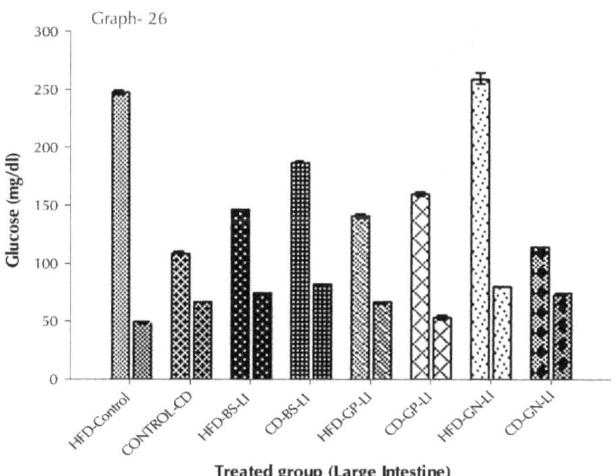

GRAPH 25–26 Assessment of Serum Glucose in various treatment groups coated with Eudragit L100-55 (graph 25) and Eudragit S100 (graph 26). Data are expressed as Mean ± SE of 3 animals.

As shown in graph 25 HFD-GN-SI and CD-GN-SI treated group of rats showed lower glucose level compared to control rats, while HFD-GP-SI is higher than control indicating the predominance of gram positive and gram negative bacteria respectively. While broad spectrum antibiotic treated group had lower blood glucose than control. Similarly in CD-GN-LI and HFD-GN-LI treated group of rats glucose level was higher and HFD-GP-LI glucose level higher than control rats broad spectrum treated group of rats showed higher level of glucose compared to control group (Graph 26).

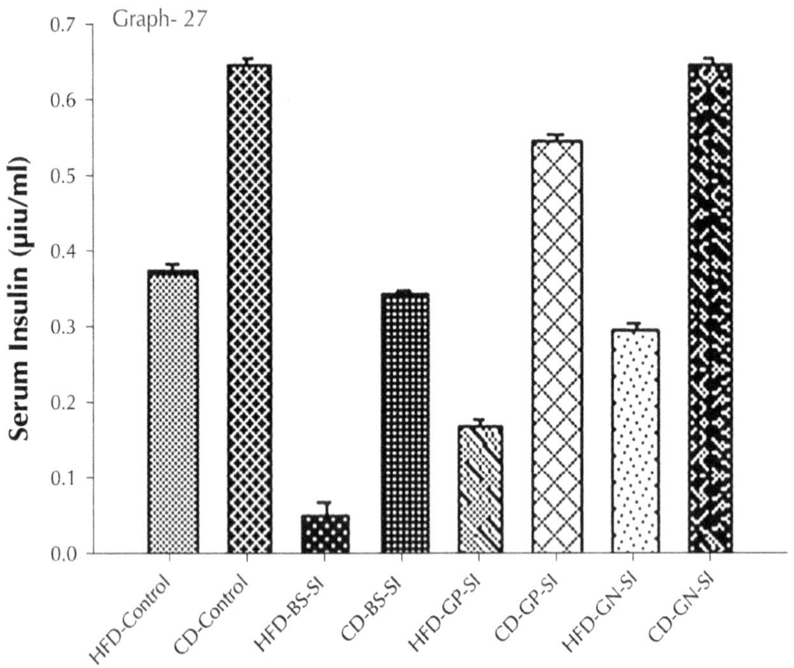

GRAPH *(Continued)*

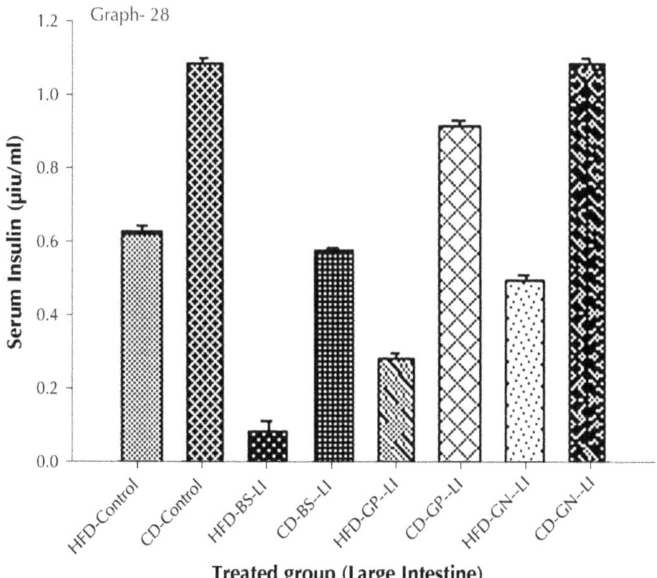

GRAPH 27–28 Assessment of serum Insulin in various treatment groups coated with Eudragit L100-55 (graph 27) and Eudragit S100 (graph 28). Data are expressed as Mean ± SE of 3 animals.

In CD-GN-LI group insulin level is higher compared to control rats while glucose level is normal this could be possibly due to presence of gram positive bacteria. In CD-GP-LI, CD-GP SI, HFD-GP-LI, and HFD-GP-SI group of rats insulin level is low and glucose level is high on 15 days treatment this could be due to predominance of gram negative bacteria. In CD-BS-LI, CD-BS-SI, HFD-BS-SI, and HFD-BS-LI group of rats insulin level is low compared to control rats and glucose level is high. So, since insulin production is low therefore, blood glucose levels are higher than the control rats.

In HFD-GN-LI insulin is high compared to control rats but glucose level is also high, but since in fructose fed rats hyperinsulinemia is reported (Julie et al., 1980) but since it is much higher than control rat as it can be seen in graph 28 so this could also be attributed to predominance of gram positive bacteria.

10.4.4 ORAL GLUCOSE TOLERANCE TEST (OGTT)

After 10 day treatment in HFD-BS-LI, HFD-BS-S, I CD-GN-LI, and CD-BS-LI group of rats the glucose value were in range of 140–200 mg/dl as shown in graph 35 and 36 meaning at increased risk of developing diabetes.

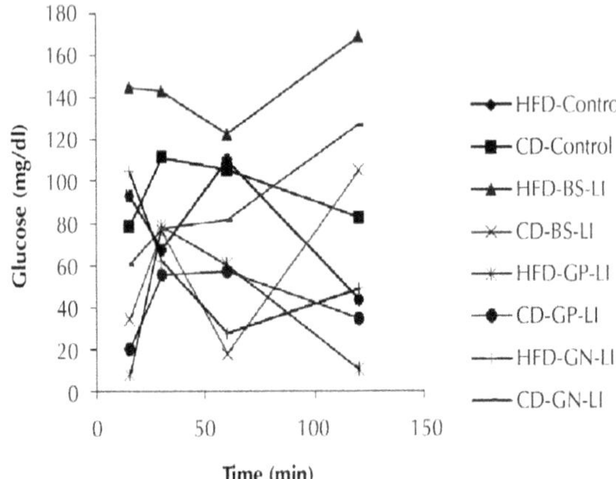

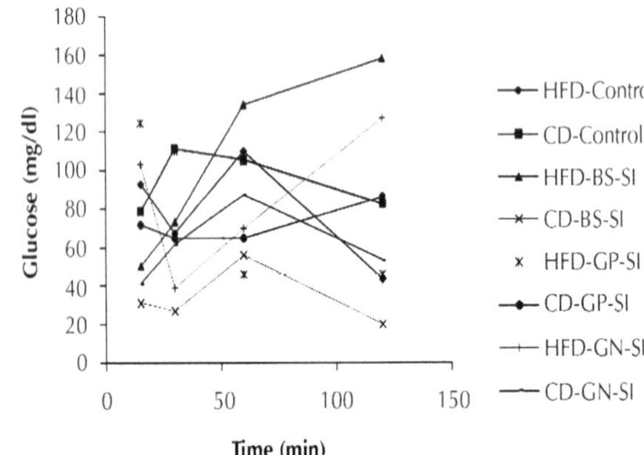

GRAPH 29–30 Assessment of serum OGTT in various treatment groups coated with Eudragit L100-55 (graph 29) and Eudragit S100 (graph 30). Data are expressed as Mean ± SE of 3 animals.

Gut microbiota modulation and effect on adiposity was seen and CD-GP-LI (control diet administered with linezolid coated with Eudragit S100) treated group had higher total fat pad compared to control rats in spite of having same body weight due to predominance of gram negative bacteria In CD-GN-LI (Control diet administered with cefdinir coated with Eudragit S100) group, increased levels of liver glycogen was observed, this may be due to partial removal of gram negative bacteria and presence of predominately useful gram positive bacteria like *lactobacilli* and *bifidobacteria* which may be responsible for accumulation of glycogen.

Antibiotic treatment had the protective effect on HDL-C as in HFD-GN-SI and CD-GN-SI group on 15th day. It was lower than the control rats but after 30 days, HDL-C value increased indicating the positive effect of gram positive bacteria. But HFD-GP-SI values were lower after 30 days treatment indicating the negative effect of gram negative bacteria. Total cholesterol levels of HFD-GP-SI and CD-GP-SI were significantly higher than the control rat which is expected due to the presence of gram negative bacteria.

While value of liver cholesterol HFD-GN-LI and CD-GN-LI were slightly higher or equal to control rats because of the predominance of gram positive bacteria and values of CD-GP-SI and HFD-GP-SI were much higher compared to the control rats and this may be due to predominance of gram negative bacteria. Similarly values of CD-GP-LI and HFD-GP-LI were significantly higher than control rats.

In all treated group of small intestine, urea level was higher than control rats. High urea levels suggest impaired kidney function. In total protein test of treated groups of large intestine that is, CD-GN-LI were slightly lower than control rats. Low total protein levels can suggest a liver disorder, a kidney disorder, or a disorder in which protein is not digested or absorbed properly. Aspartate transaminase (AST) or SGOT tests showed that CD-GN-LI and HFD-BS-LI were much higher compared to the control rats indicating liver damage. Billirubin levels of CD-BS-LI, HFD-GP-LI, CD-GP-LI, and HFD-GN-LI are higher compared to control rats indicating liver damage. Similarly, for HFD-GN-SI, HFD-GP-SI, and HFD-BS-SI are higher than the control rats indicating liver damage.

Serum triglycerides of HFD-GN-LI, CD-GN-LI, HFD-GN-SI, and CD-GN-LI were lower than control rats and HFD-GP-LI, CD-GP-LI,

HFD-GP-SI, and CD-GP-SI were higher than the control rats due to predominance of gram positive and gram negative bacteria respectively. Similarly, glucose levels of HFD-GN-LI, CD-GN-LI, HFD-GN-SI, and HFD-GN-LI were lower than control rats and HFD-GP-LI, CD-GP-LI, HFD-GP-SI, and CD-GP-SI were higher than the control rats.

10.5 CONCLUSION

The modulation of gut microbiota by using pH specific antibiotics with a view to increase gram positive bacteria especially bifidobacteria may lead to reduced endotoxaemia and improved metabolic parameters, as well as reducing inflammation development in high fructose diet-fed rats. Together, these findings suggest that the gut microbiota contribute to the pathophysiological regulation of endotoxaemia and set the tone of inflammation. Thus, specific strategies for modifying gut microbiota in favor of *bifidobacteria* and *lactobacilli* could be useful tools for reducing the impact of high-fat feeding on the occurrence of metabolic diseases.

KEYWORDS

- **Antibiotic**
- **Eudragit**
- **Fructose diet**
- **Gut Micro flora**
- **Large Intestine**
- **Small Intestine**

REFERENCE

1. Amar, J., Burcelin, R., Ruidavets, J. B., Cani, P. D., Fauvel, J., and Alessi, M. C. *Am. J. Clin. Nutr.*, **87**, 1219–23 (2008).
2. Anderson, P. D., Mehta, N. N., Wolfe, M. L., Hinkle, C. C., Pruscino, L., and Comiskey, L. L. *J. Clin. Endocrinol. Metab.*, **92**, 2272–9 (2007).
3. Backhed, F., Manchester, J. K., Semenkovich, C. F., and Gordon, J. I. *Proc. Natl. Acad. Sci. USA*, , **104**, 979–84 (2007).
4. Basu, S. K. and Adhiyaman, R. *Tropical J. Pharm. Res.*, **7** (3), 1033–1041 (2008).
5. Bazari, H. Approach to the patient with renal disease. In: L. Goldman, D. Ausiello, (Eds), *Cecil Medicine*. 23rd ed. Saunders Elsevier, Philadelphia,, p. 115 (2007).
6. Berk, D. R., Mallory, S. B., Keeffe, E. B., and Ahmed, A. *Clin. Gastroenterol. Hepatol.*, **5**, 142–151 (2007).
7. Bolke, E., Jehle, P. M., Storck, M., Nothnagel, B., Stanescu, A., and Orth, K. *Clin. Chim. Acta.*, **303**, 49–53 (2001).
8. Brugman, S., Klatter, F. A., Visser, J. T. J., Wildeboer-Veloo, A. C. M., and Harmsen, H. J. M. *Diabetologia*, **49**(9), 2105–8 (2006).
9. Cani, P. D., Bibiloni, R., Knauf, C., Waget, A., Neyrinck, A. M., and Delzenne, N. M. *Diabetes*, **57**, 1470–81 (2008).
10. Cani, P. D., Neyrinck, A. M., Fava, F., Knauf, C., Burcelin, R. G., Tuohy, K. M., Gibson, G. R., and Delzenne, N. M. *Diabetologia*, **50**, 2374–83 (2007).
11. Clarkson, M. R., Friedewald, J. J., and Eustace, J. A. Acute kidney injury. In, B. M. Brenner, S. A. Levine, eds. *Brenner & Rector's the kidney*. 8th ed. Philadelphia, Pa: Saunders Elsevier, pp 943–986 (2008).
12. Dibaise, J. K., Zhang, J., Crowell, M., Brown, K., Decker, A., and Rittmann, B. E. *Mayo, Clin. Proc.*, **83**, 460–469 (2008).
13. Dumas, M. E., Wilder, S. P., Bihoreau, M. T., Barton, R. H., Fearnside, J. F., Argoud, K., D'Amato, L., Wallis, R. H., Blancher, C., Keun, H. C., Baunsgaard, D., Scott, J., Sidelmann, U. G., Nicholson, J. K. and, Gauguier, D. *Nat. Genet.*, **39**, 666–672 (2007).
14. Erridge, C., Attina, T., Spickett, C. M., and Webb, D. J. *Am. J. Clin. Nutr.*, **86**, 1286–92 (2007).
15. Finberg, W., Moellering, R. C., Tally, F. P., Craig, W. A., Pankey, G. A., Dellinger, E. P., West, M. A., Joshi, M., Linden, P. K., Rolston, K. V., Rotschafer, J. C., and Rybak, M. J. *Clin. Infect. Dis.*, **39**, 1314–20 (2004).
16. Gaudier, E., Rival, M., Buisine, M. P., Robineau, L., and Hoebler, C. *Physiol. Res.*, **58**, 111–119 (2009).
17. Gerard, P., Beguet, F., Lepercq, P., Rigottier-Gois, L., Rochet, V., Andrieux, C., and Juste, C. *FEMS Microbiol. Ecol.*, **47**, 337–343 (2004).
18. Goto, T., Eden, S., Nordenstam, G., Sundh, V., Svanborg-Eden, C., and Mattsby-Baltzer, I. *Clin. Diagn Lab. Immunol.*, **1**, 684–8 (1994).

19. Hasday, J. D., Bascom, R., Costa, J. J., Fitzgerald, T., and Dubin, W. *Chest*, **115**, 829–35 (1999).
20. Hoverstad, T., Carlstedt, D. B., Lingaas, E., Midtvedt, T., Norin, K. E., Saxerholt, H., and Steinbakk, M. *Scand. J. Gastroenterol.*, **21**, 621–626 (1986).
21. Jakobsson, H. E., Jernberg, C., Andersson, A. F., Karlsson, M. S., Jansson, J. K., and Engstrand, L. *Plos one*, **5**(3), e9836 (2010).
22. Jernberg, C., Löfmark, S., Edlund, C., and Jansson, J. K. *ISME J.*, **1**, 56–66 (2007).
23. Klein, A., Friedrich, U., Vogelsang, H., and Jahreis, G. *Eur. J. Clin. Nutri.*, **62**(5): 584–593 (2008).
24. Larsen, N., Vogensen, F. K., Van-den-Berg, F. W. J., Nielsen, D. S., Andreasen, A. S., Pedersen. B. K., Al-Soud, W. A., Sørensen, S. J., Hansen, L. H., and Jakobsen, M. *PLOS One*, **5**(2), e9085 (2010).
25. Ley, R. E., Turnbaugh, P. J., Klein, S., and Gordon, J. I. *Nature*, **444**, 1022–3 (2006).
26. Löfmark, S., Jernberg, C., Jansson, J. K., and Edlund, C. J. Antimicrob. Chemother., **58**, 1160–1167 (2006).
27. Mayes, P. A. *Am. J. Clin. Nutr.*, **58**, 754S–765S (1993).
28. Mazumder, R., Nath, L. K., Haque, A., Maity, T., Choudhury, P. K., Shrestha, B., Chakraborty, M., and Pal, R. N. *Int. J. Pharm. Pharmaceut. Sci.*, **2**(1): 211–219 (2010).
29. Membrez, M., Blancher, F., Jaquet, M., Bibiloni, R., Cani, P. D., Burcelin, G., Corthesy, I., Mace K., and Chou, C. J. *FASEB J.*, **22**, 2416–2426 (2008).
30. Peng, L., Li, Z. R., Green, R. S., Holzman, I. R., and Lin, J. *J. Nut.*, **139**, 1619–1625 (2009).
31. Pratt, W. B., Maithel, S. K., Vanounou, T., Huang, Z. S., Callery, M. P., and Vollmer, C. M. *Jr. Ann. Surg.*, **245**, 443–451 (2007).
32. Reaven, G. M., Chen, Y. D., Jeppesen, J., Maheux, P., and Krauss, R. M. *J. Clin. Invest.*, **92**, 141–146 (1993).
33. Snanoudj, R., Timsit, M. O., Tricot, L., Loupy, A., Hiesse, C., Zuber, J., Kreis, H., Martinez, F., Thervet, E., Méjean, A., Lebret, T., Legendre, C., Delahousse, M. *Am. J. Transplant.*, **8**, 219 (2008).
34. Turnbaugh, P. J., Ley, R. E., Mahowald, M. A., Magrini, V., Mardis, E. R., Gordon, J. I. *Nature*, **444**, 1027–31 (2006).
35. Vander Vries, J. Biochem. J. 1954, 57: 410-416.
36. Wiedermann, C. J., Kiechl, S., Dunzendorfer, S., Schratzberger, P., Egger, G., and Oberhollenzer, F. J. *Am. Coll. Cardiol.*, **34**, 1975–81 (1999).
37. Wu, X., Ma, C., Han, L., Nawaz, M., Gao, F., Zhang, X., Yu, P., Zhao, C., Li, L., Zhou, A., Wang, J., Moore, J. E., Millar, B. C., and Xu, J. *Curr. Microbiol.*, **61**(1), 69–78 (2010).
38. Xie, N., Cui, Y., Ya-Ni, Y., Xin, Z., Jun-Wen, Y., Zheng-Gen, W., Nian, F., Yong, T., Xue-Hong, W., Xiao-Wei, L., Chun-Lian, W., and Fang-Gen, L. *BMC Complement. Altern. Med.*, **11**, 53–64 (2011).
39. Yadav, S., Boddula, R., Genitta, G., Bhatia, V., Bansal, B., Kongara, S., Julka, S., Kumar, A., Singh, H. K., Ramesh, V., and Bhatia, E. *Indian J. Med. Res.*, **128**, 712–720 (2008).

40. Yap, I. K. S., Li, J. V., Saric, J., Martin, P. F., Davies, H., Wang, Y., Wilson, I. D., Nicholson, J. K., Utzinger, J., Marchesi, J. R., and Holmes, E. *J. Proteome Res.*, **7**, 3718–3728 (2008).
41. Zhang, C., Zhang, M., Wang, S., Han, R., Cao, Y., Hua, W., Mao, Y., Zhang, X., Pang, X., Wei, C., Zhao, G., Chen, Y., and Zhao, L. *ISME J.*, **4**(2), 232–41 (2010).

CHAPTER 11

PREVALENCE OF DIABETES MELLITUS IN PATIENTS PRESENTING WITH ACUTE MYOCARDIAL INFARCTION

MEEAKSHI NARKHEDE, SATYANARAYAN DURGAM, HARSHAL BHITKAR, SWAPNIL YADAV, and DILIP MHAISEKAR

CONTENTS

ABSTRACT

The coronary heart disease (CHD) is common in people with diabetes mellitus (DM). In people with diabetes, CHD causes almost 60% of their deaths. They have a two- to three-fold increased risk for CHD and two- to four-fold higher CHD morbidity and mortality rates. Diabetic patients with myocardial infarction (MI) have a two- to three fold higher mortality than do their non-diabetic counterparts. The most important factor for this is increased left ventricular failure which may be due to a "diabetic cardiomyopathy" that is not related to the atherosclerosis. Another possible factor is the higher prevalence of silent ischemia that can lead to delayed diagnosis of CHD in people with diabetes. Diabetic patients with MI also have worse long-term prognosis than do their non-diabetic counterparts. The present observational and prospective study was conducted in the intensive care unit of a tertiary care centre and Government Medical College, Nanded. The aim of this chapter was to study the prevalence of DM in patients presenting with acute myocardial infarction (AMI). The objectives of this study were to compare clinical outcome in diabetic *versus* non diabetic patients with AMI, to study the role of some risk factors in AMI patients associated with DM. All the patients presenting with AMI admitted in the Intensive Cardiac Care Unit (ICCU) from July 2011 to January 2012 were studied. Patients were diagnosed to have DM as per American Diabetes Association (ADA) Guidelines. Study population was divided into two groups, patients having diabetes and not having diabetes. Detail present, past, and family history along with clinical examination of every patient was collected and entered in a performa prepared specially for collection of data. Glycosylated hemoglobin was not done due to non-affordability of patients, being a resource limited setting. Consecutive patients having ST elevation MI (As per World Health Organization criteria) who were treated with Streptokinase at the time of admission in MICU were included in the study. Patients coming after 12 hr of chest pain and patients suffering from type 1 diabetes mellitus (T1DM) were excluded from the study. A total of 176 patients were included in the study. One hundred thirty three were male and 43 females. In diabetics 71 (78.7%) out of 91 patients ($p< 0.0001$) and in non-diabetics 28 (33.2%) out of 85 patients developed complications during their ICCU stay. Diabetics have more complications as compared to non-diabetics, recurrent chest pain (64.1% *versus* 33.1%, $p< 0.0001$), heart failure (36.6% *versus* 18.82%, $p< 0.0001$), arrhythmias (43.6% *versus* 17.6%, $p< 0.0001$), and mortality (4.3% *versus* 1.17%, $p< 0.05$). Smoking (42.1%) and alcohol consumption (56.5%) were found to be significant in diabetic group as compared to the non-diabetic group. Hypertension was found more common in diabetic ($p< 0.05$) as compared to non-diabetic study population.

Prevalence of diabetes among patients admitted with AMI was found to be 51.7%. Male patients showing slightly higher (52.63%) prevalence of diabetes as compared to females (50.00%). The AMI patients having diabetes encounter more adverse clinical outcome in the form of complications. More number of patients having AMI and diabetes were alcoholics and smokers.

11.1 INTRODUCTION

The type 2 diabetes mellitus (T2DM) is a chronic metabolic disorder also known as non-insulin dependent diabetes or adult onset diabetes. It is characterized by impaired insulin secretion, insulin resistance, hyperglycemia, and relative insulin deficiency. Long term complications of it develop gradually over the years and affect almost every organ of the body. Chronic complications of T2DM include microvascular and macrovascular complications. Microvascular complications affect eyes causing diabetic retinopathy, Kideys causing diabetic nephropathy and nerves casing diabetic neuropathy. Macrovascular complications cause cerebrovascular disease, peripheral arterial disease, and coronary heart disease. The Framingham heart study revealed a marked increase in congestive heart failure, CHD, MI, and sudden death in diabetes mellitus. The American Heart Association has designated DM as a CHD risk equivalent. The CHD is the leading cause of death in India and the leading cause of death worldwide. The CHD was previously thought to affect primarily high-income countries but now is seen to be common in low- and middle-income countries, such as India. In developed countries, ischemic heart disease is predicted to rise 30–60% between 1990 and 2020. In developing countries, prevalence rates are predicted to increase by 120% in women and 137% in men from 1990 to 2020 (Murray et al., 1997). It is also predicted that 60% of the world's patients with heart disease, including CHD, are to live in India by 2010 (Ghaffar et al., 2004).

The AMI can be considered as a potential epidemic for mankind (WHO, 1982). The incidence of coronary artery disease is rising in India. The DM is one of the six primary risk factors identified for MI, others being dyslipidemia, smoking, male gender, hypertension, and family history of atherosclerotic arterial disease. The DM is a metabolic disorder which increases the rate of atherosclerosis progression of vascular occlusion. Even after prompt thrombolysis the aftermath of diabetic patients is still worse than the non-diabetics, indicating impaired post thrombolytic left ventricular function and prognosis.

The DM is a strong risk factor for cardiovascular disorders, including coronary heart disease. The DM has been diagnosed in 10–24% of patients with AMI.

The prevalence of diabetes is rapidly rising all over the globe at an alarming rate. Over the past 30 years, the status of diabetes has changed from being considered as a mild disorder of the elderly to one of the major causes of morbidity and mortality affecting the youth and middle aged people. It is important to note that the rise in prevalence is seen in all six inhabited continents of the globe. Although, there is an increase in the prevalence of T1DM also, the major driver of the epidemic is T2DM which accounts for more than 90% of all diabetes cases.

India leads the world with largest number of diabetic subjects and being termed the "diabetes capital of the world". According to the Diabetes Atlas 2006 published by the International Diabetes Federation, the number of people with diabetes in India was around 40.9 million in 2006 is expected to rise to 69.9 million by 2025 unless urgent preventive steps are taken. The so called "Asian Indian Phenotype" refers to certain unique clinical and biochemical abnormalities in Indians which include increased insulin resistance, greater abdominal adiposity that is higher waist circumference despite lower body mass index, lower adiponectin, and higher high sensitive C-reactive protein levels. This phenotype makes Asian Indians more prone to diabetes and premature coronary artery disease. At least a part of this is due to genetic factors.

As per World Health Organization (WHO's), the *World health statistics 2012* report, one in six adults obese, one in 10 diabetic, and one in three has raised blood pressure. Dr Margaret Chan, Director-General of WHO says "this report is further evidence of the dramatic increase in the conditions that trigger heart disease and other chronic illnesses, particularly in low, and middle-income countries. In some African countries, as much as half the adult population has high blood pressure."

Many studies have reported that DM is associated with increased CHD morbidity and mortality. Compared with the general population, diabetic individuals have a twofold increase in CHD mortality, and it is estimated that CHD accounts for 30–50% of all diabetic deaths after 40 years of age. The prevalence of diabetes is increased in patients suffering a MI and both the short- and long-term prognosis after an Ml is poorer among diabetic individuals. In chapter, there is evidence that diabetic women have a poorer prognosis than diabetic men after an Ml.

Thrombolysis is still the most preferred treatment in resource limited settings. And in the ICCU's evaluation of ST segment changes are considered to be cost effective way to assess coronary reperfusion. Whereas coronary angiogram is a marker for epicardial reperfusion, ST segment resolution offers a better reflection of micro vascular reperfusion. Although, successful thrombolysis of the epicardial vessel is necessary for good prognosis but the micro-vascular flow more strongly correlates with the outcome. The ST segment is therefore a better indicator of prognosis, and provides information which cannot be assessed on basis of coronary angiogram alone.

The T2DM patients without a prior MI have a similar risk for coronary artery related events as non-diabetic individuals who have had a prior MI. Because of the extremely high prevalence of underlying cardiovascular disease in individuals with diabetes (especially in T2DM), evidence of atherosclerotic vascular disease (e.g., cardiac stress test) should be sought in an individual with diabetes who has symptoms suggestive of cardiac ischemia or peripheral or carotid arterial disease.

The screening of asymptomatic diabetic individuals for CHD is controversial, and recent studies have not shown a clinical benefit. Silent ischemia or absence of chest pain is common in persons with diabetes, and a thorough cardiac evaluation should be considered in individuals undergoing major surgical procedures. It is also observed that prognosis of individuals with diabetes having CHD or MI is worse than that of non-diabetics. Multivessel coronary involvement is more likely in diabetics than non-diabetics.

It Improve glycemic control immediately after the diagnosis of diabetes reduces cardiovascular and microvascular complications in DM. The glycemic goal for individuals with long-standing diabetes remains unclear. In both the DCCT (T1DM) and the UKPDS (T2DM), cardiovascular events were not reduced by intensive treatment during the trial but were reduced at follow up 10–17 years later. This effect has been termed legacy effect or metabolic memory. In the DCCT trial, an improvement in the lipid profile of individuals in the intensive group, lower total and LDL cholesterol, lower triglycerides was noted. In various trials to examine whether very aggressive glycemic target, HbA_{1C} near 6% reduce cardiovascular events in T2DM did not show a survival benefit of reducing the A_{1C} below 7% (and in one trial, the outcome was worse). Current recommendations do not suggest more aggressive glucose lowering in this patient population. The possibility of atherogenic potential of insulin is suggested by the data in non-diabetic individuals showing higher serum insulin levels (indicative of insulin resistance) in association with greater risk of cardiovascular morbidity and mortality. Treatment with insulin and OHA, the sulfonylureas did not appear to increase the risk of cardiovascular disease in diabetics.

Antiplatelet treatment reduces cardiovascular events in diabetics having CHD. Current ADA recommendations include the use of aspirin for secondary prevention of coronary events and the consideration of primary use of Aspirin in diabetic individuals with an increased cardiovascular risk.

Diabetes is a chronic disease and need lifelong therapy. It is treatable and can be kept under control. But even when glucose levels are under control it greatly increases the risk of heart disease and stroke. That is because people with diabetes, especially T2DM, often have associated risk factors that contribute for developing cardiovascular disease like hypertension. The various studies across the globe report a positive association between hypertension and insulin resistance. When patients have both hypertension and diabetes their risk for cardiovascular disease doubles.

Abnormal cholesterol and high triglycerides Patients with diabetes often have high LDL ("bad") cholesterol, low HDL ("good") cholesterol, and high triglycerides. Abnormal body mass index, Obesity and sedentary life style along with diabetes are a major risk factor for cardiovascular disease and have been strongly associated with insulin resistance. Life style modification and weight loss can improve cardiovascular risk, decrease insulin resistance, and increase insulin sensitivity. Obesity and insulin resistance also have been associated with other risk factors like hypertension. Poorly controlled diabetes also increases risk of CHD.

As per various studies MI is the most common cause of mortality in diabetics which is twice that of nondiabetics. The mechanism for the "diabetic factor" underlying increased MI-related mortality in diabetic patients is unclear. The excess mortality due to MI in diabetic patients is independent of commonly recognized comorbid clinical conditions, including the extent of myocardial injury, left ventricular contractile dysfunction or coronary artery patency after reperfusion therapy. Improved understanding of molecular mechanisms and pathways that promote death in diabetic patients after MI is a major goal of biomedical science. Diabetes increases oxidant stress and doubles the risk of dying after MI but the mechanisms underlying increased mortality are unknown. In a research published in the journal of clinical research authors observed that Mice with streptozotocin-induced diabetes developed profound heart rate slowing and doubled mortality compared with controls after MI. They observed that oxidized Ca2+/calmodulin-dependent protein kinase II (ox-CaMKII) was significantly increased in pacemaker tissues from diabetic mice compared with that in non-diabetic mice after MI. It is also found that Streptozotocin-treated mice had increased pacemaker cell ox-CaMKII and apoptosis, which were further enhanced by MI. They developed a knock-in mouse model of oxidation-resistant CaMKIIδ (MM-VV), the isoform associated with cardiovascular disease. The findings suggest that activation of a mitochondrial/ox-CaMKII pathway contributes to increased sudden death in diabetic patients after MI. Diabetes can cause blood sugar to rise to dangerous levels. Treatment may be necessary to manage abnormal blood sugars.

Smoking and tobacco intake in diabetic patients increases the risk of MI. So, the modifiable factors should be corrected by keeping blood pressure, blood sugars and lipid levels under strict control, along with changes in life style.

11.2 MATERIALS AND METHODS

To find out prevalence of diabetes in patients admitted with AMI the present study was planned which included 176 patients presenting with AMI admitted in the ICCU from July 2011 to January 2012. Patients were diagnosed to have DM as per ADA Guidelines. The aims and objectives of the study were to study the prevalence of DM in patients of AMI, to compare clinical outcome in diabetic versus non diabetic patients with AMI and to study the role of some risk factors in AMI patients associated with diabetes mellitus.

All cases of AMI with the diagnosis based on WHO criteria that is, presence of any two of the following were included.1) chest pain consistent with AMI of less than 24 hr duration, 2) electrocardiography (ECG) changes that is, ST-segment elevation >0.2mv in at least two contagious chest leads or >0.1mv in at least two contiguous limb leads, 3) new or presumably new left bundle branch block on electrocardiogram, and 4) raised levels of cardiac enzymes CPK-MB more than double of the reference value or positive Troponin I test done with commercially available kits of Trop I. In all the patients CPK-MB levels were done but being a resource limited setting Troponin test was not done. The patients admitted in the ICCU within 12 hr of chest pain, with ST elevation on the ECG and having elevated CPK-MB levels, received Streptokinase on presentation. Patients coming after 12 hr of chest pain and suffering from T1DM were excluded.

In this study population was divided into two groups, GROUP-A— non-diabetics (n=85) and GROUP-B— diabetics (n=91). Only those patients, who were known cases of diabetes or in whom it was established during hospital stay by repeated blood glucose estimation, were included in Group B.

A detailed history was taken, particularly of age, sex, occupation, address, history of smoking, diabetes mellitus, hypertension, and family history of ischemic heart disease. The time from onset of chest pain to presentation in emergency was noted through the history. Complete physical examination of patients was done upon presentation in emergency department and important parameters, such as pulse and blood pressure were noted. Patients were followed up daily. Pulse, ECG changes, and complications if any were monitored till death or discharge of the patient.

Repeat ECG was performed after 60 min of administration of Streptokinase (SK) in every patient. The ST resolution was observed in the lead with the maximum ST elevation. ST resolution was defined as a reduction of >50% ST segment elevation after thrombolysis. Informed written consent of the patient/attendant was taken. Follow up was conducted for each patient throughout his/her hospital stay.

Patients were diagnosed to have DM as per Amarican diabetes association, 2011. The symptoms of diabetes (Polyurea, polydipsia, polyphagia) plus random blood glucose concentration 200 mg/dL (11.1 mmol/L) *or* Fasting plasma glucose 126 mg/dL (7.0 mmol/L) *or* A1C > 6.5% *or* Two-hour plasma glucose 200 mg/dL (11.1 mmol/L) during an oral glucose tolerance test. Patients previously diagnosed to have diabetes were also included in the study. Blood sugar levels were done immediately on admission. Fasting plasma glucose was recorded from all patients, in the morning of day following hospital admission. For differentiating new cases of diabetes, stress hyperglycemia, and non-diabetic, fasting plasma glucose measurements were repeated in stable condition prior to discharge from hospital.

Patients were continuously monitored in the ICCU and assessed for any complications. Major complications assessed were— recurrent ischemic chest pain, heart failure, arrhythmias, and death. Recurrent ischemic chest pain was assessed on the basis of history and ECG, heart failure was assessed on the basis of clinical examination, chest X-ray, and echocardiography.

11.2.1 STATISTICAL ANALYSIS

All the collected data was analyzed in the statistical package for social sciences (SPSS) version 12.0 for windows. Chi-square test was used to compare the demographic characteristics and complication in both groups with 0.05% level of significance.

11.3 DISCUSSION

In this study they found 51.7% prevalence of diabetes among patients admitted with AMI. They compared their results with various studies done in different countries. Several authors report on the prevalence of diabetes in AMI patients ranging from 8% to 18%. Some authors report that diabetes increases the risk of AMI. According to one study, diabetes as a risk factor was present in 10–24% of patients with AMI. Among patients with AMI, the percentage of diabetes in an ethnic group was 54%, whereas in another one it ranged from 21.6% to 33%.

Therefore, there is an extreme inconsistency in the prevalence of diabetes among AMI patients worldwide, data are ranging between 9.7% to 25.6%. Probably due to different parameters used for diagnosing diabetes.

In this study, prevalence of diabetes among patients admitted with AMI was found to be 51.7% which is comparable to other studies conducted at Delhi by Bansal et al. (2005), that shows prevalence rate of diabetes as 31.67%. Male patients showed slightly higher (52.63%) prevalence of diabetes as compared to females (50.00%) ,this is in contrast with the study by Baizer C.T., Cleveland (2006), that shows more number of diabetic females as compared to males.

Norhammar et al.studied 181 consecutive patients admitted to the coronary care units of two hospitals in Sweden with AMI, no diagnosis of diabetes, and a blood glucose <200 mg/dl (< 11.1 mmol/l) on admission. A standard 75 g glucose tolerance test was done at discharge and again 3 months later. The authors found a 31% prevalence of diabetes at the time of hospital discharge and a 25% prevalence of diabetes 3 months after discharge in this group with no previous diagnosis of diabetes.

Umpierrez et al.reported a 26% prevalence of known diabetes in hospitalized patients in a community teaching hospital. An additional 12% of patients had unrecognized diabetes or hospital-related hyperglycemia. Levetan et al.reported a 13% prevalence of laboratory-documented hyperglycemia (blood glucose >200 mg/dl (11.1 mmol) in 1,034 consecutively hospitalized adult patients. Based on hospital chart review, 64% of patients with hyperglycemia had preexisting diabetes or were recognized as having new-onset diabetes during hospitalization. Thirty-six percent of the hyperglycemic patients remained unrecognized as having diabetes in the discharge summary, although diabetes or "hyperglycemia" was documented in the progress notes for one-third of these patients.

In a study done by Muhammad Ali Khan et al, "Predicting clinical outcome in diabetics versus non-diabetics with AMI after thrombolysis, using ECG as a tool", the percentage of patients with AMI was significantly higher in the group of diabetics than in non-diabetics ($p<0.01$). The percentage of women with AMI was significantly higher among diabetics than among non-diabetics in all three study years (1991 and 1993, $p< 0.01$; 1996, $p< 0.05$). Among non-diabetics, the percentage of AMI was significantly higher in men as compared with women in all three study years ($p< 0.001$).

Recurrent chest pain was the most common complication observed in this study. A study supporting their results showed that there was a significant interaction between diabetic status and treatment strategy with respect to the occurrence of in-hospital recurrent ischemia that shows 29.5% diabetics and 23.1% non-diabetics developed recurrent ischemia after fibrinolysis, ($p< 0.001$). As shown by another study, diabetic patients may have a greater residual lesion in the infarct related artery after treatment with fibrinolytics, resulting in a higher rate of recurrent ischemia.

In this study 33(35.90%) diabetic patients had heart failure. Since most patients never had an echocardiography before this hospital admission to rule out prior heart failure, so, any indication of heart failure post thrombolysis was considered as a new development. Their results are supported by the findings of a study which showed that in-hospital heart failure was more common among diabetics after fibrinolysis.

A study on total of 2,767 consecutive patients presenting with ST-elevated myocardial infarction (STEMI) or non-ST elevated myocardial infarction (NSTEMI), an oral glucose tolerance test (OGTT) was performed at day 4 after admission. For the comparison of patients with different glucose abnormalities Kaplan–Meier plots were produced. The mean age was 66.4 years (median) and 74.6% male. Of the patients with glucose values (2536) 769 (30.5%) had normal glucose tolerance, 417 had impaired fasting glucose (16.6%), 182 impaired glucose tolerance (7.2%) and 461 had newly diagnosed diabetes (18.3). A total of 689 or 27.4% had pre-existent diabetes mellitus. Patients with abnormal glucose values were younger, more often female, had more risk factors like hypertension, increases in serum creatinine, and had a frequent history of cardiovascular events. The relative risk for death and major adverse cardiac and cerebrovascular event (MACCE) gradually increased in patients with increasing dysglycemia. Authors concluded that there was a considerable prevalence of dysglycemia in patients presenting with an AMI and leads to an increase in death rates.

In their study mortality in diabetic group was 4.3% compared to 1.17% in non-diabetic group (P< 0.015). A study supporting these findings was carried out by Timmer JR et al. According to their results, diabetes was associated with increased 30-day mortality. In diabetic patients mortality was 12.4% and in non-diabetics it was 6.9% after thrombolysis at 30 day end point.

In a study conducted by Muhammad Iqbal, et al. "Complications and mortality in ST segment elevation AMI in diabetic and non-diabetic patients", 240 patients (76 diabetic and 164 non-diabetic) suffering from ST-segment elevation AMI were included in the study. The complications of AMI and the outcome were compared between diabetics and non-diabetic patients. Among the patients admitted with STEMI, about 32% were diabetic. In overall, left ventricular failure and arrhythmia were the significant complications. Mortality at young age was significantly higher in diabetics than non-diabetics. Streptokinase reduced mortality in both diabetic (about 2.5 times) and non-diabetic (about 8.4 times) patients. Different complications studied varied significantly (P< 0.001) within diabetics, non-diabetics and in overall after controlling for diabetes. The abnormalities including cardiogenic shock (OR = 1.9; 95% CI = 0.85-4.22), left ventricular failure (OR = 2.5), re-infarction (OR = 2.2), arrhythmia (OR = 2.04), and ventricular septal defect (OR = 2.17) were 4.2, 4.7, 21.3, 4.2, and 85.24 times higher in diabetics, respectively.

Mortality due to STEMI in diabetics was 2.3 times higher than in non-diabetics. Mortality varied significantly between different age groups in non-diabetics and in overall after controlling for diabetes. Results of this study were similar to that of present study.

The present study was conducted over a short period and on small number of patients. There was no post hospital follow up, so, that is another weak factor of this study. Since the hospital is equipped to deal with life threatening emergencies, in-hospital death as a complication was not that high in any group.

Our study was limited by the fact that the prognosis after ST elevation AMI is affected by various factors such as age, gender, number of coronary risk factors presented by the patient, use of aspirin within 7 days, and number of angina attacks the patient's suffered . They could not assess these factors, which may correlate strongly with the mortality in their study. A multivariate analysis is required to exclude the importance of these confounding factors.

11.4 RESULTS

A total of 176 patients were investigated in this study, out of which 133 (75.56%) were male and 43 (24.43%) were females. Ninety one (51.7%) patients had diabetes. Out of these 70 (76.92%) were male and 21 (23.08%) were females, showing higher prevalence of diabetes in male as compared to female patients. The prevalence of diabetes among patients admitted with AMI was found to be 51.7%.

TABLE 1 Shows the demographic characteristics of the study population

Demographic characters	Diabetic(n = 91)	Non diabetic(n = 85)
Mean age(years)	56.66 ± 12.23	53.54 ± 11.56
Male	70 (76.92%)	63 (74.11%)
Female	21 (23.08%)	22 (25.89%)
Hypertension	44 (48.35%)	36 (42.63%)
Smoking	33 (36.26%)	51 (60.00%)
Alcohol	51 (56.7%)	49 (58.7%)
Time of thrombolysis in hours	8.18 ± 1.7	7.59 ± 1.3

As observed in the Table 1, among 91 patients having diabetes 44 (48.35%) had hypertension. 51 (56.7%) and 33 (36.26%) patients were alcoholic and smokers, respectively. Mean time from onset of chest pain to thrombolysis was 8.18 hr.

TABLE 2 Showing rate of complications among diabetics and non-diabetics

	Complications	No Complications	Total
Diabetic	71 78.30%)	20 (21.70%)	91 (100%)
Non-diabetic	28 33.60%)	57 (66.40%)	85 (100%)

Table 2 shows that 78.30% patients of AMI had some complication during the admission in the ICCU. The most common complications were recurrent ischemic chest pain, heart failure and arrhythmias.

TABLE 3 Shows different complications among diabetics and non-diabetics

Complications	Diabetic(n = 91)	Non diabetic(n = 85)	P value
Recurrent chest pain	58 (64.20%)	28 (33.87%)	P< 0.0001
Heart failure	33 (35.90%)	16 (18.82%)	P< 0.01
Arrhythmias	39 (43.10%)	15 (17.60%)	P< 0.0001
Mortality	04 (4.30%)	01 (1.17%)	P< 0.05

As observed in the Table 3, maximum number of patients had recurrent chest pain during stay in the ICCU. The 35.90% of the patients had heart failure. Commonest arrhythmias seen in these patients 43.10%, were ventricular tachycardia and ventricular fibrillation. The rate of different complications was observed to be higher in patients having diabetes than that of patients not having diabetes, and the difference is statistically significant.

11.5 CONCLUSION

The prevalence of diabetes among patients admitted with AMI was found to be 51.7%. Male patients showed slightly higher (52.63%) prevalence of diabetes as compared to females (50.00%). The 78.30% patients of AMI had some complication during the admission in the ICCU. The rate of different complications was observed to be higher in patients having diabetes than that of patients not having diabetes, and the difference is statistically significant. The most common complications were recurrent ischemic chest pain, heart failure and arrhythmias. Patients of AMI having diabetes had more percentage of alcoholics and smokers. So, the modifiable factors should be corrected by keeping blood pressure, blood sugars and lipid levels under strict control, also life style modification.

KEYWORDS

- **Acute myocardial infarction**
- **Coronary heart disease**
- **Diabetes mellitus**

REFERENCES

1. Alajbegović, S. and Metelko, Z. *Diabetologia Croatica*, **75**, 35–4, 2006,
2. Angeja, B. G. and de Lemos, J. *American Heart Journal*, **144**, 649–56 (2002).
3. Bajzer, C. T. *Medicine index*, Cleveland Clinic Foundation, pp. 222–6.
4. Carlsson, J. and Kamp, U. *Herz*, **24**, 440–7 (1999).
5. Clement, S. and Braithwaite, S. S. *American Diabetes Association*, Impact factor: 8.1 (2011).
6. De Lemos, J. A. and Braunwalo, E. *Journal of American College of Cardiology*, **38**, 1283–94 (2001).
7. *Diabetes care*, Management of Diabetes and Hyperglycemia in Hospitals.
8. *Diabetes Spectrum*, **12**(2), 80–83 (1999).
9. Gitt, A., Bramlage, P., Towae, F., Papp, A., Deeg, E., Senges, J., Zeymer, U., Zahn, R., Fleischmann, H., Boehler, S., Schnell, O., Standl, E., and Tschöpe, D. *J Am Coll Cardiol.*, **61**, 1096–1097 (March, 2013).
10. Harrisons online, Chapter 344, *Diabetes Mellitus*.
11. Health.india.com World Health Statistics 2012: One in six adults obese, one in three hypertensive, one in 10 diabetic Sep 29, 2012 at 8:30 AM.
12. Huffman, D. M., *Coronary heart disease in India*, Northwestern University Feinberg School of Medicine, Chicago, USA and Centre for Chronic Disease Control, New Delhi, India.

13. Karlson, B. W. and Herlitz, J. *Diabetic Medicine*, **10**, 449–454 (1993).
14. Khan, M. A. *Journal of Pakistan Medical Association*, (October, 2011).
15. Mak, K. H. and Moliterno, D. J. *J Am Coll Cardiol.*, **30**(1), 171–9 (Jul, 1997)
16. Min Luo;Xiaoqun Guan;Elizabeth D;Luczak;Di Lang;William Kutschke;Zhan Gao;Jinying Patric, Y. Samuel, G., Sossalla;Paari D. Swaminathan;Robert M. Weiss;Baoli Yang5;Adam G. Rokita;Lars S. Maier;Igor R. Efimov;Thomas J. Hund, and Anderson, M. E. *J Clin Invest.*, **123**(3), 1262–1274 (2013).
17. Mohan, V., Sandeep, S., Deepa, R., Shah, B., and Varghese, C. *Indian J Med Res*, **125**, 217–230 (March, 2007).
18. Muhammad, I. *Medical Journal of Islamic World Academy of Sciences*, **19**(2), 87–94 (2011).
19. Norhammar, A., Tenerz, A., Nilsson, G., Hamsten, A., Efendic, S., Ryden, L., and Malmberg, K. *Lancet*, **359**, 2140–2144 (2002).
20. Schröder, R. *Circulation*, **110**, 506–10 (2004).
21. Schröder, R. and Dissmann, R. *Journal of American College of Cardiology*, **24**, 384–91 (1994).
22. Sprafka, J. M. and Burke, G. L. The Minnesota Heart Survey, *Diabetes care*, **14**(7), (July, 1991).
23. Standards of medical care in diabetes. American Diabetes Association, *Diabetes Care* **34**, S11, (2011).
24. Tenerz, A., Lo □nnberg, I., Berne, C., Nilsson, G., and Leppert, J. *Eur Heart J*, **22**, 1102–1110 (2001).
25. Van 't Hof, A. W. Zwolle Myocardial infarction Study Group, *Lancet*, **350**, 615–9 (1997).
26. Woodfield, S. L. And Lundergan, C. F. *Journal of American College of Cardiology*, **28**, 1661–9 (1996).
27. www.heart.org/HEARTORG/.../Diabetes/WhyDiabetesMatters/American Heart Association.

CHAPTER 12

DEVELOPMENT OF THERAPEUTIC STRATEGY TO RESTORE CORONARY MICROCIRCULATION AND VEGF SIGNALING CASCADE IN DIABETES: A NOVEL APPROACH TO PREVENT CARDIAC COMPLICATION IN DIABETES

SUBRINA JESMIN, ARIFUR RAHMAN, ABDULLAH AL MAMUN, FARZANA SOHAEL, SHAMIMA AKTER, YOSHIO IWASHIMA, NOBUTAKE SHIMOJO, NAOTO YAMAGUCHI, MICHIAKI HIROE, TARO MIZUTANI, and MASAO MOROI

CONTENTS

ABSTRACT

The microcirculatory disturbances in diabetic heart and the consequences: Abnormal coronary microcirculation is an integral part of the pathophysiology of both ischemic and nonischemic cardiomyopathies, and is not only a unique tool to aid diagnosis and determination of prognosis, but also to guide interventions and management. Microcirculatory dysfunction is well documented, even in the pre-diabetic state; it involves alterations in coronary circulation, globally as well as regionally, even in absence of large coronary obstructive lesions. Authors background to Diabetic coronary microcirculation research: they and other research groups found that disturbances in the levels of microcirculatory growth factor are central key in the development and progression of diabetic cardiomyopathy. Most recently their research group has focused on findings ways of correcting altered microcirculation in diabetic heart. Vascular endothelial growth factor (VEGF), a major vascular factor involved in all three types of vascular growth (angiogenesis, arteriogenesis and atherogenesis), acts as a central trigger myocardium leading to all the structural and functional changes in diabetic myocardium, such as decreased abnormal coronary collaterals development, abnormalities in coronary flow reserve, coronary microvascular rarefaction, myocardial hypertrophy, myocyte death, and varying degrees of fibrosis, impaired myocardial function, defective cardiac progenitor cell growth, and myocyte formation. Thus, a diagnostic tool based on coronary microcirculation in diabetic subjects and the therapeutic approach for the restoration of VEGF, as well as coronary microcirculation, is crucial for the prevention and treatment of diabetic cardiac complication. They previously have used pharmacological intervention in diabetic model and systematically assessed the effects of drug on the development and progression of various complications in diabetes including diabetic cardiomyopathy. They found that endothelin (ET) blockade is effective, systematically, to prevent the development, and progression of various diabetic complications including those localized in the heart through the modification of respective microcirculation and the associated signal transduction. Systemic administration of ET blocker prevents diabetic cardiomyopathy through restoration of VEGF, prevents diabetes-mediated erectile dysfunction through VEGF upregulation, and prevents the development of diabetic retinopathy and nephropathy through VEGF inhibition. Their ongoing study uses statin and has beneficial effect on heart.

12.1 INTRODUCTION

The diabetes-induced heart failure is alarmingly, an epidemic that has increased dramatically in recent times, both at the international and national level (Aneja et al., 2008). Diabetic subjects carry up to eight times the risk of cardiovascular events compared with non-diabetic individuals, making cardiovascular disease the largest cause of mortality worldwide (Grundy et al., 1999). In addition, the incidence of subclinical diabetic heart disease (abnormal myocardial function in patients with diabetes mellitus (DM) but without overt heart disease) is also gradually increasing. Abnormal coronary microcirculation is an integral part of the pathophysiology of both ischemic and nonischemic cardiomyopathies, and is not only a unique tool to aid diagnosis and determination of prognosis, but also to guide interventions and management. Diabetic cardiomyopathy is characterized by microvascular pathology, independent of coronary disease, leading to progressive heart failure (De Boer et al., 2003; Factor et al., 1980; Fein et al., 1985). Microcirculatory dysfunction is well documented, even in the pre-diabetic state; it involves alterations in coronary circulation, globally as well as regionally, even in absence of large coronary obstructive lesions. A microvascular changes lead to reduced perfusion and mismatch of myocardial supply and demand and contributes to adverse cardiovascular events in the diabetic patient (McDonagh and Hokama, 2000; Nahser et al., 1995*)*. However, epidemiology, pathogenesis, and nature of microcirculatory alterations remain obscure. In this chapter, we will discuss the microcirculatory disturbances in diabetic heart and the therapeutic strategies to restore them. Although, growth factor or cell-based angiogenic therapies are an attractive therapeutic option for diabetic patients, a better understanding of pro and antiangiogenic influences in diabetic patients is crucial to maximize the effects of such therapies.

12.2 MICROCIRCULATORY DISTURBANCES IN DIABETIC HEART

The DM is associated with macro and microvascular complications in multiple organ systems (Grundy et al., 1999). A large body of epidemiological and pathological data demonstrates that diabetes is an independent risk factor for cardiovascular disease in both men and women (Grundy et al., 1999), and coronary artery disease is considered the leading cause of morbidity and mortality in patients with diabetes (Heller, 2005). The microcirculation is an important system, containing resistance arterioles, capillaries, and venules, whose main function is to transport oxygen and nutrients to the tissues (Cicco and Cicco, 2010). Microcirculation and tissue oxygenation are very important factors strongly linked to hemorheology, especially in cardiovascular patients, and their alterations could cause impairment, or initiate cardiovascular pathologies (Cicco and Cicco, 2010). Diabetic microangiopathy is responsible for an important rate of morbidity and mortality related to the disease. Microvascular rarefaction (loss of capillary), a major cause of end-stage organ failure in diabetes, which results in a decreased coronary blood flow reserve rendering the myocardium vulnerable to ischemia and exacerbation of heart failure. Severe micro vascular rarefaction has been detected in the myocardium of diabetic patients and animal models of diabetes (Sasso, 2005; Schiekofer et al., 2005). The progressive microvasculature rarefaction is related to the duration of diabetes (Messaoudiet al., 2009; Yoon et al., 2005). The reduction in capillary density leads to cardiac dysfunction following myocardial ischemia (Yoon et al., 2005), and its preservation improves recovery of left ventricular (LV) function in diabetes (Messaoudiet al., 2009). These studies strongly suggest that insufficient angiogenesis and microvascular rarefaction may represent one of the most critical mechanisms involved in the pathogenesis and progression of diabetic cardiac dysfunction. Thickening of the capillary basement membrane has been reported in mice (Giacomelliand Wiener, 19790), rats (Okruhlicova et al., 2005), and humans (Fischer et al., 1984, Silver et al., 1977). Thompson (Thompson and Proc, 1994) quantified the effect of diabetes on different components of the myocardial microvasculature in rats, by demonstrating a decrease in mean capillary diameter by 11% after 12 weeks and 22% after 26 weeks of diabetes. Moreover, stereological analysis showed a significant progressive decrease in capillary density, which after 26 weeks of diabetes reached 77% of the value seen in non-diabetic age-matched control rats (Thompson and Proc, 1994). Ultrastructural signs of angiogenesis have also been reported and are characterized by alterations in endothelial and pericyte shape (Okruhlicova, 2005). A study of human diabetic myocardium (Fischer et al., 1984) found two characteristic abnormalities in myocardial capillaries: endothelial swelling and/or degeneration and thickening of the capillary basement membrane.

This is the pathological hallmark of diabetic microangiopathy and occurred in an uneven, patchy, segmental manner (Fischer et al., 1984). Cardiac remodeling in streptozotocin (STZ)-diabetic rats can include myocyte loss and compensatory hypertrophy that would reduce the vascular area density of even a constant number of microvessels (Ashoff et al., 2012). In the recent study, the coronary capillary morphology obtained from lectin staining represented that STZ-induced diabetes resulted in an evident reduction in coronary capillaries in LV sections (Jesmin et al., 2007; Jesmin et al., 2006; Jesmin et al., 2006). The total capillary density determined by the lectin method showed a 25% reduction in diabetes (Figure 1). Representative micrographs of coronary capillaries of LV sections in control and diabetic rats obtained from lectin and double enzymatic staining to differentiate coronary capillaries were shown (Figure 1A, B).

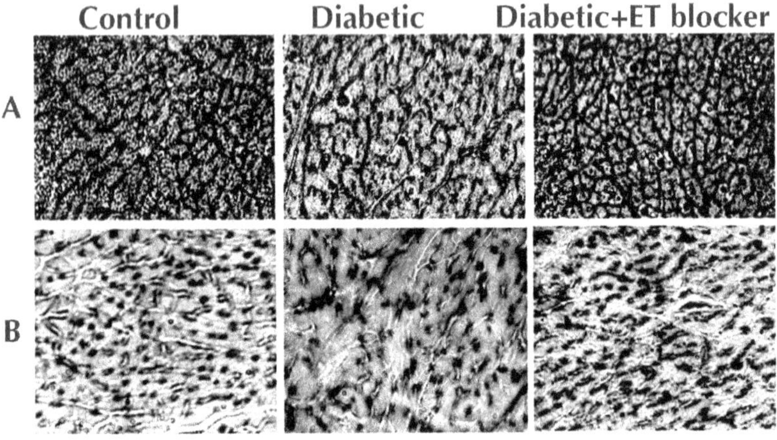

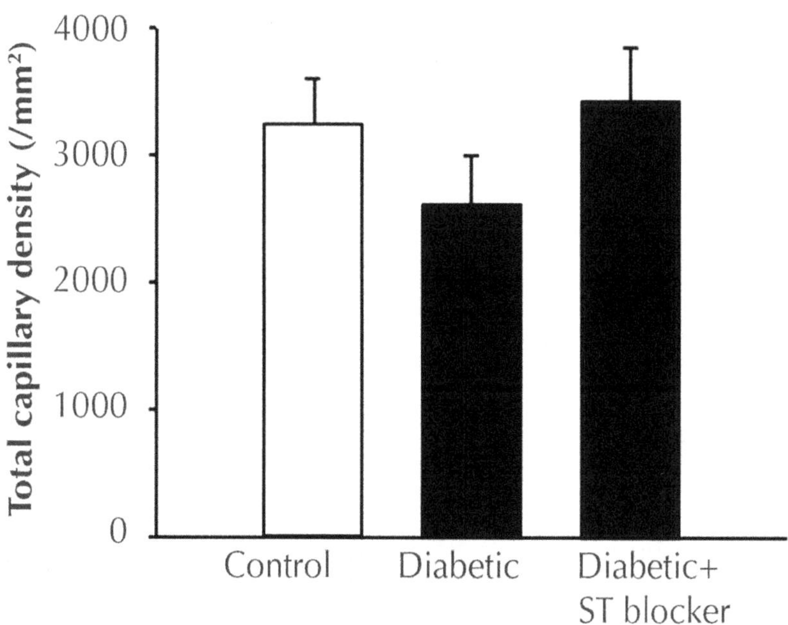

FIGURE 1 Evaluations of morphologically existing coronary capillaries in LV sections of non-diabetic control, diabetic, and dual ET blocker-treated diabetic rats. A: photomicrographs showing capillaries detected by staining the endothelium with lectin (brick red color) (upper panel), Magnification ×400; B: photomicrographs of subendocardial LV sections from double staining. Arteriolar, intermediate, and venular capillaries were stained blue, violet, and red, respectively. Magnification × 400. C: bar graph summarizing the total capillary density, obtained by the lectin staining method. Values are means ± SD (30 fields × 17 samples). $P < 0.05$ vs. non-diabetic control (*) and vs. diabetic (#).

The venular capillary portion, which stained red, was evidently remarkable in control rats, whereas the intermediate and arteriolar capillary portions, which stained violet and blue, respectively, were much pronounced in diabetic rats (Jesmin et al., 2006). Diabetic myocardial capillary microangiopathy has also been shown by others (Cameron 1973; Kilo 1972). Table 1 summarizes the microvascular alterations seen in various models of diabetic cardiomyopathy (taken from several published articles).

TABLE 1 Summary of the major microvascular changes in experimental and human diabetic cardiomyopathy (taken from published articles) STZ, Strptozotocin; Biobreeding (BB); Otsuka Long Evans Tokushima Fatty (OLETF); Zucker diabetic fatty (ZDF);

Diabetes type	Model	Microvascular changes
Type 1 diabetes	STZ rat	Decreased capillary diameter and density Decreased venular capillary, increased arteriolar and intermediate capillary subtypes
		Narrow capillary lumen with endothelial swelling
		Basement membrane thickening (201)
	Alloxan rat	Decreased capillary lumen
		Endothelial swelling
		Basement membrane thickening
	BB Wister rat	No changes
Type 2 diabetes	OLETF rat	Depending on diabetes stages, capillary density alters
		Perivascular fibrosis
	KK Mice	No changes
	ZDF	Perivascular fibrosis
	ob/ob Mice	Basement membrane thickening
Type 1 and 2 diabetes humans		Decreased coronary capillary density
		Basement membrane thickening

12.3 DIABETES MELLITUS AND CORONARY COLLATERIZATION

The DM has been found to be an inhibiting factor on coronary collateral development in a small clinic (Morimoto et al., 1989) and a postmortem study (Ramirez et al., 1983) (Figure 2). Another study with a large number of patients shows the relationship between DM and collateral vessel development. It demonstrates that collateral vessel development is poorer in

DM than in non-diabetic patients (Abaci et al., 1999) (Figure 2). We can speculate that DM is an important factor among the factors affecting the development of coronary collaterals.

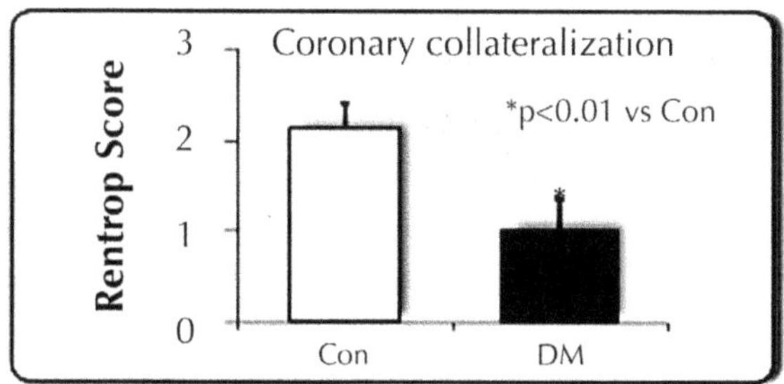

FIGURE 2 Coronary collateralization, as quantified by rentrop scoring, in non-diabetic (Con) *vs.* diabetic (DM) patients.

12.4 ROLE OF VASCULAR ENDOTHELIAL GROWTH FACTOR (VEGF) IN CORONARY MICROCIRCULATION IN DIABETES

There are various mechanisms have been postulated to explain the impaired angiogenic response in diabetes. First, the presence of vascular dysfunction, characterized by both endothelial and vascular smooth muscle impairments, is a well-documented phenomenon in this setting (Caballero et al., 1999; Momose et al., 2002; Papaioannou et al., 2004; Rosen et al., 1996). Second, exposure to chronic hyperglycemia leads to the nonenzymatic glycation of proteins and in particular, glycation of the extracellular matrix has been shown to impair the formation of new blood vessels (Kuzuya et al., 1998; Tamarat et al., 2003). Lastly, the presence of diabetes is associated with abnormalities in growth factor signaling, which have been under intense research investigation recently, in the myocardium. The VEGF, an endothelial cell-specific mitogen that is important in neovascularization under both physiological and pathophysiological conditions, plays a crucial role in developmental blood vessel formation and regulation of hypoxia-induced tissue angiogenesis (Banai et al., 1994; Ferrara and Davis-Smyth, 1997). The following two high-affinity VEGF tyrosine kinase receptors have been identified: fms-like tyrosine kinase

1 (FLT-1) and fetal liver kinase 1 (FLK-1), both of which are expressed almost exclusively in endothelial cells (Neufeld et al., 1999). A significant increase in VEGF levels can be observed after myocardial infarction in non-diabetic patients (Shinohara et al., 1996), consequently leading to the development of collateral vessels in the advanced stages of coronary atherosclerosis (Abaci et al., 1999). Diabetic microvascular complications are considered to be influenced by angiogenic factors, including VEGF, as a response to both ischemia and hyperglycemia. In diabetic patients, however, there is inadequate collateral vascular formation in response to ischemia that ultimately results in increased cardiovascular morbidity and mortality rates (Abaci et al., 1999). Thus, diabetic patients suffering from coronary artery disease have a less favorable outcome compared with non-diabetic patients, including a three- to fourfold increase in mortality risk (Smith et al., 1984, Stone et al., 1989). Interestingly, a previous study showed that myocardial expression levels of messenger ribonucleic acid (mRNAs) for VEGF and its receptors, FLT-1 and FLK-1, were significantly decreased in nonischemic short-term STZ-induced diabetic rats, and a twofold reduction in VEGF and FLK-1 was observed in autoptic ventricular specimens from diabetic patients compared with non-diabetic subjects who died from myocardial infarction (Chou et al., 2002). Early downregulation of VEGF and vascular endothelial growth factor receptor 2 (VEGFR-2) could play a key role for initiating the pathophysiological cascade that leads to the onset of diabetic cardiomyopathy (Yoon et al., 2005). Similar findings were obtained in the recent study (Jesmin et al. 2007; Jesmin et al., 2006; Jesmin et al., 2006). enzyme-linked immunosorbent assay (ELISA) and Western blot analysis showed a 40% decrease in VEGF protein in heart after 5 weeks of diabetes compared with non-diabetic controls (Figure 3) (Jesmin et al, 2007).

A similar reduction was also observed at its gene level in LV of diabetic rats, which was obtained from real-time quantitative polymerase chain reaction (PCR) (Figure 1) (Jesmin et al, 2007). In the same study, LV expression levels of FLK-1 and FLT-1 proteins were reduced by 42 and 33%, respectively, in diabetic rats (Figure 4) (Jesmin et al, 2007). The decrease in protein expression of these VEGF receptors in LV of diabetic rats correlated with their mRNAs (Figure 4) (Jesmin et al, 2007). In addition, the phosphorylation level of the VEGF angiogenic receptor, FLK-

1, was significantly lower in LV tissues of diabetic rats than in controls (Jesmin et al., 2007).In this study (Jesmin et al., 2007), both expression levels of phosphorylated and nonphosphorylated FLK-1 were decreased in the diabetic heart, which was consistent with the previous report (Sasso et al., 2005).

Serial clinicopathological investigation of DM rats revealed (Yoon et al., 2005) that the decrease of VEGF expression in the myocardium was the initial event, followed by endothelial cell apoptosis, decreases in capillary density, and decreases in circulating endothelial progenitor cell (EPC) counts in STZ-induced diabetic rat. These changes were followed by diastolic dysfunction, cardiomyocyte apoptosis, myocardial degeneration, replacement fibrosis, and finally systolic dysfunction (Yoon et al., 2005). This temporal sequence and its reversal by VEGF gene therapy provide evidence that implicates disordered VEGF homeostasis in the pathophysiology of diabetic cardiomyopathy (Yoon et al., 2005).

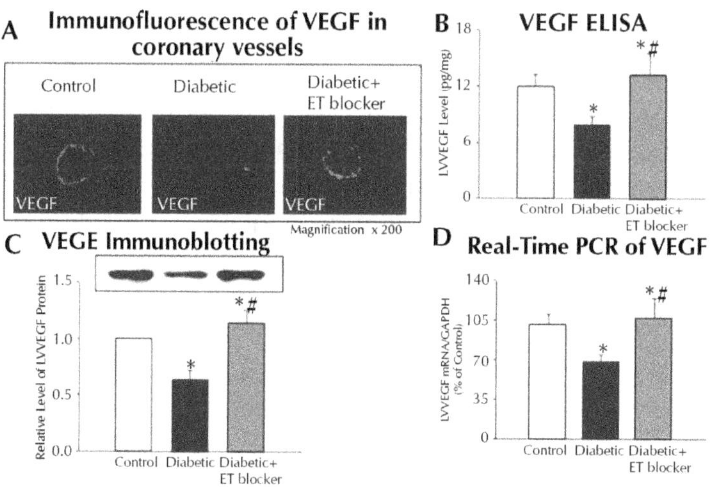

FIGURE 3 Protein and gene expression levels of vascular endothelial growth factor (VEGF) in LV tissues of non-diabetic control, diabetic, and dual endothelin (ET) blocker-treated diabetic rats. Immunofluorescence staining (A); ELIZA (B) and Immunoblot analysis (C) were performed for protein expression of VEGF. For immunoblot analysis, in each of the experiments, the band obtained in the non-diabetic control is normalized to 1.0. D: total RNA isolated from LV was analyzed by real-time quantitative PCR. Values are means ± SD. P< 0.05 vs. non-diabetic control (*) and vs. diabetic (#); n = 17 rats.

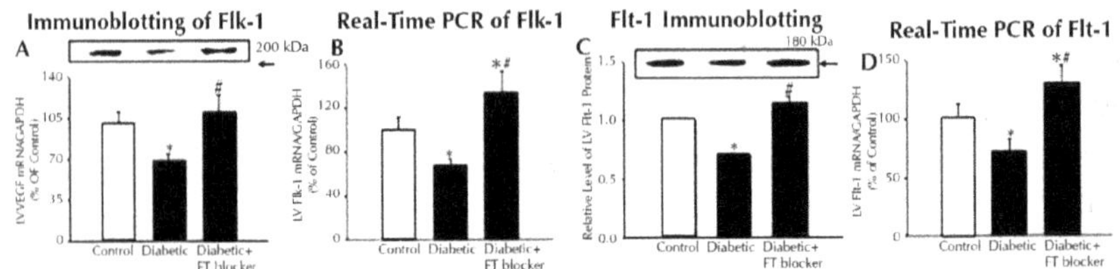

FIGURE 4 Protein and gene expression levels of fetal liver kinase 1 (FLK-1; A and B) and fms-like tyrosine kinase 1 (FLT-1; C and D) in LV tissues of non-diabetic control, diabetic, and dual endothelin (ET) blocker-treated diabetic rats. Western blot analysis was performed for protein expression, and immunoreactive Flk-1 (A) and Flt-1 (C) were detected as a single band with a molecular mass of 200 and 180 kDa, respectively. For immunoblot analysis, in each of the experiments, the band obtained in the non-diabetic control is normalized to 1.0. Total RNA isolated from LV was analyzed by real-time quantitative PCR (B and D). Values are means ± SD. $P< 0.05$ vs. non-diabetic control (*) and vs. diabetic (#); n = 17.

The decrease in capillary density in diabetic heart is accompanied by decreased myocardial perfusion, a direct indicator of myocardial ischemia, and by progressive LV dysfunction (Yoon et al., 2005). In a well-recognized mouse model of diabetes, a significant reduction in microvessel density, reduced expression of selected VEGF isoforms, and an increase in oxidative stress in myocardium were observed (Han et al., 2009). These changes were apparently linked and were statistically associated with measures of LV performance. Another recent study showed that LV angiotensin II in spontaneously diabetic tori (SDT) rats at 8 and 16 weeks induces cardiomyocyte hypertrophy without affecting hyperglycemia or blood pressure, which promotes and suppresses coronary angiogenesis, respectively, *via* VEGF and thrombospondin-1 produced from hypertrophied cardiomyocytes under chronic hypoxia (Masuda et al., 2012). Collectively, the observations with other studies suggest that microvascular rarefaction contributes to diabetes-related cardiomyopathy in the absence of atherosclerosis. Here it must be mentioned that in type 2 diabetes, at the early insulin resistant phase cardiac VEGF expression is upregulated as a compensatory adaptation but with the increase in the duration of diabetes cardiac VEGF signaling is downregulated (Jesmin et al., 2002).

12.5 THERAPEUTICS TO RESTORE CARDIAC VEGF LEVEL IN DIABETES

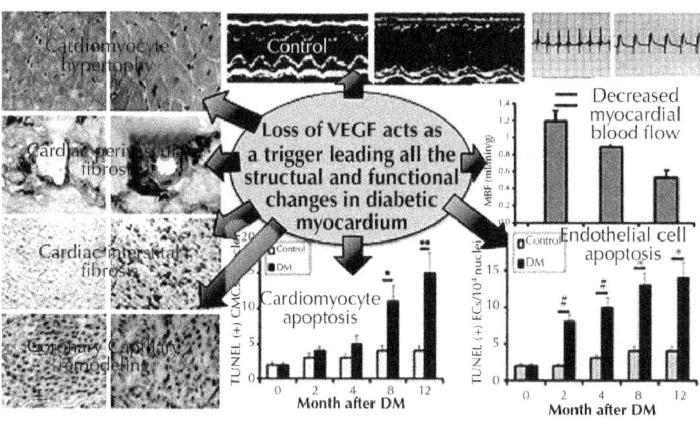

FIGURE 5 VEGF is one of the central players for the development and progression of diabetic cardiac complications (from morphology to function).

Since 1999s, Authors have been researching alterations in the microcirculation of the diabetic heart and the factors associated with abnormal collateral development and formation (microcirculation disturbances). They and other research groups found that disturbances in the levels of microcirculatory growth factor are central key in the development and progression of diabetic cardiomyopathy (Figure 5). Most recently their research group has focused on searching ways of correcting altered microcirculation in diabetic heart. The VEGF, a major vascular factor involved in all three types of vascular growth (angiogenesis, arteriogenesis and atherogenesis), acts as a central trigger leading to all the structural and functional changes in diabetic myocardiam, such as decreased and abnormal coronary collateral development, abnormalities in coronary flow reserve, coronary microvascular rarefaction, myocardial hypertrophy, myocyte death, and varying degrees of fibrosis, impaired myocardial function, defective cardiac progenitor cell growth, and myocyte formation. Thus, a diagnostic tool based on coronary microcirculation in diabetic subjects and the therapeutic approach for the restoration of VEGF, as well as coronary microcirculation, is crucial for the prevention and treatment of diabetic cardiac complication. In human autopsy and biopsy samples of heart, coronary capillary density, and VEGF signaling cascade is greatly suppressed. In their ongoing study, using the human samples of Japanese and Bangladeshi diabetic patients, they are now systematically determining the expression and activities of VEGF.

12.6 PHARMACOLOGICAL APPROACHES TO RESTORE CORONARY MICROCIRCULATION AND CARDIAC VEGF SIGNALING IN DIABETES

Authors have used pharmacological intervention in diabetic model and systematically assessed the effects of drug on the development and progression of various complications in diabetes including diabetic cardiomyopathy. They found that ET blockade is effective in restoring the decreased coronary capillary and VEGF signaling in diabetic heart. ET blocker is also effective in reversing the cardiac dysfunction in diabetes (Jesmin et al., 2003; 2006; 2006). They also found that pitavastatin is useful in reversing the decreased VEGF signaling in diabetic heart (Jesmin et al, submitted elsewhere, 2012). They are now working on other popular cardiovascular drugs to investigate their effects on coronary microcirculation in diabetes.

12.7 ENDOTHELIN BLOCKER AND DIABETIC CARDIAC MICROCIRCULATION

Evidence is now strong for a role of endothelin (ET)-1, a potent vasoconstrictor with vasoproliferative activity (Miyauchi and Masaki, 1999), in diabetes. Plasma ET-1 levels have been shown to be elevated in animal models of DM (Hopfner et al., 1999, Makino and Kamakata, 1998, Takeda et al., 1991) and in diabetic patients (Donatelli et al., 1994; Moriseet al., 1995). Furthermore, it has been reported that activity of endogenous ET-1 on ET_A receptors is enhanced in the resistance vessels of diabetic patients (Cardillo et al., 2002). Thus the ET system appears to play a key role in the development of cardiovascular complications associated with diabetes and, therefore, therapy with intervention designed to suppress the ET system may prevent the development of cardiovascular complications in diabetes.

In their recent study (Jesmin et al., 2007), they found down regulated cardiac expression levels of VEGF and its receptors, impaired cardiac VEGF signaling, decreased coronary capillary density, and cardiac dysfunctions in rats with 5 week of STZ-induced diabetes. Diabetic rats exhibited a significant increase in ET-1 in LV tissues compared with non-diabetic controls. The final goal of this study was to determine whether treatment with SB-209670, which is an antagonist against both ET_A and ET_B receptors (dual ET receptor antagonist), could improve deteriorations of the VEGF signaling pathways, coronary capillary morphology, and cardiac functions in diabetic rats.

12.8 EXPERIMENTAL ANIMALS USED

Male Sprague–Dawley rats (10 weeks and 200–250 g body wt) were used in this study. After an overnight fast, the animals received a single intraperitoneal injection of STZ (65 mg/kg). The STZ was dissolved in a citrate solution (0.1 M citric acid and 0.2 M sodium phosphate, pH 4.5). Control rats (n = 26) received an equivalent volume of citrate buffer alone. All animals injected with STZ developed diabetes, as indicated by plasma glucose levels >250 mg/dl (Glucometer Elite; Bayer) at 48 hr following the injection. After the STZ injection (1 wk), diabetic animals were randomly divided into two groups. One group of diabetic rats (n = 20) was given SB-209670 (dual ET receptor antagonist) (SmithKline Beecham Pharmaceuticals) at a dose of 1 mg/day for 4 week subcutaneously through an osmotic pump that was implanted in the back. Another group (n = 27) was given the physiological saline alone. Treatment with SB-209670 for 4 week was also conducted on some control rats. All rats were fed with the same diet and water until they were used 4 week later. All animal procedures were reviewed and approved by the Animal Experiment Committee at the University of Tsukuba.

12.9 EXPRESSION OF VEGF AND ITS RECEPTORS

ELISA and Western blot analysis showed a 40% decrease in VEGF protein after 5 week of diabetes compared with non-diabetic controls (Figure 3). A similar reduction was also observed at its gene level in LV of diabetic rats, which was obtained from real-time quantitative PCR (Figure 3). Treatment with SB-209670 (dual ET blocker) for 4 week normalized LV expression of VEGF at both protein and mRNA levels (Figure 1) (Jesmin et al., 2007). On immunoblots, LV expression levels of FLK-1 and FLT-1 proteins were reduced by 42 and 33%, respectively, in diabetic rats (Figure 4). SB-209670 (dual ET bocker) treatment greatly ameliorated downregulation of the two VEGF receptors in diabetes (Figure 4) (Jesmin et al., 2007).

12.10 VEGF SIGNALING PATHWAYS

As shown in Figure 6, the phosphorylation level of the VEGF angiogenic receptor, FLK-1, was significantly lower in LV tissues of diabetic rats than in controls. The decrease in the phosphorylated FLK-1 level was completely reversed by SB-209670 treatment (Jesmin et al., 2007). The results of immunoblot analysis revealed that total protein expression of AKT, a downstream effecter of VEGF, was unchanged by diabetes (Figure 6). However, the phosphorylated level of AKT was significantly diminished in diabetic rats (Figure 6). They found a substantial reduction in the phosphorylated level of endothelial nitric oxide synthase (eNOS) in diabetic LV tissues without any significant change in total eNOS expression (Figure 6). Treatment with dual ET receptor blocker (SB-209670) normalized the decreased phosphorylation levels of AKT and eNOS observed in diabetic LV tissues (Figure 6) (Jesmin et al., 2007).

12.11 MORPHOLOGICAL DATA

Treatment of diabetic rats with SB-209670 significantly improved the capillary density to the control level (Figure 1) (Jesmin et al., 2007). The

Figure 1 shows representative micrographs of coronary capillaries of LV sections in control, diabetic, and SB-209670-treated diabetic rats obtained by the double-staining method (Figure 1) (Jesmin et al., 2007). Treatment of diabetic rats with SB-209670 (dual ET receptor blocker) evidently reversed the decreased portion of venular capillaries in diabetic rats (Figure 1) (Jesmin et al., 2007).

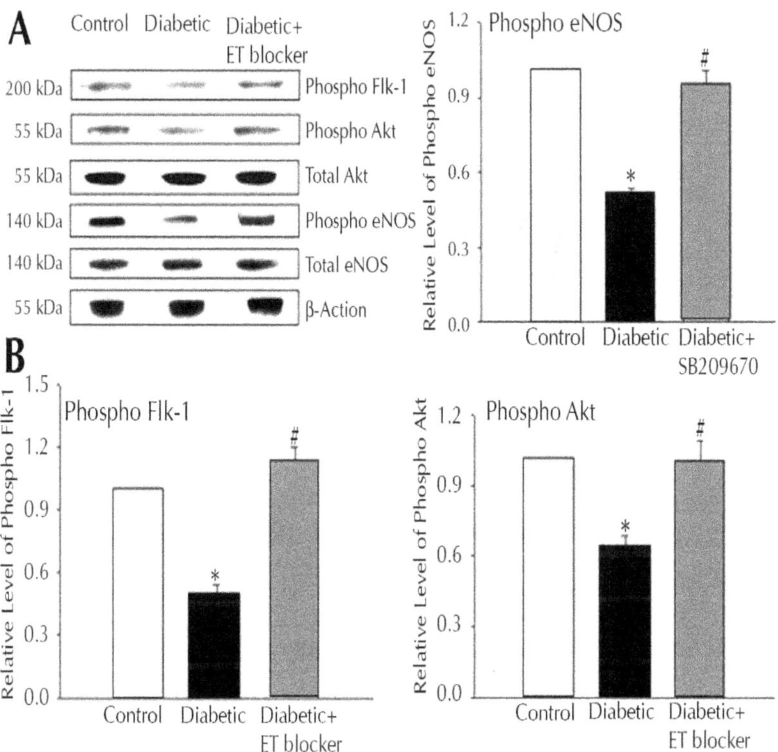

FIGURE 6 Effects of endothelin (ET) antagonism on cardiac phosphorylated important downstream molecule of VEGF angiogenic signaling. Analysis of FLK-1, AKT, and endothelial nitric oxide synthase (eNOS) phosphorylation in LV tissues of non-diabetic control, diabetic, and dual endothelin (ET) blocker-treated diabetic rats. Protein phosphorylation was analyzed by Western blot using phosphospecific antibodies. A: representative blots. Protein loading was verified using anti-β-actin antibodies. B: densitometric results. In each of the experiments, the band obtained in the non-diabetic control is normalized to 1.0. Values are means ± SD. *P< 0.05 vs. non-diabetic control; #P< 0.001 vs. diabetic; n = 17.

12.12 ASSESMENT OF CARDIAC FUNCTIONS BY ECHOCARDIOGRAPHY

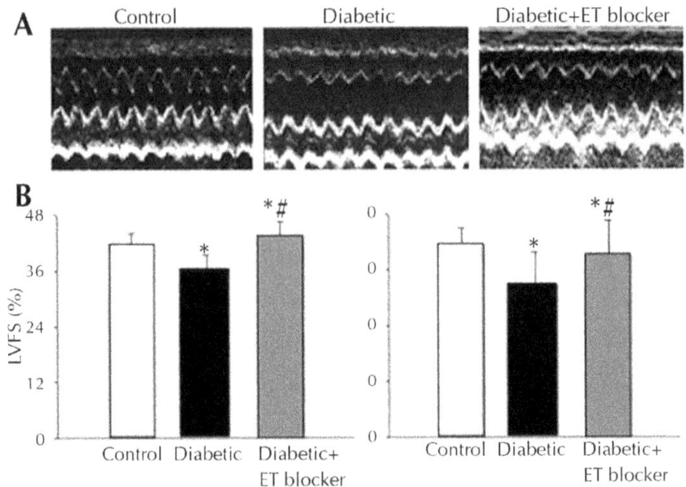

FIGURE 7 A: representative M-mode echocardiograms of non-diabetic control, diabetic, and dual endothelin (ET) blocker-treated diabetic rats. A two-dimensional short-axis view was recorded at the level of papillary muscle. B: summarized data for LV fractional shortening (LVFS) and cardiac output (CO) measured by echocardiography. Values are means ± SD. P< 0.05 vs. non-diabetic control (*) and vs. diabetic (#);n = 10–13.

Representative M-mode echocardiograms of control, diabetic, and SB-209670-treated diabetic rats are shown in Figure 7 (Jesmin et al., 2007). Left ventricular fractional shortening (LVFS) and cardiac output (CO) were significantly lower in diabetic rats compared with controls (Figure 7) (Jesmin et al., 2007). Treatment of diabetic rats with SB-209670 significantly ameliorated these cardiac function parameters (Figure 7) (Jesmin et al., 2007).

They showed that the ET-1 level in LV tissues was 1.5-fold higher in diabetic than in control rats (Jesmin et al., 2007). In diabetes, the change in balance of endothelial mediators released by endothelium may shift to angiotensin II and ET, substances that enhance proliferation of smooth muscle cells and limit the coronary reserve of myocardium (Rosen et al.,

1996; 1998). The expression levels of ET-1 and its receptors have been documented to be augmented in the hearts of rats with both short and long terms of STZ-induced diabetes (Chen et al., 2000; Lin et al., 1996; Vesciet al., 1995). Finally, chronic ET receptor blockade with bosentan has been shown to improve functional cardiac performance in STZ diabetic rats of more prolonged duration (Verma et al., 2001). A growing body of evidence thus has suggested that alterations in the ET system have a significant role in the pathogenesis of diabetic heart disease (Chen et al., 2000; Vesciet al., 1995).

The interaction between VEGF and ET-1 in vascular endothelial and smooth muscle cells is well documented (Matsuura et al., 1998). ET-1 and VEGF apparently play a complementary and coordinated role during neovascularization and malignant ascites formation in ovarian carcinoma (Salaniet al., 2000). The endothelial autocrine regulatory role of ET-1 as a putative angiogenic factor in the process of neovascularization has been recently reported (Salaniet al., 2000). In contrast with those reports, ET receptor blockade with bosentan shows a marked proangiogenic effect in an ischemic leg after femoral occlusion, and this effect appears to be directly dependent on the VEGF/AKT pathways (Iglarzet al., 2001). Bosentan was considered to modulate ischemia-induced angiogenesis by increasing the speed of revascularization and maintaining sustained activation of the process (Iglarz et al., 2001). However, several lines of evidence suggest cell mitogen and proliferating effects of ET-1 in *in vitro* studies (Hirata et al., 1989; Wren et al., 1993, Yang et al., 1999). They clearly demonstrate that ET receptor blockade with SB-209670 normalizes declined cardiac VEGF angiogenic signaling and thus impaired coronary capillary morphology in diabetic rats (Jesmin et al., 2007). In diabetes, pleural stimuli may be involved in the angiogenic response, depending on the tissue type or organ investigated. Future studies should aim to shed light to the mechanistic insight underlying the improvement of the declined cardiac VEGF signaling by ET receptor antagonism in diabetes. In the present study, blood pressure was unchanged after ET receptor blockade with SB-209670 in diabetic rats, implying the blood pressure-independent mechanism for the regulation of cardiac VEGF signaling (Jesmin et al., 2007). We confirmed that no significant change was seen in cardiac function or LV VEGF expression in non-diabetic control rats treated with SB-209670 (Jesmin et al., 2007). Furthermore, the specific effect of SB-209670 on ET receptors was supported by our preliminary experiments showing no difference in VEGF levels between cultured neonatal rat ventricular cardiomyocytes with or without treatment with SB-209670 (Jesmin et al., 2007).

12.13 STATINS AND CARDIAC VEGF SIGNALING IN DIABETES

Recently, emerging evidences suggest that statin therapy was associated with reduction in coronary events regardless of baseline cholesterol levels and comorbid cardiovascular disease (CVD) conditions in patients with diabetes (Pyorala et al., 1997; Diabetes Care 2003; Lancet 2003) and the validity of statins in the primary prevention of CVD in diabetes was subsequently established by the Collaborative Atorvastatin Diabetes Study (CARDS) (Lancet 2004). Besides, many investigators have focusing on the possibility of preventive effect on heart failure by statins (Shanes et al., 2007), especially in high-doses (Khush et al., 2007; Strandberg et al., 2009), still remains controversial though (CORONA, NEJM 2007; GISSI-HF, Lancet 2008).

Statins are the most commonly prescribed agents for hypercholesterolaemia, an essential component of diabetes, and recently known to have anti-inflammatory, anti-oxidant, anti-apoptotic, anti-fibrotic, and anti-hypertrophic features, which have been collectively referred to as pleiotrophic effects. Many of these pleiotropic effects of statins may exert beneficial effects on the pathological process of CVD and/or heart failure in patients with diabetes, but precise mechanisms are still not revealed (VanLinthout et al., 2007).

Statins is as well reported to have influences on the pathological expression of VEGF and/or VEGF related mechanisms in various organs including retina (Zheng et al., 2010; Li et al., 2010; Media et al., 2008; Al-Shabrawey et al., 2008; Bitto et al., 2008; Baraka et al., 2010; Ho et al., 2008; Zeng et al, 2005; Fujita et al., 2010), in diabetes, but intervention with statin therapy to cardiac VEGF signaling and cardiac function in diabetes has been not reported, especially from a molecular point of view.

The final goal of their study was to determine whether treatment with pitavastatin can improve deteriorations of the VEGF signaling pathways, coronary capillary morphology, and cardiac functions in diabetic rats.

The key observations made in their study are summarized as follows: 1) increase in concentration of plasma glucose and decrease in insulin levels in STZ-induced diabetes-rats are not affected by statin treatment, 2) concentration of low density lipoprotein cholesterol, high density lipoprotein cholesterol, and total cholesterol levels in the blood are not changed significantly in statin-treatment rats compared with control rats, 3) UCG imaging showed that treatment with statin ameliorated the LV hypertrophy and recovered LV dysfunction, 4) the tissue expression levels of protein and mRNA of VEGF and its receptors, FLK-1 and FLT-1, in diabetic rat heart were recovered by treatment with statin (Figure 8), and 5) in diabetes rat heart, the expression of phosphorylated AKT and phosphorylated eNOS were down-regulated, both of which were recovered by treatment with statin.

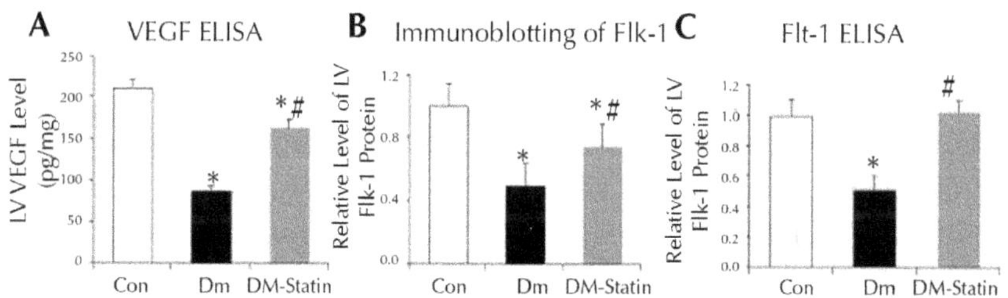

FIGURE 8 Protein expression levels of vascular endothelial growth factor (VEGF; A); fetal liver kinase 1 (Flk-1; B) and fms-like tyrosine kinase 1 (Flt-1; C) in LV tissues of non-diabetic control, diabetic, and pitavastatin (statin)-treated diabetic rats. Values are means ± SD. P< 0.05 vs. non-diabetic control (*) and vs. diabetic (#); n = 19.

The present study for the first time provides a comprehensive investigation into aspect of the VEGF, VEGF receptors, and the downstrem molecules of VEGF angiogenic signaling (AKT and eNOS) in the early STZ-induced diabetic heart treated with statin. To the best of their knowledge, this study is for the first to show that statin normalizes cardiac dysfunction and LV hypertrophy with restoration of the expression of VEGF, VEGF receptors, and its related signaling molecules. Very recently, statin is reported to be effective for preventing auto amputation of the ischemic limb of STZ-induced diabetes mice (Fujii et al., 2008), and also be effective for pancreatic beta-cell growth and regeneration associated with intra islet vasculogenesis in the STZ-induced diabetic neonatal rat (Marchand et al., 2010), though VEGF or VEGF-receptors were not examined in their studies.

12.14 DIABETIC CARDIAC COMPLICATION AND GENE THERAPY

The angiogenic growth factors are downregulated in the diabetic myocardium, in turn hampering myocardial collateral vessel formation as an adaptation to ischemia (Martin et al., 2003). Therefore, supporting the overexpression of these factors by means of gene therapy might aid in repairing the process of impaired angiogenesis in the diabetic ischemic myocardium. However, therapy using vectors encoding a single angiogenic factor has shown less significant improvement than what was expected, mainly because the biological system requires a cascade of growth factors and responsive intracellular signaling mechanisms for the development of a fully functional vascular system (Markkanen et al., 2003; Carmeliet, 2000; Risau, 1997). Therefore, therapeutic angiogenesis is currently targeting combinations of angiogenic molecules as a therapeutic measure to induce myocardial angiogenesis (Markkanen et al., 2005). In STZ-induced diabetic rat, restoration of VEGF expression with a local gene therapy approach has been shown to restore the myocardial microcirculation and cardiac function (Yoon et al., 2005). Replenishment of deficient VEGF *via* gene therapy reestablished VEGF homeostasis in the myocardium, breaking the vicious circle of endothelial cell/cardiomyocyte apoptosis, myocardial degeneration, and worsening VEGF deficiency in STZ-induced diabetic rat (Yoon et al., 2005). Angiopoietin -1 is known to modify VEGF responses to neovascularization by positively affecting vessel maturation and stability (Ylä-Herttuala and Alitalo, 2003). Recent findings have documented that intramyocardial coadministration of adenoviral vectors encoding VEGF and angiopoietin -1 induces angiogenesis and vessel maturation, thereby rendering cardioprotection against the ischemic stress induced by myocardial infarction (MI) in STZ-induced type 1 diabetic rats (Samuel et al., 2010). This therapy significantly reduced the ventricular remodeling as evidenced by the significant reduction in the collagenous fibrotic tissue and improvement in the myocardial functions in conjunction with significant increase in the levels of VEGF and its receptor FLK-1, angiopoietin 1 (Ang-1) and its receptor tyrosine kinase 2 (Tie-2), p-MK2, and anti apoptotic survivin(Samuel et al., 2010). Another recent study investigated the effect of thioredoxin-1 (Trx1) gene delivery on myocardial fibrosis, oxidative stress, cardiomyocyte and endothelial cell apoptosis, capillary and arteriolar density, and, LV remodeling in diabetic rats (Samuel et al., 2010). It has been observed that the myocardium can be rescued from diabetes-related impairment of angiogenesis, severity of functional disorder, and subsequent heart failure by Trx1 gene therapy in STZ-induced diabetic rats (Samuel et al., 2010).

There have been several attempts at preclinical and clinical levels to induce angiogenesis by overexpressing angiogenic factors in the peri-infarct zone after myocardial infarction. Most of the studies have approached this issue using a single gene as the therapeutic agent. Delivery of vectors encoding $VEGF_{165}$ (VEGF) and VEGF-2 was shown to improve collateral vascular perfusion and nourish the oxygen-depleted myocardium, thereby reducing angina and improving heart function in human clinical trials (Losordoet al., 1998; Reillyet al., 2005; Gyöngyösiet al., 2005). However, investigations into the long-term effects of sustained expression of VEGF in mice models revealed deleterious effects due to the formation of leaky immature vessels/hemangiomas and subsequent death of the experimental animal (Carmeliet 2000; Lee et al., 2000). Furthermore, transgenic mice overexpressing VEGF revealed lengthy and leaky dermal vessels with evident inflammation (Jainand Munn, 2000; Thurstonet al, 2000).

12.15 ORGAN SPECIFIC EXPRESSION AND ROLE OF VEGF IN DIABETIC COMPLICATION

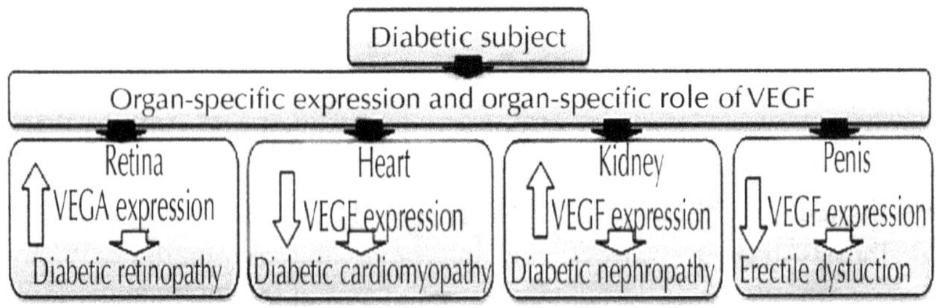

FIGURE 9 Organ specific role of VEGF in diabetic complications.

The VEGF has organ-specific expressions and roles in the pathogenesis of diabetic organ complications (Figure 9). In the last decade, many research groups including us have revealed that organ-specific aberrations in the expression of VEGF in target organs are part of the key central mechanisms that underlie microcirculatory-based organ dysfunctions in diabetes. Loss (heart, penis, brain) or over-expression (retina, kidney) of VEGF initiates signaling cascades that ultimately lead to structural and functional changes in the target organs of diabetics (Sasso et al., 2005; Yoon et al., 2005; Chou et al., 2002, Jesmin et al., 2003, 2006, 2006, 2007; Masuzawa et al., 2006; Cha et al., 2004, Tsuchida et al., 1999). However, although the role of VEGF in the development of these complications (diabetic cardiovascular/organ complications) is largely known, the factors/mechanistic processes responsible for triggering aberrant expressions of VEGF are greatly unknown, and solutions to normalizing altered VEGF expressions and function are almost non-existent. For instance, in diabetic retinopathy VEGF or VEGF receptor- based local treatment has been applied recently. However, this treatment exerts no protective effect on other target organs that will or are equally prone to be affected by diabetes. For diabetic cardiomyopathy in animals, intra myocardial VEGF therapy has been performed and proved effective. However, it is invasive, locally-restricted, and expensive. For these reasons, their group proposes development of systemic treatment options that are designed to act in an organ-, tissue-, and cell-specific manner simultaneously (Figure 10).

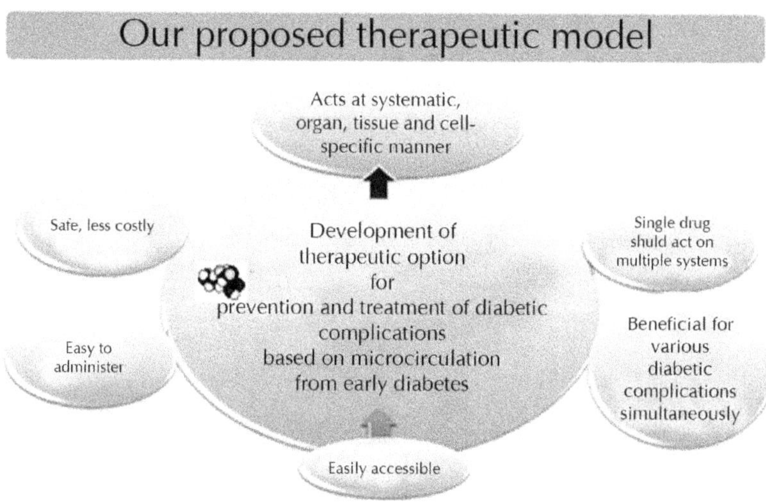

FIGURE 10 Our proposed therapeutic model for treatment and prevention of diabetic microvascular complications from early diabetes.

12.16 OUR PROPOSED THERAPEUTIC MODEL FOR DIABETIC MICROVASCULAR COMPLICATIONS

Systemic administration of ET blocker prevents diabetic cardiomyopathy through restoration of VEGF, prevents diabetes-mediated erectile dysfunction through VEGF upregulation, and prevents the development of diabetic retinopathy and nephropathy through VEGF inhibition (Figure 11). Our therapeutic approach would introduce a pharmacological therapeutic approach to normalize and prevent the microvascular-based organ complications in diabetic subjects that will works in systematic, organ, tissue, and cell-specific manner, should be beneficial for various diabetic complications like diabetic cardiomyopathy, diabetic retinopathy, diabetic nephropathy, diabetes-mediated erectile dysfunction, and diabetic neuropathy simultaneously (Figure 10). Single drug (proposed therapeutic) should act on multiple systems, signaling cascade, genetic network, biological pathways, and should be easily accessible, easy to administer, safe, and less costly (Figure 10). In developing countries use of local VEGF gene therapy or stem cell therapy would be too costly, pose safety, (like viral vectors) and technical difficulties to confer organ-specific protection in diabetes.

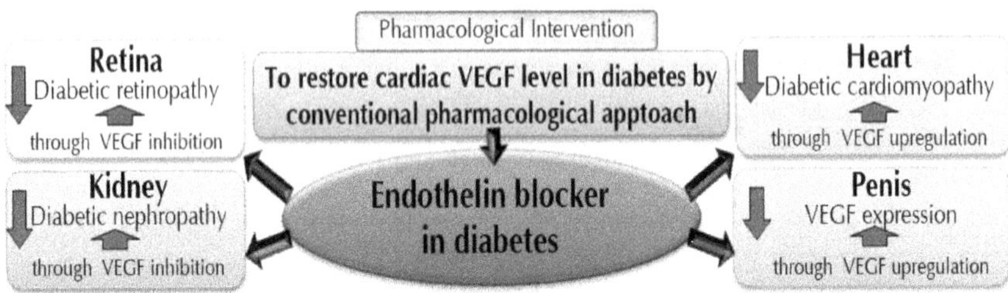

FIGURE 11 Schematic outlines of effectiveness of endothelin (ET) blocker through modulation of VEGF signaling for various diabetic complications. microvascular complications from early diabetes.

12.17 CONCLUSION

Multidisciplinary management of diabetes is of outstanding importance for the treatment and the prevention of diabetic complications, being helpful in reducing social costs and the detriment to the patient; however newer therapeutic approaches are needed. Although, still to date, the pathogenesis and treatment of diabetic heart failure are elusive, it is now convincing from a series of studies from several research groups that downregulation and deficiency of myocardial VEGF play a key role in the initiation and aggravation of diabetic cardiovascular complications and that therapeutic strategies targeted at preserving the myocardial microvasculature in DM may retard or prevent the development of diabetic cardiac complication. Our unique and promising preclinical findings of organ specific restoration of microcirculation as well as VEGF signaling therefore support the development of a pharmaceutical therapy for therapeutic myocardial angiogenesis and call for the initiation of a clinical trial to assess the efficacy of this unique therapeutic strategy in the treatment of diabetes-related human heart failure.

KEYWORDS

- **Microcirculation**
- **Nephropathy**
- **Retinopathy**
- **Signaling**
- **VEGF**

ACKNOWLEDGEMENT

Authors greatly thank the sincere technical assistance of whole research staffs of Health and Disease Research Center for Rural Peoples (HDR-CRP), Dhaka, Bangladesh. A part of this work was supported in part by a Grant-in-Aid for Scientific Research from the Ministry of Education, Culture, Sports, Science, and Technology of Japan and Japan Society for the promotion of Science. A part of this work has also been supported by research grant from Kowa pharmaceutical company (Japan). Authors also acknowledge the technical contribution of World Diabetes Foundation (WDF), Denmark through their current project to HDRCRP, Dhaka, Bangladesh on diabetes.

ABBREVIATION

DM	Diabetes mellitus
CO	Cardiac output
CVD	Cardiovascular disease
ET	Endothelin

FLK-1	Fetal liver kinase
FLT-1	Fms-like tyrosine kinase 1
LV	Left ventricular
LVFS	Left ventricular fractional shortening
MI	Myocardial infarction
VEGF	Vascular endothelial growth factor

REFERENCES

1. Abaci, A., Oguzhan, A., Kahraman, S., Eryol, N. K., Unal, S., Arinc, H., and Ergin, A. *Circulation*, **99**, 2239–2242 (1999).
2. Aneja, A., Tang, W. H., Bansilal, S., Garcia, M. J., and Farkouh, M. E. *Am J Med.*, **121**, 748–757 (2008).
3. Al-Shabrawey, M., Bartoli, M., El-Remessy, A. B., Ma, G., Matragoon, S., Lemtalsi, T., Caldwell, R. W., and Caldwell, R. B., *Invest Ophthalmol Vis. Sci.*, **49**, 3231–8 (2008).
4. Ashoff, A., Qadri, F., Eggers, R., Jöhren, O., Raasch, W., and Dendorfer, A. *J., Vasc Res.*, **49**(3), 260–6 (2012).
5. Bitto, A., Minutoli, L., Altavilla, D., Polito, F., Fiumara, T., Mrini, H., Galeano, M., Calo M, Lo Cascio P, Bonaiuto M, Migliorato A, Caputi A. P, and Squadrito F. *Pharmacol Res.*, **57**(2), 159–69 (2008).
6. Banai, S., Shweiki, D., Pinson, A., Chandra, M., Lazarovici, G., and Keshet, E., *Cardiovasc Res.*, **28**, 1176–1179 (1994).
7. Baraka, A. M., Guemei, A., and Gawad, H. A., *Biochem. Pharmacol*, **79**(11), 1634–9 (2010).
8. Caballero, A. E., Arora, S., Saouaf, R., Lim, S. C., Smakowski, P., Park, J. Y., King, G. L., LoGerfo, F. W., Horton, E. S., and Veves, A. *Diabetes*, **48**,1856–1862 (1999).
9. Cameron, D. P., Amherdt, M., Leuenberger, P., Orci L., and Stauffacher, W. *Adv. Metab. Disord.*, **2**(Suppl. 2), 257–269 (1973).
10. Cardillo, C., Campia, U., Bryant, M. B., and Panza, J. A. *Circulation*, **106**, 1783–1787 (2002).
11. Carmeliet, P. *Nat. Med.*, **6**, 1102–1103 (2000).
12. Cha, D. R., Kang, Y. S., Han, S. Y., Jee, Y. H., Han, K. H., Han, J. Y., Kim, Y. S., and Kim, N. H. *J Endocrinol*,**183**(1),183–94 (2004).
13. Markkanen, J. E., Rissanen, T. T., Kivelä, A., Ylä-Herttuala, S. Cardiovasc Res, **65**, 656–664 (2005).
14. Chen, S., Evans, T., Mukherjee, K., Karmazyn, M., and Chakrabarti, S. *J Mol Cell Cardiol*, **32**, 1621–1629 (2000).

15. Chou, E., Suzuma, I., Way, K. J., Opland, D., Clermont, A. C., Naruse, K., Suzuma, K., Bowling, N. L., Vlahos, C. J., Aiello, L. P., and King, G. L. *Circulation*, **105**, 373–379 (2002).
16. Cicco, G. and Cicco, S. *Adv. Exp. Med. Biol.*, **662**, 33–9 (2010).
17. De Boer, R. A., Pinto, Y. M., and Van Veldhuisen, D. J. *Microcirculation*, **10**, 113–126 (2003).
18. Donatelli, M., Colletti, I., Bucalo, M. L., Russo, V., and Verga, S. *Diabetes Res.*, **25**, 159–164 (1994).
19. Factor, S. M., Okun, E. M., and Minase, T. N *Engl J Med.*, **302**, 384–388 (1980).
20. Fein, F. S. and Sonnenblick, E. H. *Prog Cardiovasc Dis.*, **27**, 255–270 (1985).
21. Ferrara, N. and Davis-Smyth, T. *Endocr Rev.*, **18**, 4–25 (1997).
22. Fischer, V. W., Barner, H. B., and Larose, L. S. *Hum. Pathol.*, **15**, 1127–1136 (1984).
23. Fujii, T., Onimaru, M., Yonemitsu, Y., Kuwano, H., and Sueishi, K. *Am J Physiol Heart CircPhysiol*, **294**, H2785–H2791 (2008).
24. Giacomelli, F. and Wiener, J. *Lab Invest*, **40**, 460–473 (1979).
25. Grundy, S. M., Benjamin, I. J., Burke, G. L., Chait, A., Eckel, R. H., Howard, B. V., Mitch, W., Smith, S. C. J.r., and Sowers, J. R. *Circulation*,**100**, 1134–1146 (1999).
26. Gyöngyösi, M., Khorsand, A., Zamini, S., Sperker, W., Strehblow, C, Kastrup, J., Jorgensen, E., Tägil, K, Bøtker, H. E., Ruzyllo, W., Teresiñska, A, Dudek, D., Hubalewska, A., Rück, A., Nielsen, S. S., Graf, S., Mundigler, G, Novak, J, Sochor. H, Maurer, G., Glogar, D., and Sylven, C. *Circulation*, **112**, I157–I165 (2005).
27. Han, B., Baliga, R., Huang, H., Giannone, P. J., and Bauer, J. A. *Am J Physiol Heart Circ Physiol*, **297**, H829–35 (2009).
28. Heller, G. V. *Am J Med.*, **118**, S9–S14 (2005).
29. Hirata, Y., Takagi, Y., Fukuda, Y., and Marumo, F. *Atherosclerosis*, **78**, 225–228 (1989).
30. Ho, C., Hsu, Y. C., Tseng, C. C., Wang, F. S., Lin, C. L., and Wang, J. Y. *Ren Fail*, **30**(5), 557–65 (2008).
31. Hopfner, R. L., McNeill, J. R., and Gopalakrishnan, V. *Eur J Pharmacol*, **374**, 221–227 (1999).
32. Iglarz, M., Silvestre, J. S., Duriez, M., Henrion, D., and Levy, B. I. *Arterioscler Thromb Vasc Biol*, **21**, 1598–1603 (2001).
33. Jain, R. K. and Munn, L. L. *Nat. Med.*, **6**,131–132 (2000).
34. Jesmin, S., Sakuma, I., Salah-Eldin, A., Nonomura, K., Hattori, Y., and Kitabatake, *A. J Mol Endocrinol*, **31**(3), 401–18 (2003).
35. Jesmin, S., Miyauchi, T., Goto, K., and Yamaguchi, I. *Eur J Pharmacol*, **7**, **542**(1-3), 184-5 (2006).
36. Jesmin, S., Zaedi, S., Yamaguchi, N., Maeda, S., Shimojo, N. Masuzawa, K. Yamaguchi, I. Goto, K., and Miyauchi, T. *Exp. Biol. Med. (Maywood).*, **231**(6), 902–6 (2006).
37. Jesmin, S., Zaedi, S., Shimojo, N., Iemitsu, M., Masuzawa, K., Yamaguchi, N., Mowa, C. N., Maeda, S., Hattori, Y., and Miyauchi, T. *Am. J. PhysiolEndocrinol-Metab.*, **292**(4), E1030–40 (2007).
38. Kilo, C., Vogler, N., and Williamson, J. R. *Diabetes*, **21**, 881–905 (1972).
39. Khush, K. K., Waters, D. D., Bittner, V, et al. *Circulation*, **115**, 576–583 (2007).
40. Kuzuya, M., Satake, S, Ai, S., Asai, T., Kanda, S., Ramos, M. A., Miura, H., Ueda, M. and Iguchi, A. *Diabetologia*, **41**,491–499 (1998).

41. Li, J., Wang, J. J., Yu, Q. Chen, K., Mahadev, K., and Zhang, S. X. *Diabetes*, **59**(6), 1528–38 (2010).
42. Lee, R. J., Springer, M. L., Blanco-Bose, W. E., Shaw, R., Ursell, P. C., and Blau, H. M. *Circulation*,**102**,898–901 (2000).
43. Lin, Y. W., Duh, E., and Jiang, Z. *Diabetes*, **45**, Suppl 2, 48A (1996).
44. Losordo, D. W., Vale, P. R., Symes, J. F., Dunnington, C. H., Esakof, D. D., Maysky, M., Ashare, A. B., Lathi, K., Makino, A., and Kamata, K. *Br J Pharmacol*, **123**, 1065–1072 (1998).
45. Makino, A. and Kamata, K. *Br J Pharmacol*, **123**, 1065–1072 (1998).
46. Markkanen, J. E., Rissanen, T. T, Kivelä, A., and Ylä-Herttuala, S. *Cardiovasc Res.*, **65**, 656–664 (2005).
47. Marchand, K. C., Arany, E. J., and Hill, D. J. *Am J PhysiolEndocrinolMetab.*, **299**, E92–E100 (2010).
48. Martin, A., Komada, M. R., and Sane, D. C. *Med Res Rev.*, **23**,117–145 (2003).
49. Masuda, T., Muto, S., Fujisawa, G., Iwazu, Y., Kimura, M., Kobayashi, T., Nonaka-Sarukawa, M., Sasaki, N., Watanabe, Y., Shinohara, M., Murakami, T., Shimada, K., Kobayashi, E., and Kusano, E. *Am J Physiol Heart Circ Physiol.*, **302**, H1871–83 (2012).
50. Masuzawa, K., Goto, K., Jesmin, S., Maeda, S., Miyauchi, T., Kaji, Y., Oshika, T., and Hori, S. *Curr Eye Res.*, **31**, 79–89 (2006).
51. Matsuura, A., Yamochi, W., Hirata, K., Kawashima, S., and Yokoyama, M. *Hypertension*, **32**, 89–95 (1998).
52. Miyauchi, T. and Masaki, T. *Annu Rev Physiol.*, **61**, 391–415 (1999).
53. McDonagh, P. F. and Hokama, J. Y. *Microcirculation*, **7**, 163–181 (2000).
54. Media, R. J., O'Neill, C. L., Devine, A. B., Gardiner, T. A., and Stitt, A. W. *PloS One*, **3**(7): e2584 (2008).
55. Messaoudi, S., Milliez, P., Samuel, J. L., and Delcayre, C. *FASEB J*, **23**, 2176–2185 (2009).
56. Momose, M., Abletshauser, C., Neverve, J., Nekolla, S. G., Schnell, O., Standl, E., Schwaiger, M., and Bengel, F. M., *Eur J Nucl Med Mol Imaging.*, **29**, 1675–1679 (2002).
57. Morimoto, S., Hiasa, Y., Hamai, K., Wada, T., Aihara, T., Kataoka, Y., and Mori, H. Kokyu To Junkan, **37**, 1103–1107 (1989).
58. Morise, T., Takeuchi, Y., Kawano, M., Koni, I., and Takeda, R. *Diabetes Care*, **18**, 87–89 (1995).
59. Nahser, P. J. J.r., Brown, R. E., Oskarsson, H., Winniford, M. D., and Rossen, J. D. *Circulation*, **91**, 635–640 (1995).
60. Neufeld, G., Cohen, T., Gengrinovitch, S., and Poltorak, Z. *FASEB J*, **13**, 9–22 (1999).
61. Okruhlicova, L., Tribulova, N., Weismann, P., and Sotnikova, R. *Cell Res.*, **15**, 532–538 (2005).
52. Papaioannou, G. I., Seip, R. L., Grey, N. J., Katten, D., Taylor, A., Inzucchi, S. E., Young, L.H., Chyun, D. A., Davey, J. A., Wackers, F. J., Iskandrian, A. E., Ratner, R. E., Robinson, E. C., Carolan, S., Engel, S., and Heller, G. V. *Am J Cardiol*, **94**, 294–299 (2004).
63. Ramirez, M. L. and Fernandez de la Reguera G. *Arch Inst Cardiol Mex.*, **53**, 397–405 (1983).

64. Pyorala, K., Pedersen, T. R., Kjekshus, J., Faergeman, O., Olsson, A. G., Thorgeirsson, G. Diabetes Care 1997, 20(4), 614-620.
65. Risau, W. Nature 1997, 386, 671–674.
66. Reilly, J. P., Grise, M. A., Fortuin, F. D., Vale, P. R., Schaer, G. L, Lopez J, Van Camp J. R, Henry T, Richenbacher W. E, Losordo D. W, Schatz R. A, Isner J. M. J Interv Cardiol 2005,18:27–31
67. Rosen, P., Ballhausen, T., and Stockklauser, K. *Diabetes Res. Clin. Pract.*, **31**, Suppl, S143–S155 (1996).
68. Rosen, P., Du, X., and Tschope, D. *Mol Cell Biochem.*, **188**, 103–111 (1998).
69. Salani, D., Taraboletti, G., Rosano, L., Di Castro, V., Borsotti, P., Giavazzi, R., and Bagnato, A. *Am J Pathol*, **157**, 1703–1711 (2000).
70. Samuel, S. M., Thirunavukkarasu, M., Penumathsa, S. V., Koneru, S., Zhan, L., Maulik, G., Sudhakaran, P. R., and Maulik, N. *Circulation.*, **121**(10), 1244–55 (2010).
71. Sasso, F. C., Torella, D., Carbonara, O., Ellison, G. M., Torella, M., Scardone, M., Marra, C., Nasti, R., Marfella, R., Cozzolino, D., Indolfi, C., Cotrufo, M., Torella, R., and Salvatore, T. *J Am CollCardiol*, **46**, 827–834 (2005).
72. Schiekofer, S., Galasso, G., Sato, K., Kraus, B. J., and Walsh, K. *Arterioscler Thromb. Vasc. Biol.*, **25**, 1603–1609 (2005).
73. Shanes, J. G., Minadeo, K. N., Moret, A., Groner, M., and Tabaie, S. A. *Am Heart J*, **154**(4), 617–623 (2007).
74. Shinohara, K., Shinohara, T., Mochizuki, N., Mochizuki, Y., Sawa, H., Kohya, T., Fujita, M. Fujioka, Y., Kitabatake, A., and Nagashima, K. *Heart Vessels*, **11**,113–122 (1996).
75. Silver, M. D., Huckell, V. F., and Lorber, M. *Pathology*, **9**, 213–220 (1977).
76. Smith, J. W., Marcus, F. I., and Serokman, R. *Am J Cardiol*, **54**, 718–721 (1984).
77. Strandberg, T. E., Holme, I., Faergeman, O., Kastelein, J. J., Lindahl, C., Larsen, M. L., Olsson, A. G., Pedersen, T. R., and Tikkanen, M. J, IDEAL Study Group. *Am J Cardiol*, **103**(10), 1381–1385 (2009).
78. Stone, P. H., Muller, J. E., Hartwell, T. York, B. J., Rutherford, J. D., Parker, C. B., Turi, Z.G., Strauss H. W, Willerson J. T, and Robertson T. *J Am Coll Cardiol*, **14**, 49–57, (1989).
79. Takeda, Y., Miyamori, I., Yoneda, T., and Takeda, R. *Life Sci*, **48**, 2553–2556 (1991).
80. Tamarat, R., Silvestre, J. S., Huijberts, M., Benessiano, J., Ebrahimian, T. G., Duriez, M. Wautier, M. P., Wautier, J. L., and Levy, B. I. *Proc Natl Acad Sci U S A.*, **100**, 8555–8560 (2003).
81. Tsuchida, K., Makita, Z., Yamagishi, S., Atsumi, T., Miyoshi, H., Obara, S., Ishida, M., Ishikawa, S., Yasumura, K., and Koike, T. *Diabetologia*, **42**(5), 579–88 (1999).
82. Thompson, E. W., *Proc. Soc. Exp. Biol. Med.*, **205**, 294–305 (1994).
83. Thurston, G., Rudge, J. S., Ioffe, E., Zhou, H., Ross, L., Croll, S. D., Glazer, N., Holash, J., McDonald, D. M., and Yancopoulos, G. D. *Nat. Med.*, **6**, 460–463 (2000).
84. Van Linthout, S., Riad, A., Dhayat, N., Spillmann, F., Du, J., Dhayat, S., Westermann, D., Hilfiker-Kleiner, D., Noutsias, M., Laufs, U., Schultheiss, H. P., and Tschope, C. *Diabetologia*, **50**(9), 1977–1986 (2007).
85. Verma, S., Arikawa, E., and McNeill, J. H. *Am J Hypertens*, **14**, 679–687 (2001).
86. Vesci, L., Mattera, G. G., Tobia, P., Corsico, N., and Calvani, M. *Pharmacol Res.*, **32**, 363–367 (1995).

87. Vlahos, C. J., Aiello, L. P., and King, G. L. *Circulation*, **105**, 373–379 (2002).
88. Wren, A. D., Hiley, C. R., and Fan, T. P. *Biochem Biophys Res Commun.*, **196**, 369–375 (1993).
89. Yang, Z., Krasnici, N., and Lüscher, T. F. *Circulation*, 100, 5–8 (1999).
90. Ylä-Herttuala, S., Alitalo, K. *Nat. Med.*, **9**, 694–701 (2003).
91. Yoon, Y. S., Uchida, S., Masuo, O., Cejna, M., Park, J. S., Gwon, H. C., Kirchmair, R., Bahlman, F., Walter, D., Curry, C., Hanley, A., Isner, J. M., and Losordo, D. W. *Circulation*, **111**, 2073–2085 (2005).
92. Zheng, Z., Chen, H., Wang, H., Ke, B. Zheng, B., Li, Q., Li, P., Su. L, Gu, Q., and Xu, X. *Diabetes*, **59** (9), 2315–25 (2010).
93. Zeng, L., Xu, H., Chew, T. L., Eng, E., Sadeghi, M. M., Adler, S., Kanwar, Y. S., and Danesh, F. R. *FASEB J*, **19**(13), 1845–7 (2005).
94. The LIPID Study Group. Secondary prevention of cardiovascular events with long-term pravastatin in patients with diabetes or impaired fasting glucose: results from the LIPID trial. *Diabetes Care*, **26**, 2713–2721 (2003).
95. Heart Protection Study Collaborative Group. MRC/BHF Heart Protection Study of cholesterol-lowering with simvastatin in 5963 people with diabetes: a randomized placebo controlled trial. *Lancet*, **361**, 2005–2016 (2003).
96. The CARDS Investigators. Primary prevention of cardiovascular disease with atorvastatin in type 2 diabetes in the Collaborative Atorvastatin Diabetes Study (CARDS): multicenterrandomized placebo controlled trial. *Lancet*, **364**, 685–696 (2004).
97. The CORONA Investigators. Rosuvastatin in older patients with systolic heart failure. *N Engl J Med.*, **357**, 2248–2261 (2007).
98. Gissi-HF Investigators. Effect of rosuvastatin in patients with chronic heart failure (the GOSSI-HF trial): a randomized, double-blind, placebo-controlled trial. *Lancet*, **372** (9645), 1231–1239 (2008).

INDEX

D

E

F

G

N

O

V

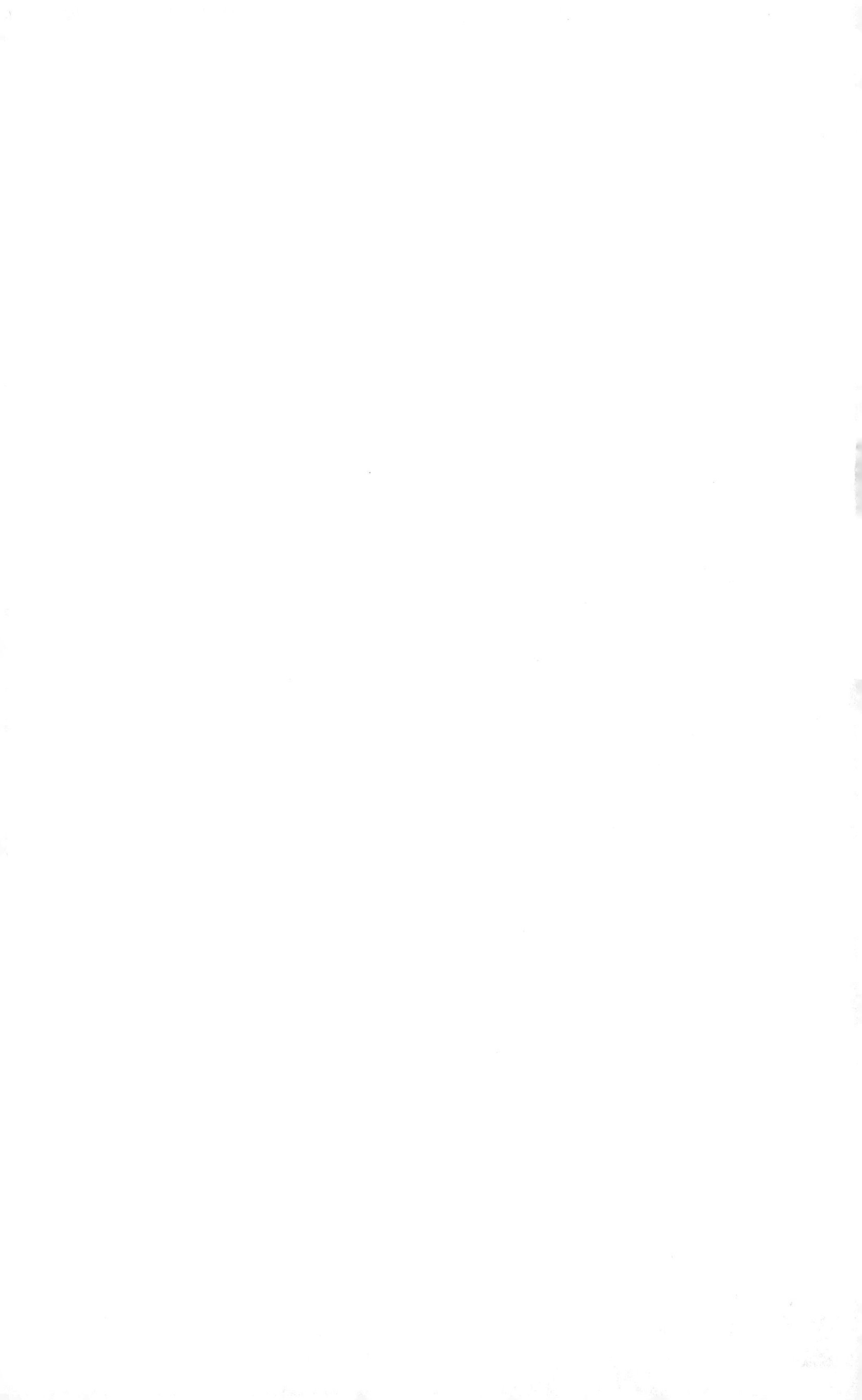

For Product Safety Concerns and Information please contact our EU representative GPSR@taylorandfrancis.com
Taylor & Francis Verlag GmbH, Kaufingerstraße 24, 80331 München, Germany

www.ingramcontent.com/pod-product-compliance
Lightning Source LLC
Chambersburg PA
CBHW060422220326
41598CB00021BA/2256

* 9 7 8 1 7 7 4 6 3 3 0 3 8 *